Breast Cancer
Immunodiagnosis
and Immunotherapy

Breast Cancer Immunodiagnosis and Immunotherapy

Edited by
ROBERTO L. CERIANI

*John Muir Cancer
and Aging Research Institute
Walnut Creek, California*

SPRINGER SCIENCE+BUSINESS MEDIA, LLC

Library of Congress Cataloging in Publication Data

International Workshop on Monoclonal Antibodies and Breast Cancer (3rd: 1988: San Francisco, Calif.)
  Breast cancer immunodiagnosis and immunotherapy / edited by Roberto L. Ceriani.
      p.   cm.
  "Proceedings of the Third International Workshop on Monoclonal Antibodies and Breast Cancer, held November 17-18, 1988, in San Francisco, California" – T.p. verso.
  Includes bibliographical references.
  ISBN 978-1-4757-1298-8   ISBN 978-1-4757-1296-4 (eBook)
  DOI 10.1007/978-1-4757-1296-4
  1. Breast – Cancer – Immunodiagnosis – Congresses. 2. Breast – Cancer – Immuno-therapy – Congresses. 3. Monoclonal antibodies – Diagnostic use – Congresses. 4. Monoclonal antibodies – Therapeutic use – Congresses. I. Ceriani, Roberto L. II. Title.
  [DNLM: 1. Antibodies, Monoclonal – diagnostic use – congresses. 2. Breast Neoplasms – diagnosis – congresses. 3. Breast Neoplasms – therapy – congresses. 4. Immunologic Tests – congresses. 5. Immunotherapy – congresses. WP 870 I614b 1988]
  RC280.B8I58   1988
  616.99'4490756 – dc20
  DNLM/DLC   89-16328
  for Library of Congress   CIP

Proceedings of the Third International Workshop on
Monoclonal Antibodies and Breast Cancer,
held November 17-18, 1988, in San Francisco, California
© 1989 Springer Science+Business Media New York
Originally published by Plenum Press, New York in 1989
Softcover reprint of the hardcover 1st edition 1989

3RD INTERNATIONAL WORKSHOP ON MONOCLONAL ANTIBODIES AND BREAST
CANCER

San Francisco, California
November 17-18, 1988

Organized by the John Muir Cancer & Aging Research Institute,
with the cooperation of the International Association for
Breast Cancer Research.

WORKSHOP CHAIRPERSON

Dr. Roberto L. Ceriani
John Muir Cancer & Aging Research Institute

ORGANIZING COMMITTEE

Chairperson: Dr. Roberto L. Ceriani

Members: Ms. Shannon Jackson
              Dr. Jerry A. Peterson
              Ms. Kelly Travers

ACKNOWLEDGEMENTS

The Organizing Committee for the 3rd International Workshop on
Monoclonal Antibodies and Breast Cancer, together with the John
Muir Cancer & Aging Research Institute, gratefully acknowledge
the support of the following in making the Workshop possible:

SPONSORS

COULTER IMMUNOLOGY, HIALEAH, FLORIDA
SANDOZ RESEARCH INSTITUTE, EAST HANOVER, NEW JERSEY
CAMBRIDGE RESEARCH LABORATORY, CAMBRIDGE, MASSACHUSETTS
ABBOTT LABORATORIES, NORTH CHICAGO, ILLINOIS
BOEHRINGER MANNHEIM GmbH, MANNHEIM, WEST GERMANY
CETUS CORPORATION, EMERYVILLE, CALIFORNIA
E.I. du PONT de NEMOURS & CO., NO. BILLERICA, MASSACHUSETTS
GENENTECH, INC., SOUTH SAN FRANCISCO, CALIFORNIA
ICI PHARMA, WILMINGTON, DELAWARE
TRITON BIOSCIENCES, INC., ALAMEDA, CALIFORNIA
CIBA-GEIGY Corporation, Summit, New Jersey
Bristol-Myers Company, Wallingford, Connecticut
Centocor, Inc., Malvern, Pennsylvania
Christian Brothers Winery, Saint Helena, California
Lilly Research Laboratories, Indianapolis, Indiana
Cytogen Corporation, Princeton, New Jersey
Miles, Inc./Bayer AG, Elkhart, Indiana
Xenetics Biomedical, Inc., Irvine, California
Bio-Rad, Richmond, California
Vector Laboratories, Inc., Burlingame, California
Xoma Corporation, Berkeley, California
John Muir Medical Center, Walnut Creek, California

PREFACE

    The convening of the 3rd International Workshop on Monoclonal
Antibodies and Breast Cancer had the character of a self-search
exercise. After almost a decade of research in the basic and
applied aspects of the use of serological means to diagnose and
possibly treat breast cancer several milestones have been reached.
Among them a clear understanding of immunopathological use and
limitations of monoclonal antibodies against breast epithelium, the
complete development and clinical use of immunoassays for
circulating breast epithelial antigens, the striking advances in the
diagnostic use of monoclonal antibodies to estrogen and progesterone
receptor proteins and the first communications on proposed
immunotherapeutic use of different conjugates of anti-breast
antibodies.

    New areas of investigation have developed in our field, some
which are reaching a full blossom while others are still facing
obstacles and at times a re-definition of their goals and
objectives. These meetings have acted in a way as a clearing house
and have permitted their attendees to derive predictions that have
helped shape future research and fine-tune objectives. But above
all, the re-evaluation of past research at these Workshops and the
renewed excitement brought to them by new information has helped
generate a momentum and enthusiasm that assures for the future large
scientific gains.

    The sustainment of interest of scientists in these Workshops has
allowed for the development of an ordered historical perspective of
the growth and development of the field of immunology and breast
cancer and how it relates to the use of serological approaches. The
ingenuity of investigators has produced an inexhaustible amount of
studies that have enlarged this area of research. As these reagents
become used in other areas of breast cancer studies, such as
immunotherapy, there will be a great need for interaction among
those dedicated to fight breast cancer and for the facilitation
provided by scientific dialogue such as the one sustained in these
Workshops.

                                                    R.L. Ceriani

CONTENTS

SESSION I

The Potential of Synthetic Tumor - Associated Glycoconjugates
     S-TAGs) for Generating Monoclonal Antibodies for Breast
     Cancer Imaging and for Specific Immunotherapy   3
  G. MacLean, A. McEwan, E. Mackie, P. Fung, C. Henningsson,
     R. Koganty, M. Madej, T. Sykes, A. Noujaim, and M. Longe-
     necker

Extracellular Keratins: An Update   13
  R. Cardiff, S. Taniuchi, and D. He

Preclinical Evaluation of MoAbs Mc5 and BrE1   19
  R.L. Ceriani, E.W. Blank, J.A. Peterson, and C. Zoellner

The Use of Human Monoclonal Antibodies to Identify and Isolate Breast
     Tumor Associated Antigens   33
  A.J. Strelkauskas and P.H. Aldenderfer

Clinical and Molecular Investigations of the DF3 Breast Cancer -
     Associated Antigen   45
  D.F. Hayes, M. Abe, J. Siddiqui, C. Tondini, and D.W. Kufe

An Assay For Cryptic Tumor Antigens in Sera of Women With Breast
     Cancer   55
  R. Kinders, J. Slota, J. Patrick, C. Plate, I. Kafer,
     W. Caminiti, H. Rittenhouse, and G. Manderino

SESSION II

Biosynthesis of the Cell Surface Sialomucin From Ascites 13762 Rat
     Mammary Adenocarcinoma Cells: Intracellular Maturation   71
  S.R. Hull, J. Spielman, and K.L. Carraway

Epithelial Mucin Antibodies and Their Epitopes: Core Protein
     Epitopes of a Polymorphic Epithelial Mucin (PEM)   81
  J. Taylor-Papadimitriou, J. Burchell, S. Gendler, M. Boshell, and
     T. Duhig

Cell Heterogeneity and Complexity of Breast Epithelial Surface
     Antigens Expression and MoAb Therapy   95
  J.A. Peterson, E.W. Blank, C. Zoellner, S. Enloe, G. Walkup, and
     R.L. Ceriani

The Oncogenic Potential of Membrane Receptor Proteins Encoded by
    Members of the Human erbB Proto-Oncogene Family   105
  M.H. Kraus

SESSION III

Estrogen and Progesterone Receptor Analysis and Action in Breast
    Cancer   119
  G.L. Greene, P. Gilna, and P. Kushner

Monoclonal Antibodies Against Steroid Receptors and Steroid-Induced
    Proteins   131
  M. Perrot-Applanat, J.F. Prud'homme, M.T. Vu Hai, A. Jolivet,
    F. Lorenzo, and E. Milgrom

Ten Year Survival Patterns in Primary Breast Cancers Compared to
    Hormone Receptor Antigen Detection by Monoclonal Antibodies   141
  D. Kiene, L. Kinsel, J. Konrath, G. Greene, G. Leight, E. Cox,
    K.S. McCarty, Jr., and K. McCarty, Jr.

Significance of Steroid Receptor Immunoassay in Breast Cancer   149
  E.J. Keenan and D. Corbin

H23 Monoclonal Antibodies Recognize a Breast Tumor Associated
    Antigen: Clinical and Molecular Studies   161
  I. Tsarfaty, S. Chaitchik, M. Hareuveni, J. Horev, A. Hizi,
    D.H. Wreschner, and I. Keydar

Complementation of Monoclonal Antibodies DF3 and B72.3 in Re-
    activity to Breast Cancer   171
  N. Ohuchi, M. Akimoto, S. Mori, D.W. Kufe, and J. Schlom

Differential Expression of DF3 Antigen Between Papillary Carci-
    nomas and Benign Papillary Lesions of the Breast   183
  N. Ohuchi, M.J. Merino, D. Carter, J.F. Simpson, S. Kennedy,
    D.W. Kufe, and J. Schlom

SESSION IV

Potentiation of Anti-Tumor Efficacy Resulting From the Combined
    Administration of Interferon α and of an Anti-Breast Epithelial
    Monoclonal Antibody in the Treatment of Breast Cancer
    Xenografts   195
  L. Ozzello, C.M. DeRosa, E.W. Blank, K. Cantell, D.V. Habif,
    and R.L. Ceriani

Immunolymphscintigraphy With BCD-F9 Monoclonal Antibody and Its
    F(ab)'$_2$ Fragments for the Preoperative Staging of Breast
    Cancers   203
  R. Mandeville, C. Schatten, N. Pateisky, M.J. Dicaire, B. Barbeau,
    and B. Grouix

Reaction of Antibodies to Human Milk Fat Globule (HMFG) With
    Synthetic Peptides   211
  P.X. Xing, J.J. Tjandra, X.L. Tang, D.F.J. Purcell, and I.F.C.
    McKenzie

Individually Specified Drug Immunoconjugates in Cancer Treatment   219
    R.K. Oldham and S.K. Liao

A Phase I Study of the Anti-Breast Cancer Immunotoxin 2609 MAB-rRA
    Given by Continuous Infusion   231
    B.J. Gould, M.J. Borowitz, E.S. Groves, and A.E. Frankel

In Vivo Studies of Radiolabeled Monoclonal Antibodies MC5 and KC4
    Human Breast Cancer   237
    P.A. Bunn, Jr., D.G. Dienhart, R.F. Schmelter, J.L. Lear,
    G. Miller, D.C. Bloedow, C. Longley, P. Furmanski, and
    R.L. Ceriani

Contributors   249

Index   255

SESSION I

THE POTENTIAL OF SYNTHETIC TUMOR-ASSOCIATED GLYCOCONJUGATES (S-TAGs) FOR GENERATING MONOCLONAL ANTIBODIES FOR BREAST CANCER IMAGING AND FOR SPECIFIC IMMUNOTHERAPY

Grant MacLean[a,c], Alexander McEwan[b], Eleanor Mackie[d,e], Peter Fung[d,e]
Carina Henningsson[d], Rao Koganty[e], Marian Madej[e], Thomas Sykes[e]
Antoine Noujaim[e,f] and Michael Longenecker[d,e]

Departments of Medicine[a] and Nuclear Medicine[b], Cross Cancer Institute
Departments of Medicine[c] and Immunology[d], Faculty of Medicine, and
Faculty of Pharmacy[f], University of Alberta; Biomira Inc.[e]; Edmonton
Alberta, Canada

THOMSEN FRIEDENREICH (TF) AND Tn ANTIGENS AS MARKERS FOR BREAST CANCER

The Thomsen Friedenreich (TF) antigen may be important for the detection and immunotherapy of a number of common cancers including breast cancer. Revealed on normal human erythrocytes by neuraminidase treatment, TF has been characterized as: ß-D-Gal-(1-3)-α-GalNAc, attached to glycophorin or other glycoproteins through O-serine or O-threonine linkages (1). Tn, the TF precursor, is reported to be α-GalNAc-O-serine/threonine. While TF is normally cryptic due to the presence of a terminal sialic acid residue, Tn is exposed in individuals with a recessive genetic disorder (2). Springer (1) has claimed expression of TF and Tn antigens on over 90% of cancers of the breast, lung and pancreas, although the nature of the molecules which bear these antigens and their exact structures has not been defined.

Our group was the first to generate monoclonal antibodies (MAbs) against TF-like antigens expressed on human cancer cells (3,4). Since then, however, we have been able to derive many different MAbs of predetermined specificity for TF-like epitopes utilizing our ability to generate synthetic tumor-associated glycoconjugates (S-TAGs) and MAbs against these. Different conformations of TF were synthesized and used as immunogens to derive MAbs which were selected for their reactivity with the S-TAGs. Several of these MAbs were also demonstrated to have in-vitro specificity for human adenocarcinomata in frozen tissue sections (5). We describe here the initial radioimmunoimaging studies with two of these radiolabelled anti-synthetic-TF MAbs, in patients with metastatic adenocarcinoma of the breast. Such studies are enabling us to probe the *in vivo* expression of TF on metastatic human adenocarcinomata, and to ask whether TF-like antigens can be used as targets for the detection of metastatic cancer.

The ease with which anti-TF MAbs could be generated demonstrated the immunogenicity of TF in mice. We thus wanted to know whether synthetic TF could be used (in an appropriate formulation) to actively induce a protective specific immune response against tumor cells? In a relevant murine mammary adenocarcinoma model (the tumor cells express TF-like structures) we recently showed that synthetic TF and Tn could be used to induce a T lymphocyte response which had protective anti-cancer reactivity (6). Further experiments, reported here, have probed strategies to optimize both the cellular and humoral immune responses to synthetic TF, asking whether synthetic TF has potential for active specific immunotherapy.

Thus, our aim has been to identify human tumor-associated glycoconjugate antigens, synthesize them, and test whether these synthetic glycoconjugates have potential both as immunogens for active specific immunotherapy (ASI), and as immunogens to derive relevant MAbs for localizing (radioimmunoimaging) cancers. Successful radioimmunoimaging in humans would validate a particular synthetic glycoconjugate, while the animal model would be used to study the potential of the same antigen for ASI. We recently summarized this approach to cancer therapy and detection with TF S-TAGs and their corresponding MAbs (7).

In addition to the potential of TF as a target antigen of breast cancer, there is evidence that TF and Tn antigens may be functional markers of malignancy. Investigators studying the expression of TF in human bladder cancers have shown a relationship between TF expression and likelihood of invasive recurrence (8,9). Springer and colleagues have extensively studied TF and Tn antigen expression on human breast carcinomas (1,10) and claim that the ratio of expression of Tn to TF correlates with the aggressiveness (and degree of dedifferentiation) of the cancer. Howard and Batsakis (11) analysed 22 breast carcinomas, and found that the 17 well differentiated tumors expressed TF antigen, while the remaining 5 undifferentiated tumors lacked TF antigen.

Yuan and coworkers (12) used one of our TF MAbs (3) to study the early expression of TF antigens on premalignant polyps and colon adenocarcinomas (normal adult mucosa was not marked by the MAb) and showed that this MAb marked pre-malignant polyps as well as adenocarcinoma. We have also confirmed this. This MAb also marked fetal colon tissue, suggesting that TF may be an oncodevelopmental antigen in human colon cancer.

Perhaps the best evidence for a functional role of the TF system in malignancy is provided by a genetic disorder which results in a selective loss of 3-ß-D-galactosyl-transferase activity and the appearance of Tn positive RBCs and hematopoietic stem cells (the Tn syndrome). This disorder is associated with a high incidence of leukemia and other hematopoietic disorders. This suggests that Tn expression might be indicative of deregulation of pleuripotent stem cells, with a proliferative advantage for Tn^+ cells (2).

The first question to be answered then was whether the TF S-TAGs were identical to the TF-like structures expressed on human cancers *in vivo*.

SUCCESSFUL *IN VIVO* IMAGING OF METASTATIC HUMAN BREAST CANCER, USING MAbs 155H.7 AND 170H.82 GENERATED USING SYNTHETIC TF GLYCOCONJUGATES

Two monoclonal antibodies (MAbs), designated 155H.7 and 170H.82, were generated against synthetic TFß conjugated to HSA, and were shown to react strongly *in vitro* with most adenocarcinomata with little or no obvious tumor heterogeneity (very few negative cancer cells) (5). Of relevance here is that 27/27 adenocarcinomata of the breast reacted with the MAb 155H.7. Reactivity with normal tissues and other malignancies was limited, so it was proposed to study the reactivity of these two MAbs *in vivo*, in clinical radioimmunoimaging.

It proved possible to radiolabel each of these without loss of immunoreactivity. Phase 1 radioimmunoimaging studies were instituted, prior to the development of Phase 2 and 3 imaging trials. Because of the unique development of these MAbs - being derived against S-TAGs - the pilot studies have been designed to answer the following questions:
1) Are the radiolabeled anti-S-TAGs toxic?
2) Are the compounds stable *in vivo*? Do they bind to known sites of adenocarcinomata *in vivo* ?
3) Can a dose response be demonstrated, with improved imaging efficacy at increasing doses of antibody?

The underlying questions were:
a) Can MAbs derived against synthetic glycoconjugates bind to human cancers *in vivo* ? and
b) Are the S-TAGs being developed for specific immunotherapy (and which were used to derive the MAbs for imaging) relevant to human cancers?

The first clinical imaging study used MAb 155H.7. This pilot study included a comparison between the MAb radiolabeled with Iodine-131 and with Indium-111. Iodination was performed carefully over no more than two minutes (to avoid loss of immunoreactivity) using an Iodogen method. Indium labeling was accomplished by pre-chelating the MAb with 4-6 chelate groups via the DTPA anhydride reaction, with free chelate removal by diafiltration. The addition of Indium-111 in citrate buffer resulted in >98% binding to the chelated MAb 155H.7 after 30 minutes. All radioimmunoconjugates for clinical imaging are tested for immunoreactivity, sterility and apyrogenicity prior to clinical use.

As the MAb had shown a broad range of reactivity with adenocarcinomata *in vitro*, patients with a similar range of adenocarcinomata were entered into the study, including patients with adenocarcinomata of the breast, endometrium, ovary, colon and lung. As this was a pilot study, only sites of known tumor were evaluated, and the results of the immunoimaging study were compared with the results of conventional clinical and imaging investigations. No attempt has been made to define sensitivity and specificity in this phase 1 protocol. Included in this study were six patients with metastatic breast cancer evaluated with the Iodine-131 label, and two evaluated with the Indium-111 label.

Limited imaging efficacy was seen at the lower dose levels utilized (4 and 8 mg). However at increasing doses of antibody (16 and 32 mg) increasing imaging sensitivity was demonstrated, with 32 mg offering the most effective images.

It was clear from the study that Indium-111 was the more effective imaging label at all MAb dose levels used. This isotope also offers the opportunity of SPECT (single photon emission computed tomography) imaging which greatly increases diagnostic efficacy, image quality, resolution and the ability to detect presence of cancer in nodes defined as "normal" on C.T. SPECT imaging was performed using a GE 400 AT Tomographic camera interfaced to a Picker PCS 512 computer, with data acquisition on a 128*128 matrix and stored for later reconstruction analysis.

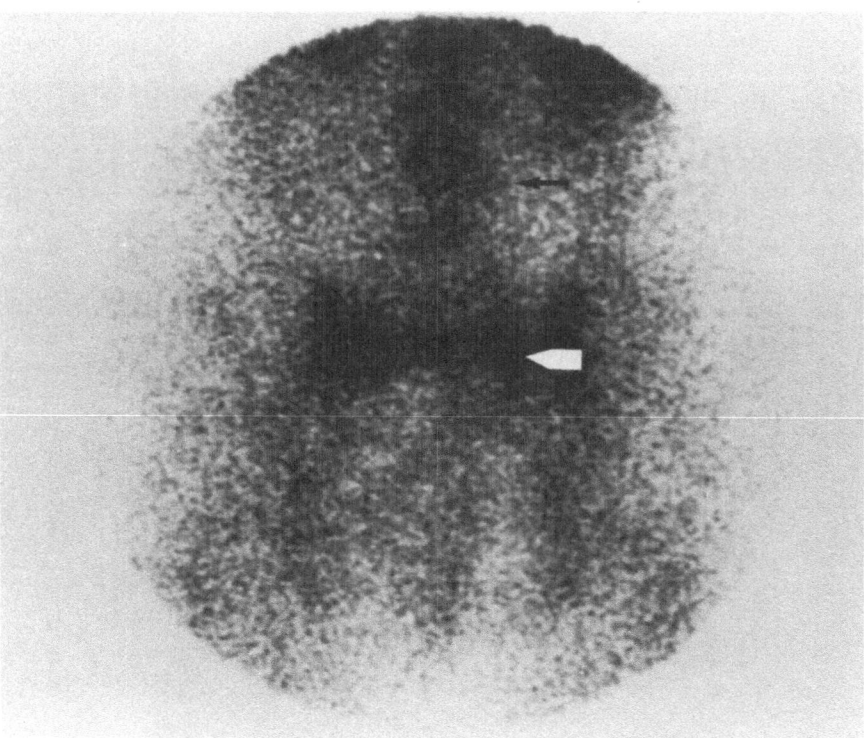

Figure 1. ^{131}I.155H.7: Uptake in metastases to bone.

A wide range of known metastatic sites in patients with breast cancer were successfully imaged, including lymph nodes, lung and bone. Figure 1 is a planar posterior abdominal image of a patient with metastatic breast cancer, using 32 mg MAb 155H.7 labeled with 2 mCi Iodine-131. Tracer uptake is seen in the known bone metastases in the right sacro-iliac joint and in the lumbar vertebrae. Figure 2 shows selected chest SPECT images of a patient with metastatic breast cancer, imaged 6 days after the infusion of 32 mg MAb 155H.7 labeled with 5 mCi Indium-111. Uptake can be clearly seen in the metastatic mass in the mediastinum.

While clinical accuracy was not the primary purpose of this study, particularly without surgical and histological confirmation of positive tracer uptake, there was a high concordance demonstrated between the findings on radioimmunoscintigraphy and the findings on CT scanning, ultrasonography and clinical examination.

A current study is investigating the diagnostic potential of radioimmunolympho-scintigraphy using [111]In.155H.7 injected into the finger web spaces of patients with breast cancer, to detect regional lymph node metastases. Tracer activity is seen in supraclavicular nodes within one hour, with retention of activity in nodes which are definitely abnormal clinically (enlarged, hard, and irregular). The next phase in this study is to biopsy these nodes for surgical/histological confirmation of the specificity of the binding of the immunoconjugate in these "involved lymph nodes".

A second pilot study has now commenced to evaluate the other anti-TF MAb, 170H.82. Although the immunogen used to derive this MAb is identical to that used to derive the MAb 155H.7, the immunoreactivity of the two MAbs with both synthetic glycoconjugates and tissue sections is different. The next study is therefore designed to compare the imaging efficacy of the two MAbs.

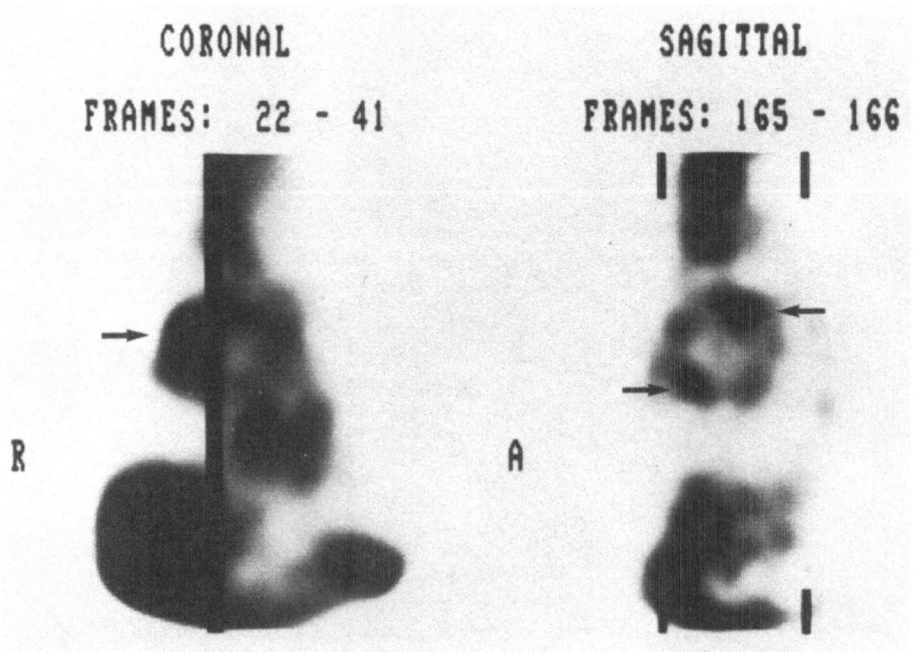

CORONAL

FRAMES: 22 - 41

SAGITTAL

FRAMES: 165 - 166

R

A

Figure 2. [111]In.155H.7; SPECT: Uptake in metastasis to mediastinum.

In this protocol Indium-111 has been used as the radiolabel, and SPECT imaging has been performed in all patients. Of the seven patients imaged to date with [111]In.170H.82, two patients have metastatic breast cancer. Figure 3 shows chest SPECT of a patient with breast cancer, imaged using 8 mg MAb and 3 mCi Indium-111. Disease is detected within the left hemi-thorax, left supraclavicular fossa and right axilla.

The data on imaging metastatic breast cancer are limited, being extracted from two pilot studies in patients with a wide variety of metastatic adenocarcinomata. However, the evidence from all the data is that these murine MAbs of predetermined specificity, derived using synthetic glycoconjugates as immunogens, have clinical potential for detection of metastatic adenocarcinoma including breast cancer. Larger prospective studies are being planned.

Based on our wider experience in patients with metastatic adenocarcinomata arising from the female genital organs (ovary, fallopian tube, uterus and cervix) we predict an expanding clinical role for radioimmunoscintigraphy in:
(1) screening for metastatic disease;
(2) in vivo analysis of radiologically detected "lesions";
(3) in vivo prediction of tumor response to treatment;
(4) intra-operative localization of metastatic disease.

If the initial, encouraging results are validated, the next phase of development will be the evaluation of a dose response protocol for targetted therapy in patients with breast and gynecologic cancers.

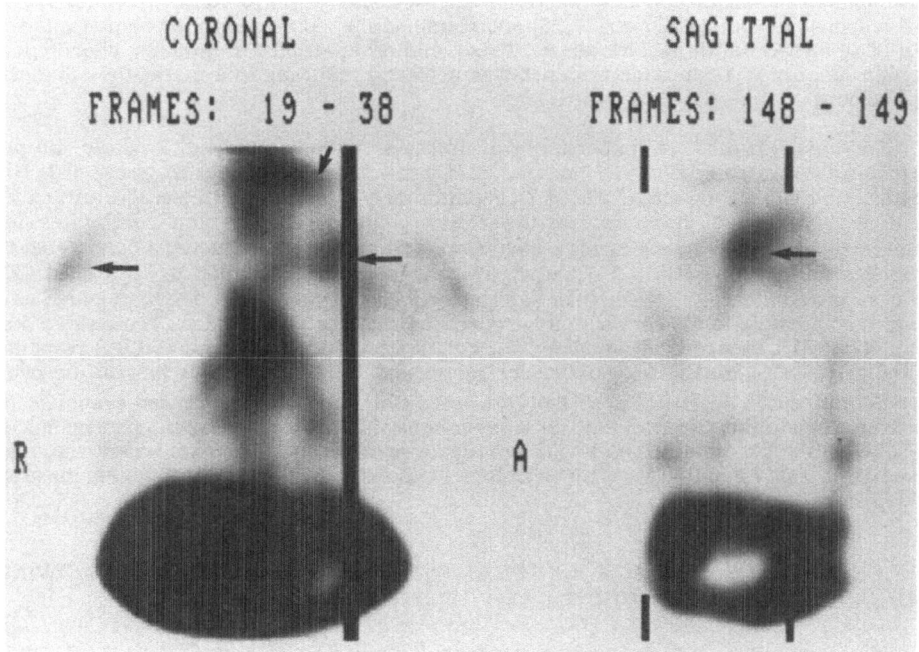

Figure 3. [111]In.170H.82; SPECT: Uptake in metastases in nodes and lung.

In addition to demonstrating the imaging potential of these MAbs, these studies have also demonstrated that TF-like antigens are expressed *in vivo* on metastases of breast cancer, that these antigens are accessible to the immune system, and that the epitopes of the synthetic glycoconjugates are identical to the epitopes expressed on cancers. Can these same S-TAGs then be used to induce a protective immune response - for immunotherapy?

IMMUNE RESPONSE TO CARBOHYDRATE ANTIGENS

In planning active specific immunotherapy we should consider and seek to measure the likely humoral and cellular immune responses to the specific antigens. Antibodies to carbohydrates (CHOs) generally have a peculiar isotype distribution and are usually of relatively low affinity. The major isotype response is IgM in both humans and mice (13). In our experience in the generation of several thousand MAbs to TF, Tn and sialated Lewis[a] haptens conjugated to HSA, greater than 90% of the clones produced IgM antibodies despite prolonged immunization. In general, the IgG anti-CHO response is predominantly IgG_2 in humans (14,15) and IgG_3 in mice (16-18). However, exceptions to these rules have been published, suggesting that the variation depends on the particular carbohydrate used for immunization or the age of the responder (17,19).

Immune responses to most polysaccharides have been classically referred to as "T-independent" since they can apparently trigger B cells to produce antibody in the absence of T-helper cell activity (20-22) and T-suppressor cells may even inhibit responses to these antigens (23-25). Immune responses to T-independent antigens are usually restricted to IgM and immunization with these antigens often fails to stimulate the production of memory cells (26).

Proteins are typical T cell-dependent antigens capable of producing a booster response and of causing a progressive switch of IgM to IgG antibodies of increasing affinities after repeated injections. Many attempts to generate IgG anti-carbohydrate antibodies have involved the conjugation of the polysaccharide to a protein carrier. This conjugation is meant to convert the polysaccharide from a T-independent to a T-dependent antigen. Such polysaccharide-protein conjugates have been used in the development of vaccines against bacterial diseases and found to markedly enhance the IgG response in young children (27,28) and young adults, compared to the response to the purified polysaccharide vaccine alone. These, and other studies in humans, show that a certain amount of thymus-dependence was achieved resulting in a markedly enhanced IgG response.

Previous studies in experimental animals have employed keyhole limpet hemocyanin (KLH) as the carrier protein. KLH has a molecular weight in excess of 7×10^6 daltons and is a strong stimulator of T cell immunity. Thus high titres of IgG antibodies against a variety of haptens may be achieved using KLH-hapten conjugates for immunization. Some recent studies have employed carbohydrate haptens conjugated to KLH as immunogens (29,30). Particularly revealing was a recent report by Tittle et al. (30) who compared the antibody response to nigerose [α(1,3)diglucoside] when it appeared as a hapten conjugated to KLH or as a native constituent of dextran. Dextran is considered to be a classical T-independent antigen. The conjugate induced a substantial IgG response with IgG_1, IgG_{2a} and IgG_{2b} subclasses increasing by 2-3 orders of magnitude over pre-immunization levels. These isotypes were not found in the *in vivo* response to dextran. In addition, dextran induced a predominant lambda response in naive splenic B cells while the pre-immunization with conjugate resulted in a dramatic kappa response to dextran, suggested that B cells can become responsive to T-independent antigens after T-dependent activation.

SUCCESSFUL GENERATION OF HIGH TITRE IgG RESPONSES FOLLOWING IMMUNIZATION OF MICE WITH TFα–KLH CONJUGATES

Mice which were immunized intraperitoneally with TFα–KLH in CFA gave IgG titres which ranged from 1:5,120 - 1:320,000 following the third immunization. The substitution of CFA by Ribi adjuvant composed of trehalose dimycolate (TDM) and monophosphyl Lipid A (MPLA) gave equivalently high IgG titres (see Table 1).

Table 1. Range of Titres[1] in CB6F1/J Mice Immunized With TF Alpha-KLH

Immunizing Antigen/ Concentration	n[*]	Second Immune Bleed IgG	IgM	Third Immune Bleed IgG	IgM
100 ug. TFα-KLH 860 haptens + CFA	5	1,280-80,000	80-5,120	20,480-330,000	80-1,280
100 ug. TFα-KLH, 3100 haptens + CFA	5	320-20,480	80-20,480	40,000-160,000	20-5,120
25 ug. TFα-KLH, 3100 haptens + CFA	5	320-20,480	< 20-1,280	5,120-330,000	<20-1,280
100 ug. TFα-KLH, 860 haptens, + Ribi (TDM + MPLA)	15	<20-81,920	80-1,280	320-330,000	320-5,120

1. Titres given as reciprocals of 4-fold dilutions beginning with 1:20.
2. Test antigen is TF alpha-HSA (0.2 ug/well, 27 haptens/mole HSA).
3. Titre against HSA also done: Range is < 20-320.
4. Immunizations were 3 I.P. injections, 2 weeks apart with tail bleeds taken 12 d after each injection.
5. [*] - "n" is the number of mice in each experiment.

SUCCESSFUL GENERATION OF DIRECT DELAYED TYPE HYPERSENSITIVITY (DTH) REACTIONS TO TFα FOLLOWING SUBCUTANEOUS IMMUNIZATION WITH A CANCER-ASSOCIATED MUCIN

In our previous studies (6), DTH responsiveness and effector cells specifically capable of recognizing and responding to epiglycanin (a murine cancer-associated mucin, see below) or the synthetic tumor-associated glycoconjugates (S-TAGs), were generated by co-culturing primed spleen cells with epiglycanin or the S-TAG molecules for 6 days. Although interesting for the generation of future T-cell clones, we felt that it was more clinically relevant to develop a reproducible method for induction of direct DTH reactions *in vivo*. Recently we developed a direct *in vivo* priming method to induce DTH responsiveness and effector cells to epiglycanin and S-TAGs. With this method, we succeeded in demonstrating that mice immunized subcutaneously with epiglycanin[+] CFA

Table 2.   Direct DTH Responsiveness to TFα

Pre-immunization	Foot-pad Antigen Challenge	Net foot-pad swelling (mm ± S.D.)[*] 24 hr	48 hr
Epi + CFA	Epi	0.53 ± 0.04	0.15 ± 0.07
	TFα-HSA	0.43 ± 0.18	0.30 ± 0.21
	HSA	0.03 ± 0.03	0.03 ± 0.06
Epi + Ribi	Epi	0.33 ± 0.04	0.18 ± 0.04
	TFα-HSA	0.40 ± 0.014	0.38 ± 0.11
	HSA	0.02 ± 0.03	0.03 ± 0.03

Epi - epiglycanin, the mucin bearing TF-like epitopes (see text below).
CFA - complete Freund's adjuvant, the standard immune adjuvant.
Ribi - Ribi adjuvant (see text above).
[*] Average of 3 mice.

or epiglycanin[+] Ribi compound (containing trehalose dimycolate and monophosphoryl lipid A emulsions) developed strong and specific DTH responses when footpad tested with either epiglycanin or S-TAGs on Day 7, after the initial immunization (Table 2). In addition, DTH responsiveness to the same antigens could be adoptively transferred to naive syngeneic recipients (data not shown).

THE TA3-Ha MURINE MAMMARY ADENOCARCINOMA, A MODEL FOR IMMUNOTHERAPY OF A MUCIN SECRETING CANCER

Most adenocarcinomas secrete mucin-like molecules which appear in the blood and which contain altered carbohydrate antigenic determinants. We have much experience with the murine adenocarcinoma TA3-Ha (6,7) which we believe provides an excellent tumor model closely approximating the human clinical situation. The TA3-Ha tumor is a spontaneous murine mammary adenocarcinoma derived originally from the A/J mouse (31-33). This tumor produces a glycocalyx containing a mucin called epiglycanin (Epi), a 500,000 m.w. glycoprotein composed of 75-80% carbohydrate, containing multiple TF and Tn determinants (34). Epi is also secreted into body fluids and resembles many tumor-associated mucin-like molecules of human tumors (35-37). Epi is believed to provide protection for the highly lethal TA3-Ha tumor against immunological attack, allowing permissive growth even in allogeneic and some xenogeneic hosts (31,38).

We have demonstrated that TF and Tn S-TAGs can be used to immunize hosts to inhibit the growth of TA3-Ha cells and that DTH effector T cells recognizing the TF antigens on epiglycanin (isolated from the TA3-Ha tumors) can be generated following immunization with synthetic antigen conjugated to protein carriers (6).

With these encouraging findings we have proceeded with an intensive, systematic investigation of the use of carbohydrate S-TAGs as defined anti-cancer "vaccines". It should be clarified at this point that the future intended use of these "vaccines" is really as active, specific immunotherapeutics in cancer patients in clinical remission, but with a high chance of recurrence. Nevertheless, the term "vaccine", rightly or wrongly, is used widely to describe this class of compounds.

INDUCTION OF EFFECTIVE ANTI-BREAST ADENOCARCINOMA IMMUNITY FOLLOWING IMMUNIZATION WITH TFα-KLH CONJUGATES

Most recently, we have designed a very effective protocol, using TFα-KLH and S-TAG conjugates, to pre-immunize mice to achieve nearly 100% long term survival following an otherwise uniformly lethal TA3-Ha challenge.

SUMMARY

Our approach is to investigate the potential of specific well defined antigens both for the generation of MAbs which can localize metastatic cancer, and for use in active specific immunotherapy. This approach is possible by the generation of well-defined synthetic glyconjugates. We describe here the studies with one of these, the "TF" antigen. We have shown, for the first time, that high titre IgG, DTH and effective anti-cancer immunity can be generated using synthetic glycoconjugates related to the Thomsen Friedenreich (TF) antigen, using the TA3-Ha murine mammary adenocarcinoma model. This model appears relevant for immunotherapy, as TA3-Ha is a mucin secreting cancer carrying tumor-associated TF determinants. Our parallel radioimmunoimaging studies in human breast cancer patients, using MAbs derived using TF S-TAGs, demonstrate the potential of anti-TF MAbs for localizing metastatic cancer, and also demonstrate the relevance of TF antigens as targets for the immune system in humans. Thus, in addition to further exploring the potential of anti-TF MAbs for cancer detection and targetted therapy, we are also encouraged to begin Phase I clinical trials of active specific immunotherapy in adenocarcinoma patients, using some of our synthetic TF glycoconjugates.

REFERENCES

1. G.F. Springer. Science 224: 1198 (1984).
2. W. Vainchenker, G. Vinci, U. Testa, A. Henri, A. Tabilio, M. Fache, H. Rochant and J. Cartron. J. Clin. Invest. 75: 541 (1985).
3. B.M. Longenecker, A.F.R. Rahmann, J. Barrington-Leigh, R.A. Purser, A.H. Greenberg, D.J. Willans, O. Keller, P.K. Petrik, T.Y. Thay, M.R. Suresh and A.A. Noujaim. Int. J. Cancer 33: 123 (1984).
4. F.R. Rahman and B.M. Longenecker. J. Immunol. 129: 2021 (1982).
5. B.M. Longenecker, D.J. Willans, G.D. MacLean, S. Selvaraj, M.R. Suresh and A.A. Noujaim. J. Natl. Cancer Inst. 78: 489 (1987).
6. C.M. Henningsson, S. Selvaraj, G.D. MacLean, M.R. Suresh, A.A. Noujaim and B.M. Longenecker. Cancer Immunol. Immunother. 25: 231 (1987).
7. B.M. Longenecker, G.D.MacLean, A.J.McEwan, T.Sykes, C.Henningson, M.R.Suresh, and A.A.Noujaim. In: Altered Glycosylation in Tumor Cells. Alan R. Liss, Inc. UCLA Symposium on Molecular and Cell Biology 79: 307 (1988).
8. J.S. Coon, R.S. Weinstein and J.L. Summers. Amer. J. Clin. Pathol. 17: 692 (1982).
9. H. Ohoka, H. Shinomiya, M. Yokoyama, K. Ochi, M. Takeuchi and S. Utsumi. Urol. Res. 13: 47 (1985).
10. G.F. Springer, P.R. Desai, M.S. Marthy, H. Tegetmeyer and E.F. Scanlon. Prog. Allergy 26: 42 (1979).
11. D.R. Howard and J.G. Batsakis. Science 210: 201 (1980).
12. M. Yuan, S.H. Itzkowitz, C.R. Boland, Y.D. Kim, J.T. Tomita, A. Palekar, J.L. Bennington, B.F. Trump and Y.S. Kim. Cancer Res. 46: 4841 (1986).
13. O. Mäkelä, P. Mattila, N. Rautonen, I. Seppälä, J. Eskola and H. Käyty. J. Immunol. 139: 1999 (1987).
14. W.F. Riesen, F. Skvaril and D.G. Braun. Scand. J. Immunol. 5: 383 (1976).
15. D.J. Barrett and E.M. Ayoub. Clin. Exp. Immunol. 63: 127 (1986).
16. R.M. Perlmutter, D. Hansburg, D.E. Briles, R.A. Nicolotti and J.M. Davie. J. Immunol. 1221: 566 (1978).
17. C. Moreno and J. Esdaile. Eur. J. Immunol. 13: 262 (1983).
18. H.O. Sarvas, L.M. Aaltonen, F. Peterfy and O. Makela. Eur. J. Immunol. 13: 409 (1983).
19. L. Hammarstrom, M.A.A. Persson and C.I.E. Smith. Immunology 54: 821 (1985).
20. D.H. Katz and B. Benacerraf. Adv. Immunol. 15: 1 (1972).
21. J.G. Howard, G.H. Christie, B.M. Courtenay, E. Leuchars and A.J.S. Davies. Cell Immunol. 2: 64 (1971).
22. B. Andersson and H. Blomgren. Cell Immunol. 2: 411 (1971).
23. W.D. Armstrong, E. Diener and G.R. Shellam. J. Exp. Med. 129: 393 (1969).
24. P.J. Baker, P.W. Stashak, D.F. Amsbaugh, B. Prescott and R.F. Barth. J. Immunol. 105: 1581 (1970).
25. P.J. Baker, N.D. Reed, P.W. Stashak, D.F. Amsbaugh and B. Prescott. J. Exp. Med. 1431 (1973).
26. P.J. Baker, P.W. Stashak, D.F. Amsbaugh and B. Prescott. Immunology 20: 469 (1971).
27. C. Lee. Molecular Immunol. 24: 1005 (1987).
28. H. Kayhty, J. Eskola, H. Peltola, M.G. Sout, J.S. Samuelson and L.K. Gordon. J. Inf. Dis. 155: 100 (1987).
29. J.A. Benjamins, R.E. Callahan, I.N. Montgomery, D.M. Studzinski and C.A. Dyer. J. Neuroimmunol. 14: 325 (1987).
30. T.V. Tittle, A. Mawle and M. Cohn. J. Immunol. 135: 2582 (1985).
31. S. Friberg. J. Natl. Cancer Inst. 48: 1436 (1972).
32. G. Klein. Exp. Cell Res. 2: 518 (1951).
33. B.H. Sanford, J.F. Codington, R.W. Jeanloz and P.D. Palmer. J. Immunol. 110: 1233 (1973).
34. D. Van den Eijden, N.A. Evans, J.F. Codington, V. Reinhold, C. Silber and R.W. Jeanloz. J. Biol. Chem. 254: 12153 (1979).
35. H.G. Rittenhouse. Lab. Med. 16: 556 (1985).
36. C.R. Boland, C.K. Montgomery and Y.S. Kim. P.N.A.S. 79: 2051 (1982).
37. J.L. Magnini, L. Steplewski, H. Koprowski and V. Ginsburg. Cancer Res. 43: 5489 (1983).
38. M.M. Lippmann, J.M. Venditti, I. Kline and D.L. Elan. Cancer Res. 33: 679 (1973).

EXTRACELLULAR KERATINS: AN UPDATE

Robert D. Cardiff, Shoichiro Taniuchi, and Daer He

Department of Pathology
University of California School of Medicine
Davis, California 95616

INTRODUCTION

Four years ago we announced the production of a series of monoclonal antibodies which react with the major epithelial keratins of MCF7 and other breast cancer cell lines (1). One of the antibodies, UCD/PR 10.11, has proven to be an excellent reagent, when used in the immunoperoxidase technique, for the diagnosis of epithelial malignancies (2). UCD/PR 10.11 reacts with CK 8 and 18. It has a superb signal-to-noise ratio in staining almost all simple epithelia and is thought by some to be one of the best diagnostic monoclonal anti-keratin available for immunopathology (3). It is now commercially available through Triton Biosciences, Inc.

At the same time, we also announced that some of the same set of monoclonal antibodies identified keratin-like epitopes which can be detected outside of the cell (1). One of the extracellular keratins was found shed into the media of MCF7 cells and the other was found attached to the external surface of the same cells (1,4). Since keratins were thought to be exclusively insoluble, intracellular proteins, the identification of a potentially extracellular form of these proteins was unexpected (1). In the intervening period, we have found that keratins-like epitopes appear to be arranged on the surface of certain malignant cells and are shed by other epithelial malignancies. Since these observations have some immediate clinical implications, it is appropriate to evaluate the data.

SHED KERATINS

In-vitro Studies

The shed-keratin antigen was first detected in the supernatant of MCF7 cells by western blot using the monoclonal antibodies UCD/AB 6.01 and 6.11 (4). The antigen is released through an as yet undetermined mechanism by MCF7 and a variety of carcinoma cell lines (5). The antigen has been found to contain epitopes related to the keratins 8, 18, and 19 (5). However, the antigen has a lower molecular weight and is more acidic than any of the three intracellular keratins (5). Furthermore, the soluble antigen has an amino acid composition similar to that expected for any keratin and a peptide map consistent with keratins 8 and 18 (5). The conversion of the intracellular keratins into the more soluble extracellular form is partially inhibited by the addition of chelating agents such as EDTA to the media of sodium azide treated cells (5). This is consistent with the hypothesis that a calcium dependent protease is responsible for the bio-conversion of the antigen into a soluble form (5,6).

In order to more thoroughly study the release of the antigen into the supernatant, an immunoradiometric assay for cytokeratin was developed (5,7). This assay uses UCD/PR 10.11 as the "catch" antibody to detect keratin in the experimental solution and UCD/AB 6.11 is used as the signal antibody. The assay detects as little as 1ng keratin/ml. and is quantitative between 10 and 100 ng keratin/ml. The assay in this configuration detects purified keratin 18 but no other intermediate filaments (7). The assay is, therefore, referred to as IRMAK 18.

The IRMAK 18 has been used to detect the release of keratin 18 from a variety of epithelial cell lines. The release of keratin 18 differs from line to line (5). However, all of the epithelial cell lines that have been studied release keratin 18. The mechanism of the release is unknown. On an experimental basis, the treatment of cells with sodium azide destroys them and results in the release of massive quantities of keratin 18. Therefore, cell death is at least one possible mechanism. However, all of the keratin shed cannot be attributed to the death of cells in culture. Others have suggested that the release of keratin-like epitopes is related to a high mitotic rate (8).

In-vivo Studies

The release of keratin from viable cultured tumor cells suggested that in-vivo tumors may also release soluble keratin. The sera of nude mice bearing transplants of MCF7 tumor cells were studied (9). The majority of the mice contained detectable levels of circulating keratin. The keratin generally did not appear in the sera until the tumors became quite large. However, the size of the tumor mass was not directly proportional to the level of circulating keratin. The level of keratin seemed to relate to the presence of tumor necrosis (9).

The sera of patients with breast cancer, benign breast disease, and a variety of malignancies were compared with samples of sera from control patients. Very few patients in any of the groups contained detectable levels of circulating keratin.

Soluble keratin was sought in other body fluids. The urine of normal individuals and most urological patients in our clinics have low levels of detectable keratin (7,10,11). However, 50% of the patients with transitional cell carcinoma of the urinary bladder have elevated urinary keratin 18 detectable with the IRMAK 18 (10). The elevation of keratin in these patients corresponds to the stage and grade of the disease.

Patients with a past history of transitional cell carcinoma of the urinary bladder frequently have detectable levels of urinary keratin (10). Approximately 20% of these patients have elevated levels of urinary keratin. We are currently studying a cohort of 102 patients who have had a past history of bladder cancer to determine whether the urinary keratins will have prognostic significance.

SURFACE KERATIN-LIKE EPITOPES

A second form of extracellular keratin appears on the surface of cells and in the region of desmosomes. The monoclonal antibody UCD/AB 6.01 identifies keratin 8 in purified extracts of cellular keratin from MCF7, A431, and EJ24 cells (5). However, it also identifies a protease sensitive antigen on the surface of most epithelial cells. The antigen is concentrated at the junction between cells and can be observed on the desmosomes of frozen sections of squamous cell carcinomas.

Acetone fixed cells have the UCD/AB 6.01 epitope on the surface of cells such as MCF7, EJT24, and A431 cells. However, the same acetone fixed cells do not have the 6.01 epitope internally on the cytoskeleton. In contrast, the antibodies UCD/AB 6.11 and UCD/PR 10.11, against keratins 8 and 18, decorate the classical intermediate filament network in the same cells fixed with acetone.

At the present time we do not know the precise nature of the antigen on the cell surface. The weight of evidence supports the notion that the antigen is a keratin-like epitope or that some keratins have an extracellular domain. Based on the morphological distribution of the antigen, we support the hypothesis that keratin 8 is primarily on the cell surface and has an extracellular domain. We would suggest that keratin 8 has a special role in anchoring the other cytoskeletal proteins to the cell membrane. This hypothesis is supported by Diaz and colleagues who have discovered that the sera of patients with pemphigus sometimes have antibodies which identify keratin 10 and binds to desmosomes (12). These auto-antibodies destroy the cell-to-cell adhesions of desmosomes and lead to bullous excoriation of the victim's skin.

The antibody UCD/AB 6.01 has been used as a radiolabelled molecule for the imaging of metastatic breast cancer (13). We have recently conjugated UCD/AB 6.01 to the photosensitizer hematoporphyrin (14) When live cells with the 6.01 epitope are incubated with the conjugated antibody and exposed to light, they are destroyed. This cytotoxic effect is dependent upon the light dose and the hematoporphyrin concentration.

To determine whether the antibody will differentially bind to the surface of tumor cells UCD/AB 6.01 conjugated with hematoporphyrin was placed on the surface of tumor bearing laryngectomy and cystectomy specimens. After washing the specimen thoroughly, the entire sample was exposed to a black lamp. The regions of the tumors fluoresce while the undisturbed normal epithelium does not suggesting that the antibody preferentially binds to certain types of tumor cells. We hope that these observations will lead to the development of an effective means of identifying and treating epithelial neoplasms.

SUMMARY

Immunological analysis of keratins have suggested that these proteins are not exclusively intracellular, soluble molecules. On one hand, soluble keratins appear in the sera of tumor bearing nude mice and in the urine of tumor bearing humans. Although the exact mechanism for the release of these antigens is not understood, their release into body fluids make them potential markers for neoplastic disease.

It now appears that keratin, or keratin-like, domains appear at the surface of epithelial cells. Our morphological data suggests that the keratin 8 molecule is almost exclusively found on the cell surface of epithelial cells. If this observation can be verified, it suggests that certain keratins and, perhaps keratin 8, represent a subset of molecules responsible for the interaction of the intermediate filament network with the cell membrane and with adhesion plaques of all types (15). Our clinical observations suggest that these elements are rearranged in some neoplasms, giving them unique immunological characteristics which may be exploited for therapeutic purposes.

Acknowledgements

This work was sponsored, in part, by a grant from Triton Biosciences, Inc, Alameda, California. The authors gratefully acknowledge the contributions of Kelly Cant, Heather Kerr, Paul Rossitto, and Kathleen Hendrix to various phases of this research.

Bibliography

1. R. Chan, P.V. Rossitto, B.F. Edwards and R.D. Cardiff. Intracellular and extracellular keratins of human mammary epithelial cells. In: "Monoclonal Antibodies and Breast Cancer," R.L. Ceriani, ed., M. Nijhoff Publishing. Dordrecht and Lancaster, Boston, (1985).
2. R. Chan, B.F. Edwards, R. Hu, P.V. Rossitto, B.H. Min, J.K. Lund, and R.D. Cardiff. Characterization of two monoclonal antibodies in an immunohistochemical study of keratin 8 and 18 expression. Am. J. Clin. Path. 89:472-480 (1988).

16

3. H. Battifora, Diagnostic uses of antibodies to keratins. A review and immunohistochemical comparison of seven monoclonal and three polyclonal antibodies. In: "Progress in Surgical Pathology," Vol. VIII. C. Fenoglio, M. Wolff, eds., Field and Wood, Inc., Philadelphia, 1987.

4. A.B. Brabon, J.F. Williams and R.D. Cardiff. A monoclonal antibody to a human breast cancer protein released in response to estrogen. Cancer Res. 44:2704-2710 (1984).

5. R. Chan, P.V. Rossitto, B.F. Edwards and R.D. Cardiff. Presence of proteolytically processed keratins in the culture medium of MCF-7 cells. Cancer Res. 46:6353-6359, (1986).

6. P.E. Bowden, R.A. Quinlan, D. Breitkreutz, and N.E. Fusenig. Proteolytic modification of acid and basic keratins during terminal differentiation of mouse and human epidermis. Eur. J. Biochem. 142:29-36 (1984).

7. P.V. Rossitto, R. Chan, M. Strand, C.H. Miller, Wm. C. Baker, A.D. Deitch, R. deVere White and R.D. Cardiff. Characterization of urinary keratin number 18 using a new assay. J. Urol. 140:431-435 (1988).

8. B. Bjorklund, and V. Bjorklund. Specificity and basis of the tissue polypeptide antigen. Cancer Detect. Prev. 6:41-50 (1983).

9. P.V. Rossitto, R. Chan, B.F. Edwards and R.D. Cardiff. A quantitative immunoradiometric assay that detects a soluble form of cytokeratin no. 18 in serum. 2nd International Workshop on Monoclonal Antibodies and Breast Cancer. November, 1986.

10. W. C. Baker, R. deVere White, P.V. Rossitto, B.H. Min and R.D. Cardiff. Quantitative analysis of keratin 18 in urine of patients with bladder cancer. J. Urol. 140:436-439 (1988).

11. B.F. Edwards, P.V. Rossitto, W.C. Baker, R.D. Cardiff, M. Strand, A.D. Deitch and R. deVere White. Transitional cell cytokeratins as a second parameter in flow cytometry of bladder cancer. World J. Urol. 5:123-126 (1987).

12. L.A. Diaz, S.A.P. Sampaio, C.R. Martins, et.al. An autoantibody in pemphigus serum, specific for the 59KD keratin, selectively binds the surface of keratinocytes: Evidence for an extracellular keratin domain. J. Invest. Dermatol. 89:287-295 (1987).

13. S.J. DeNardo, G.L. DeNardo, L.F. O'Grady, J-S. Peng, D.J. Macey, S.L. Mills, R.D. Cardiff and A.L. Epstein. Human kinetic distribution of I^{123} $F(Ab^1)_2$ and FAB compared to the parent I^{123} intact antibody. Society of Nuclear Medicine 32nd Annual Meeting, June 2-5, 1985.

14. D. He, S. Taniuchi, C.H. Sun, M.W. Berns, P.J. Donald, and R.D. Cardiff. Monoclonal antibody-photosensitizer conjugates (MAPS:PS) versus surface epitopes attach to and photoinactivate tumor cells. Canadian and United States Academy of Pathology, Annual Meeting, San Francisco, CA. March 1989.

15. S.D. Georgatos, and G. Blobel. Two distinct attachment sites for vimentin along the plasma membrane and the nuclear envelope in avian erythrocytes: A basis for a vectorial assembly of intermediate filaments. J. Cell Biology 105:105-115 (1987).

PRECLINICAL EVALUATION OF MoAbs Mc5 AND BrE1

Roberto L. Ceriani[1], Hector Battifora[2], Edward W. Blank[1], Jerry A. Peterson[1], and Cindy Zoellner[1]

[1]John Muir Cancer & Aging Research Institute, 2055 North Broadway, Walnut Creek, CA 94596

[2]City of Hope National Medical Center, 1500 East Duarte Road, Duarte, CA 91010-0269

INTRODUCTION

Breast epithelial cells possess antigenic glycoprotein components which are, if not unique, characteristic to this tissue (1). Some of these antigens are shared with other epithelial tissues of the body. In addition, neoplastic breast epithelial cells possess certain epitopes on their glycoproteins that could be oncofetal in nature and are considered tumor specific by others. They are epitopes that are made more available as a result of a lack of oligosaccharide maturation. These previously unavailable epitopes are made available, by non-lethal glycosyltransferase deletions introduced by neoplasia. As a result of these deletions inner-core saccharide sequences previously blocked by terminal monosaccharides are exposed as well as epitopes of the polypeptide previously shielded by completely synthesized oligosaccharides.

Thus, the antigens and respective epitopes in the breast epithelial cells can be divided with regard to their specificity as: class I, normal antigens shared with cells of most other tissues (2); class II, antigens shared with cells of a few other tissues but with a preponderance in the breast, that could be referred to as characteristic of the breast (1); class III, antigens present only in the gland itself, being truly breast tissue specific such as casein; class IV, breast tumor antigens shared with other tumors of the organism (3); and finally, class V, specific breast epithelial tumor antigens.

Class II antigens on the cell surface of breast epithelial cells were first evidenced by immunization of rabbits and production of polyclonal antisera made specific after repeated absorptions (1). Later on, monoclonal antibodies (MoAbs) were produced to several different components of the breast epithelial cells (4-8) which vary in molecular weight from above 400K down to below 50K (5).

Both polyclonal antibodies and MoAbs against breast epithelium have been used for immunohistochemistry (9), the detection of circulating antigens released by the tumor (10-12), and in vivo imaging (13,14). Ability to image and high breast tumor uptake of MoAbs meant their use in radioimmunotherapy (RIT) was warranted.

High uptake of the intact radioiodinated MoAb Mc5 was also shown by its F(ab)'$_2$ fragments (15). This MoAb (5) and others were initially tested for tumoricidal effectiveness. With only few exceptions, all the experimental attempts of therapy with MoAbs of breast tumors had been performed in nude mice. The few clinical trials available where systemic therapy was administered to breast cancer patients consisted in a small series of patients treated with unconjugated MoAbs against breast epithelia, MoAb KC4 (16) and a ricin-A chain conjugated MoAb (17). The former trial reported one partial response and the latter had to be interrupted due to high toxicity of the conjugate. In addition, intracavitary immunotherapy with radioactively labeled MoAbs in human breast tumors has been attempted in a small number of cases with ^{131}I-anti-milk fat globule MoAbs (18). In these studies, the authors described cytotoxic effects of the tagged MoAbs on pleural effusion cancerous cells (18) and some partial responses.

In contrast, a considerable amount of experimental therapy with unconjugated and conjugated MoAbs was performed in immunosuppressed hosts carrying human breast tumors. In early studies unconjugated MoAbs were used with some success by some investigators (19-22). In these studies, a single unconjugated MoAb could show therapeutic effectiveness in already established breast tumors, but even more effective were mixtures or "cocktails" containing two or more unconjugated anti-breast MoAbs (22).

Alternatively, in immunodeficient mice, it was clearly shown that MoAbs tagged with ^{131}I, either by themselves or in mixtures, were effective in destroying human breast tumors with much higher efficacity than unconjugated MoAbs (23). The doses of conjugated MoAbs administered were one hundred times smaller than those of unconjugated ones but their anti-tumor action was surprisingly much higher.

However, it should be pointed out that MoAbs used so far in all these studies have been MoAbs that were originally not selected for therapy or any other special criteria, and were used in therapy studies simply because they were available. These MoAbs used in experimental therapy to date are the result of early unplanned, haphazard immunizations with breast epithelial antigens of different types. With the knowledge and new technological approaches accumulated in the last 4 years and the arsenal of MoAbs already created and characterized for breast cancer treatment, it is possible now to propose a sequence of how to select a MoAb with the most desirable characteristics.

Thus, in the selection of the appropriate MoAb the following issues must be addressed: a) antigenic distribution as shown by immunohistopathology in human tissues; b) immunochemical properties of the MoAb to include: i) resistance to denaturation; ii) resistance to label conjugation; iii) Ig subclass; c) ease of production and purification, d) development of a MoAb containing a small percentage of unreacting or partially reacting Ig contamination; e) good distribution in nude mouse model grafted with human breast tumors.

Additionally, the following issues should be considered important in the selection of the radioconjugate for a MoAb: a) good binding of the conjugate to the MoAb; b) mild conjugation methodology; c) the lowest possible breakdown of the MoAb-conjugate linkage; d) good distribution of free conjugate in the nude mouse model, with least accumulation in vital organs (liver, bone marrow, lymphoid system, etc.); e) the highest possible ionizing radioactive particle.

Finally, at the therapeutic level the selected MoAb conjugate should have: a) the highest tumor incorporation and tumor to tissue differential uptake and the lowest whole body irradiation. (The latter is a combination of rate of catabolism of the MoAb conjugate and the biological half life of the radioisotope); b) should produce a long arrest of tumor growth; and, c) if attainable, should eradicate the tumor. Alternatively, measurable tumor volume reduction should be seen in the nude mouse model within a week of administration and it must be possible to administer repeated maximal tolerated therapeutic doses.

Thus, the present paper attempts to delineate the strategy for the selection of appropriate anti-breast MoAbs and its best conjugate from a pool of antibodies to be used in RIT of human breast tumors. In this case, as an example, the MoAbs to be compared (Mc5 and BrE-1) react with the 400,000 molecular weight mucin-like glycoprotein of the HMFG present on the cell surface of the breast epithelial cells.

MATERIALS AND METHODS

Histopathological distribution of MoAbs Mc5 and BrE-1 was performed in normal and neoplastic tissues after formaldehyde fixation, paraffin-embedding, sectioning at 5 μ thick, and antigen visualization with the corresponding MoAb by immunoperoxidase staining with the ABC method (Vector Labs, Burlingame, CA) and hematoxylin counter stain. Multitissue blocks (sausage system) were prepared and processed as reported (24). For flow cytometric analysis of transplantable breast tumors, single cell suspensions were prepared by mechanical dispersion, and stained with MoAbs tagged with fluorescein. Single cell suspensions of the breast carcinoma cell lines were prepared as described previously (25). The stained cells were run on a EPICS 753 and the histograms were analyzed on the EASY 88 IMMUNO Analysis program using fluoresceinated nonspecific IgG_1 MoAb stained cells as a control for determining percentage positive, relative intensity, and coefficient of variation.

Transplantable human breast tumor MX-1 was provided by A. E. Bogden, (EG&G Mason Research Institute, Worchester, MA). Immunodeficient nude mouse housing, tumor grafting MoAb distribution, and radioimmuno- therapy studies were performed as we previously described (23).

The MoAb Mc5 was created and characterized previously by us (5); while MoAb BrE-1 was created after the injection of delipidated HMFG to BALB/C mice, that provided spleen cells for fusion. Screens were performed first on HMFG and then the clones secreting MoAbs binding to it were tested for specificity vs. HMFG and membranes of the cell lines: Hela, HT-29 (a human colon carcinoma), Bris-8 (a human lymphoma), WI-38 (human fetal fibroblast line), and normal breast fibroblasts, as described (5).

Upscale production of the MoAbs, their purification, and radioiodination were already reported (23).

Post-radioiodination binding was tested as we described (23), and Ig class and subclasses by use of a MoNoAB-Screen System, Zymed, South San Francisco, CA.

RESULTS

The histopathological distribution of binding with MoAbs Mc5 and BrE-1 was performed on different normal human and neoplastic tissues. Table 1 shows the normal tissue distribution for binding of MoAb Mc5 demonstrating its multiepithelial distribution. It has been previously pointed out by ourselves (5) and others (26) that the heavy molecular weight mucin, that we call nonpenetrating glycoprotein or NPGP (5), or if not epitopes carried by NPGP and present in other cellular components, are expressed in several, if not most, secretory human epithelia. It is noteworthy that on the normal breast epithelial cell, as well on the other positive normal epithelia, binding of Mc5 is of an apical nature, that is, it binds on the membrane that interfaces with the intraluminal space (9). Upon the advent of neoplasia, it is not uncommon to see staining with MoAb Mc5 in the cytoplasm of breast tumor cells (9). Thus, breast tumors may have a heightened expression of Mc5 antigen both at the membranous and cytoplasmic level as has been shown for other anti-breast MoAbs (27). The distribution of MoAb Mc5 in different human tumors is shown in Table 2 where MoAb Mc5 binds to every human breast tumor as well as a high percentage of lung, pancreas, endometrial, and prostate tumors. Here again, the pan-epithelial nature of this antibody is evidenced. Tumors of the mesothelial layer of the organism have been generally negative.

Table 1. Normal tissue distribution of MoAb Mc5.

Breast	+	Brain	–
Lung	+	Bladder	–
Kidney	+	Muscle	–
Esophagus	+	Myocardium	–
Pancreas	+	Skin (Epider.)	–
Salivary Gland	+	Small Intestine	–
Thyroid	+	Spleen	–
Sebaceous and		Lymph Node	–
Apocrine Glands	+	Adrenal	–
Stomach	–	Liver	–

Table 2. Neoplastic tissue distribution of MoAb Mc5.

Tissue		Tissue	
Breast CA (form)*	155/163	Pancreatic CA	11/14
Breast CA (Etoh)**	48/48	Prostatic CA	1/15
Breast CA(frozen)***	40/40	Renal Cell CA	5/15
Cervical CA	2/3	Salivary CA	1/2
Cholangio CA	1/1	Salivary Adenoma	0/5
Colon CA	5/14	Warthins Tumor	2/2
Ret. Embryonal CA	1/1	Salivary Mixed Tumor	1/1
Endometrial CA	12/13	Stomach CA	4/6
Hepatoma	1/5	Thyroid	6/6
Lung CA	15/15	Undiff. CA	10/29
Ovarian CA	15/17	Mesothelioma	5/10

* Formaldehyde 10%
** Absolute ethanol
*** Frozen sections

Characteristics of MoAb antibody Mc5 have been depicted in Table 3. It is important to highlight the murine origin of the MoAb, its subclass IgG$_1$, and the important fact for radioimmunotherapy that its post radioiodination reactivity is approximately 100%. The high prevalence, of this antigen in breast tumors and its high content per cell, had a corresponding expression in the breast patient serum, which has high levels of free Mc5 antigen (28). This antibody, in summary, recognizes a very prevalent antigen present in high concentrations in breast tumors as well as in other epithelial tumors and at a much lower level on luminal areas of several normal secretory epithelia including breast.

Table 3.   Characteristics of MoAb Mc5.

Hybridoma: mouse/mouse

Hybridoma free of murine viral infection and mycoplasma contamination.

Class, subclass: IgG_1

Purified by affinity chromatography on native antigen and HPLC.

Post-iodination reactivity: 85-100%.

Upscale production both by ascites and serum-free forced perfusion fermentor (Opticell, Charles River).

Antigen present in breast cancer patient serum, highly sensitive assay available.

Most tumors carry antigen (98%).

In contrast to Mc5, MoAb BrE-1, has a much narrower histopathological distribution in normal tissues, such that it only binds some areas of the epithelial lining of the lung and scattered distal convoluted tubules of the kidney, with no apparent histopathological binding to normal breast and many other normal secretory epithelia (Table 4). In contrast, a high percentage of several human tumors, including breast, endometrium, lung, ovary, and pancreas bind MoAb BrE-1 intensely (Table 5). This characteristic of BrE-1 makes it nearly a pan-carcinoma MoAb. In summary, it can be highlighted that MoAb BrE-1 is again a murine MoAb of a different subclass (IGg_{2a}) than MoAb Mc5 (IgG_1) (Table 6). As MoAb Mc5, it has a high post-radioiodination reactivity and its antigen is present in the sera of patients although at lower levels than the antigen of MoAb Mc5.

Table 4.   Normal tissue distribution of MoAb BrE-1.

Normal Breast	0/26	Lymph Node	–
Lung, Alveolar Lining	+	Myocardium	–
Kidney Tubules	+	Ovary	–
Adrenal	–	Pancreas	–
Brain	–	Spleen	–
Bladder	–	Stomach	–
Colon	–	Thyroid	–
Liver	–	Testis	–

Table 5. Tissue distribution in histopathological sections of antigens identified by the monoclonal antibody BrE-1 on a panel of breast and non-breast tumors.

Breast CA	144/182	Neuroblastoma	0/2
Colon CA	3/27		
Duodenum CA	0/1	Oncocytoma	1/1
Endometrium CA	7/14		
Kidney CA	0/11	Paraganglioma	0/10
Lung CA	41/47		
Ovary CA	20/26	Pleoadenoma	0/7
Pancreas CA	9/15		
Prostate CA	0/2	Sarcomas	
Salivary gland CA	0/3		
Stomach CA	2/7	Unclassified	0/1
Thyroid CA	0/7	Alveolar	0/1
Gallbladder CA	0/1	Angiosarcoma	0/1
		Clear cell	0/2
		Cystosarcoma	0/1
		Epithelioid	5/12
		Ewing's	0/1
		Fibrosarcoma	0/1
Carcinoid	3/10	Leiomyoma	0/2
		Liposarcoma	0/1
Cholangio CA	7/17	Mal. Fib. Histiocyt.	0/2
		Synovial	0/7
		Spindle cell CA	5/16
		Undifferentiated	1/9
Embryonal CA	0/6		
Endodermal Sinus CA	0/2		
Fibroadenoma	0/10	Schwannoma	0/3
Gliomas	0/7	Seminoma	0/4
Hepatocholangio CA	8/33	Lung Small cell CA	1/7
Islet cell CA	0/2	Lung Sq. cell CA	5/12
Lymphoma	0/20	Teratoma	0/3
Melanoma	0/23	Thymoma	0/8
Meningioma	0/5	Transitional CA	5/10
Merkel cell CA	4/9	Undifferentiated CA	7/29
Mesothelioma	1/11	Warthin's tumor	0/1

Table 6. Characteristics of MoAb BrE-1.

Hybridoma: mouse/mouse

Class, Subclass: IgG_{2a}

Purified by affinity chromatography on native antigen and HPLC.

Post-iodination reactivity: 70-100%.

Upscale production by both ascites and serum-free forced perfusion fermentor (Opticell, Charles River).

Antigen present in breast cancer patient serum, sensitive assay available.

Breast tumor binding: 83%.

For the radioimmunotherapy experimentation transplantable human breast tumor MX-1 (23) was used. The MX-1 transplantable human mammary tumor grows at a steady pace after the implantation of a subcutaneous 1 mm^3 tumor graft (28). This steady pace of growth is maintained even after arriving to high volumes of the tumor, however, central necrosis develops starting at tumor volumes of approximately 150 mm^3. For that reason, tumors of approximately 100 mm^3 in size were used in immunotherapy experiments. Cells of MX-1 are intensely ladened with antigen detectable by MoAb Mc5 in immunohistopathological studies (29). Both cytoplasmatic and membranous staining are clearly detected. This can be quantitatively studied by flow cytofluorimetry where, as seen in Fig. 1, a wide distribution of antigenic content is seen in the tumor cell population both for the surface staining, Fig. 1A, and in the cytoplasm, Fig. 1B. Live unfixed cells represent only surface antigenic content (Fig. 1A) while with fixed cells (Fig. 1B) both surface and cytoplasmic antigen were stained. MoAb BrE-1 also shows surface staining but has considerable amounts of antigen in the cytoplasm (Fig. 2A and 2B).

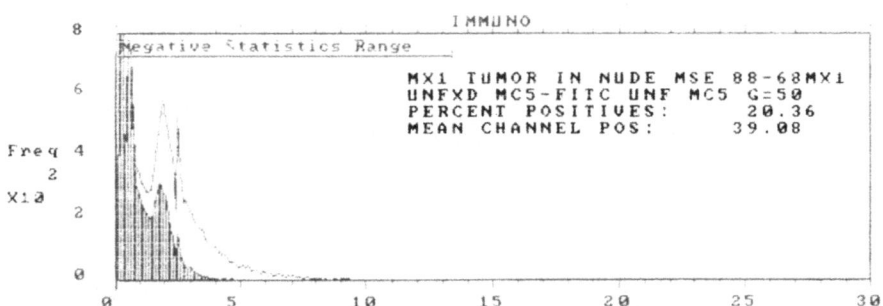

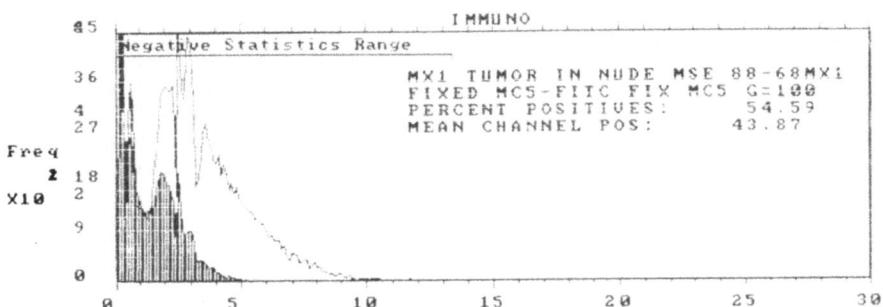

Fig. 1. Flow cytometric analysis of surface and cytoplasmic expression of an epitope identified by MoAb Mc5 in the human breast carcinoma MX1 transplanted in nude immunodeficient mice. (A) unfixed (unfxd) cells corresponding to surface staining. (B) Ethanol fixed cells corresponding to surface and cytoplasmic staining. Shaded histogram represents staining with a fluoresceinated nonspecific IgG, MoAb. Profiles were analyzed by EASY88 IMMUNO Analysis program.

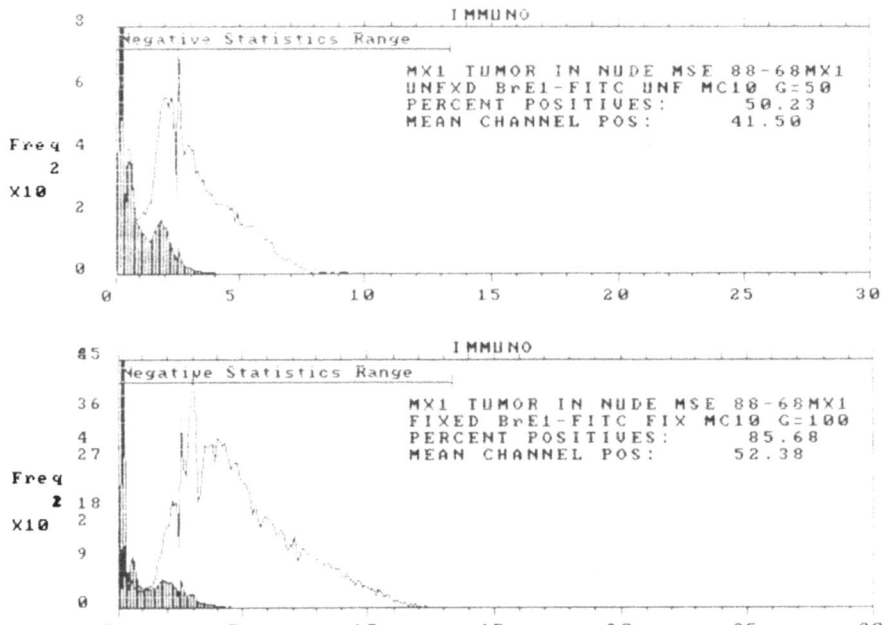

Fig. 2. Flow cytometric analysis of surface and cytoplasmic
expression of an epitope identified by MoAb BrE1 in the
human breast carcinoma MX1 transplanted in nude
immunodeficient mice. (A) unfixed (unfxd) cells
corresponding to surface staining. (B) Ethanol fixed
cells corresponding to surface and cytoplasmic
staining. Shaded histogram represents staining with a
fluoresceinated nonspecific IgG, MoAb. Profiles were
analyzed by EASY88 IMMUNO Analysis program.

As mentioned above, immunoreactivity is retained by MoAb Mc5 after
radioiodination. In Table 7 the biodistribution of ^{125}I-labeled MoAbs
Mc5 after injection in nude mice carrying MX-1 is shown where a sum of
intercompartmental distribution, catabolism and dehalogenation join
together to show a high uptake on the human breast tumor, and fast blood
decline, that is mimicked by the swift decline of uptake of other organs,
thus indicating a positive uptake by the human breast tumor, as reported
elsewhere (23). Distribution of MoAb, BrE-1 shows that it clears from
plasma slower than Mc5 but incorporates at a higher percentage into
breast tumors (Table 7). All levels in subsequent days declined (not
shown).

Maximal tolerable dose (MTD) studies for these MoAbs and their
different conjugates were performed. These studies also indicate the
effectiveness of breast tumor therapy of tagged MoAbs at their respective
MTDs' and thus help rank MoAbs and their different radioconjugates.
Maximal tolerated dose for MoAb Mc5 was shown to be 1500 µCi of
[131]I-conjugate, 750 µCi for ^{125}I-conjugate and 250 µCi of [90]Y -
conjugate (via DTPA), Table 8. For MoAb BrE-1 the MTDs were 1100 µCi
for ^{131}I-conjugate and 150 µCi for ^{90}Y conjugate. ^{125}I-BrE-1
conjugate was not tested. At these MTDs' the therapeutic effectiveness
was determined using the formula for % inhibition of growth (%IG), as
follows:

$$\%IG = (1 - \frac{Tn}{To} / \frac{Cn}{Co}) \times 100 \quad (30)$$

Table 7. Blood and tissue distribution of MoAbs Mc5 and BrE-1

	^{131}I-Mc5 Day 1	^{131}I-BrE-1 Day 1
Blood	6.30±0.80	13.03±0.35
Tumor	3.82±0.27	4.00±0.45
Skin	1.60±0.21	3.50±0.25
Spleen	1.93±0.23	2.65±0.09
Kidney	1.91±0.26	3.27±0.24
Liver	2.12±0.24	2.79±0.35
Lung	2.69±0.21	3.96±0.43
Stomach	2.56±0.37	2.06±0.18
Intestine	0.99±0.16	1.75±0.17
Bone	0.71±0.10	1.40±0.17
Brain	0.48±0.11	0.36±0.01
Muscle	0.85±0.25	0.07±0.16

Table 8. Maximum tolerable dose (MTD) of different radiolabeled conjugates of MoAb Mc5 and BrE-1.

Radiolabeled Conjugate	MTD
^{90}Y-Mc5	250 μCi
^{125}I-Mc5	750 μCi
^{131}I-Mc5	1,500 μCi
^{131}I-BrE-1	1,100 μCi
^{90}Y-BrE-1	150 μCi

In Table 9 the %IG of the two MoAbs and their different conjugates at day 15 and 30 is presented. The highest tumoricidal effectiveness is shown for ^{131}I-Mc5. This fact is associated with its high tumor binding prevalence (100% of breast tumors bind Mc5) and its fast body clearance (which anticipates lower whole body irradiation and hence less residual whole body irradiation allowing for increased repeated treatments), make ^{131}I-Mc5 the choice between the conjugates tested. As the result of preceding MoAb Mc5 is identified as the most desirable in our proposed testing scheme.

Table 9. Percent inhibition of growth of Mc5 and BrE-1 radioconjugates.

	Day 15	Day 30
[131]I-Mc5	90.6%	99.6%
[131]I-Mc10	90.5%	95.1%
[90]Y-Mc5	72.3%	53.2%
[90]Y-Mc10	85.6%	77.6%

DISCUSSION

Identifying the most appropriate conjugate for MoAb RIT of breast cancer can be conducted a priori under the scheme proposed, where characteristics of MoAbs and their different conjugates are first tested for histopathological tissue distribution, then in tracer uptake studies and finally their tumoricidal efficacy confirmed by actual experimental immune therapy experiments in nude mice. It is obvious, however, that future clinical trials with the selected MoAbs will help evaluate the appropriate weight that each parameter now studied in these model systems has in the choice made. In this regard, first, clinical trials will demonstrate if results obtained experimentally, such as MoAb tissue distribution in histopathological sections, are truly matched by patient tissue uptakes of MoAb conjugate after systemic delivery. Some preliminary studies published seem to deny this (31). Similarly, nude mice MoAb-tracer distribution studies used with the aim of predicting future human systemic distribution have to be seen in the same light. Second, once these unknowns above are resolved, what needs to be understood next is the corresponding value that final tumor therapeutic effectiveness studied in preclinical trials has in the evaluation of the MoAb conjugate tumoricidal effectiveness in human therapy. However, the value of therapeutic effectiveness found in in vitro and nude mice studies will have to wait unfortunately for eventual correlation with Phase II studies of breast cancer patient RIT. Thus, we are now far from having a proven way by which to select and introduce MoAb conjugates into clinical trials. Thus, development of evaluation studies to be then continued and followed up at the clinical level, such as the present one, are needed. In fact, it can be safely said that from the information available now, little is known about the required characteristics for a MoAb conjugate to be selected over another to be tested clinically. Teleologic interpretations have so far dominated this issue.

Thus, in view of the present state of affairs it seems in accordance with scientific principles to obtain as many parameters as possible of the action of the conjugates available, and considering the cost and effort required for the testing of each MoAb conjugate, to proceed objectively and select those MoAb conjugates excelling in those tests available. However, keeping in mind that it would be valuable to test also the less desirable MoAb conjugates (considered such as a result of all this preclinical testing) to compare and evaluate the present criteria. Hence, as information accumulates from clinical trials with different MoAb conjugates, were the present criteria for selection a faulty one, a wide range of conflicting results will be obtained with the chosen MoAbs. Clearly, only the final matching of criteria for MoAb conjugate selection, (as described here), and efficacity of patient therapy will establish true and definite criteria.

In the present experimentation, two MoAbs, Mc5 and BrE-1, were studied for their characteristics related to eventual RIT. Both MoAbs bind the heavy molecular weight mucin complex or NPGP (5) of the milk fat globule and breast epithelial cell at different epitopes (unpublished results, R.C.). Given this fact, and others shown in Tables 3 and 6, their conjugates with similar radioisotopes have comparable high tumoricidal efficacity (^{131}I-Mc5 and ^{131}I-BrE-1). In contrast, the ^{90}Y – conjugates showed higher uptake in liver and bone marrow and smaller MTD and %IG. Complete dosimetric studies will be desirable in this experimental model, with considerations concerning size and nature of the host. This could well be accomplished with local implantation of microdosimeters (32).

Both ^{131}I – conjugates of Mc5 and BrE-1 showed higher therapeutic effectiveness (%IG at days 15 and 30); however, ^{131}I – Mc5 was higher. This could be attributed to the higher MTD that could be achieved with ^{131}I-Mc5. Among facts that could condition this higher MTD for ^{131}I-Mc5, one that could have relevance is the fast clearance from the nude mouse model which could be the cause for lower whole body irradiation when compared to ^{131}I-BrE-1.

The reason for the slower clearance for ^{131}I-BrE-1 can be sought in its different Ig subclass (IgG$_{2a}$) and possible in the low levels of circulating free antigen compared to the high levels found for the Mc5 antigen (unpublished results).

In summary, both MoAbs tested have high breast tumor prevalence, are resistant to conjugation-produced denaturation, have good human breast tumor uptake in the nude mouse model, and, in this same testing host, both had good tumorostatic efficacity, however ^{131}I-Mc5 seems, under the present testing conditions the most effective, while BrE-1 seems the more breast tumor restricted.

REFERENCES

1. R. L. Ceriani, K. E. Thompson, J. A. Peterson and S. Abraham, Surface differentiation antigens of human epithelial cells carried on the human milk fat globule. Proc. Natl. Acad. Sci. USA 74:582-586 (1977).

2. R. L. Ceriani and J. A. Peterson, Characterization of differentiation antigens of the mouse mammary epithelial cell (MME antigens) carried on the mouse milk fat globule. Cell Differentiation 7:355-366 (1978).

3. A. Thor, N. Ohuchi, C. A. Szpak, W. W. Johnston and J. Schlom, Distribution of oncofetal antigen tumor-associated glycoprotein-72 defined by monoclonal antibody B72.3. Cancer Res. 46:3118-3124 (1986).

4. J. Taylor-Papadimitriou, J. A. Peterson, J. Arklie, J. Burchell, R. L. Ceriani and W. F. Bodmer, Monoclonal antibodies to epithelial-specific components of the human milk fat globule membrane: production and reaction with cells in culture. Int. J. Cancer 28:17-28 (1981).

5. R. L. Ceriani, J. A. Peterson, J. Y. Lee, F. R. Moncada and E. W. Blank, Characterization of cell surface antigens of human mammary epithelial cells with monoclonal antibodies prepared against human milk fat globule. Somat. Cell Genet. 9:415-427 (1983).

6. C. S. Foster, P. A. Edwards, E. A. Dinsdale and A. M. Neville, Monoclonal antibodies to the human mammary and extra mammary tissues. Virchows Arch (Pathol. Anat.) 394:279-293 (1982).

7. D. Colcher, P. H. Hand, M. Nuti and J. Schlom, A spectrum of monoclonal antibodies reactive with human mammary tumor cells. Proc. Natl. Acad. Sci. USA 78:3199-3203 (1981).

8. L. D. Papsidero, G. A. Croghan, M. J. O'Connell, L. A. Valenzuela, T. Nemoto and T. M. Chu, Monoclonal antibodies (F36/22 and M7/105) to human breast carcinoma. Cancer Res. 43:1741-1747 (1983).

9. R. L. Ceriani, D. L. Hill, L. Osvaldo, C. Kandell and E. W. Blank, Immunohistochemical studies in breast cancer using monoclonal antibodies against breast epithelial cell components and with lectins, in: "Immunohistochemistry in Tumor Diagnosis," J. Russo, ed., Martinus Nijhoff Publishing, Boston, p. 233-263 (1985).

10. R. L. Ceriani, M. Sasaki, H. Sussman, W. M. Wara and E. W. Blank, Circulating human mammary epithelial antigens in breast cancer. Proc. Natl. Acad. Sci. USA 79:5420-5424 (1982).

11. J. Hilkens, V. Kroezen, J. M. G. Bonfrer, M. De Jong-Bakker and P. F. Bruning, MAM-6 antigen, a new serum marker for breast cancer monitoring. Cancer Res. 46:2582-2587 (1986).

12. D. F. Hayes, H. Sekine, T. Ohno, M. Abe, K. Keefe and D. W. Kufe, Use of a murine monoclonal antibody for detection of circulating plasma DF3 antigen levels in breast cancer patients. J. Clin. Invest. 75:1671-1678 (1985).

13. T. Wilbanks, J. A. Peterson, S. Miller, L. Kaufman, D. Ortendahl and R. L. Ceriani, Localization of mammary tumors in vivo with ^{131}I-labeled Fab fragments of antibodies against mouse mammary epithelial (MME) antigens. Cancer 48:1768-1775 (1981).

14. A. A. Epenetos, K. E. Britton, S. Mathers, J. Shepherd, M. Granowska, J. Taylor-Papadimitriou, C. C. Nimmon, H. Darbin, L. R. Hawkins, J. S. Malpas and W. F. Bodmer, Targeting of iodine-123-labelled tumor-associated monoclonal antibodies to ovarian, breast, and gastrointestinal tumors. Lancet ii:999-1003 (1982).

15. R. L. Ceriani, J. A. Peterson and E. W. Blank, Breast cancer diagnosis with human mammary epithelial antigens and the prospective use of antibodies against them in therapy, in: "Mechanism of Cancer Metastases," V. K. Hohn, W. E. Powers and B. F. Sloanne, eds., Martinus Nijhoff Publishing, Boston, p. 235-258 (1986).

16. D. Hofheinz, D. Dienhart, G. Miller, S. Healy, P. Furmanski, S. Sedlacek, C. Longley, P. Bunn, K. Kortright, Monoclonal antibody, KC4G3, recognizes a novel widely expressed antigen on human epithelial cancers. 78th Annual Meeting of the AACR. Proc. AACR, 28:391, #1552 (1987).

17. B. Gould, M. Borowitz, E. Groves and A. Frankel, A phase I study of the anti-breast cancer immunotoxin 260F9 MAB-rRa given by continuous infusion, in: "Immunological Approaches to Diagnosis and Therapy of Breast Cancer II," R. L. Ceriani, ed., Plenum Press, New York, in press (1989).

18. H. P. Kalofonos and A. A. Epenetos, Antibody guided diagnosis and therapy of patients with breast cancer, in: "Immunological Approaches to the Diagnosis and Therapy of Breast Cancer," R. L. Ceriani, ed., Plenum Press, New York, p. 245-257 (1987).

19. P. M. Capone, L. D. Papsidero, G. A. Croghan and T. M. Chu, Experimental tumoricidal effects of monoclonal antibody against solid tumors. Proc. Natl. Acad. Sci. USA 80:7328-7332 (1983).

20. P. M. Capone, L. D. Papsidero and T. M. Chu, Relationship between antigen density and immunotherapeutic response elicited by monoclonal antibodies against solid tumors. J. Natl. Cancer Inst. 72:673-677 (1984).

21. R. L. Ceriani and E. W. Blank, An experimental model for the immunological treatment of breast cancer, in: "Monoclonal Antibodies and Breast Cancer," R. L. Ceriani, ed., Martinus Nijhoff, Boston, p. 248-268 (1985).

22. R. L. Ceriani, E. W. Blank and J. A. Peterson, Experimental immunotherapy of human breast carcinomas implanted in nude mice with a mixture of monoclonal antibodies against human milk fat globule components. Cancer Res. 47:532-540 (1987).

23. R. L. Ceriani and E. W. Blank, Experimental therapy of human tumors with ^{131}I-labeled monoclonal antibodies prepared against the human milk fat globule. Cancer Res. 48:4664-4672 (1988).

24. H. Battifora, The multitumor (sausage) tissue block: Novel method for immunohistochemical antibody testing. Lab Invest 55:244 (1986).

25. J. A. Peterson, J. S. Bartholomew, M. Stampfer and R. L. Ceriani, Analysis of expression of human mammary epithelial antigens in normal and malignant breast cells at the single cell level by flow cytofluorimetry. Exp. Cell Biol. 49:1-14 (1981).

26. L. D. Papsidero, G. A. Croghan, P. M. Capone and E. A. Johnson, Ductal carcinoma antigen: characteristics, tissue distribution and capacity to represent a target for monoclonal antibody therapy, in: "Monoclonal Antibodies and Breast Cancer," R. L. Ceriani, ed., Martinus Nijhoff Publishing, Boston, p. 293-302 (1985).

27. P. H. Hand, M. Nuti, D. Colcher and J. Schlom, Definition of antigenic heterogeneity and modulation among mammary carcinoma-cell populations using monoclonal antibodies to tumor-associated antigens. Cancer Res. 43:728-735 (1983).

28. R. L. Ceriani, E. H. Rosenbaum, M. Chandler, T. T. Trujillo, B. Myers and M. Sakada, Role of circulating human mammary epithelial antigens (HME-Ags) as serum markers for breast cancer, in: "Tumor markers and their significance in the management of breast cancer," Ip, C., ed., A. R. Liss, p. 3-19 (1986).

29. R. L. Ceriani, M. Sasaki, D. Orthendahl and L. Kaufman, Localization of human breast tumors grafted in nude mice with a monoclonal antibody directed against a defined cell surface antigen of human mammary epithelial cells. Breast Cancer Res. Treat. 12:177-189 (1988).

30. K. Inoue, S. Fujimoto and M. Ogawa, Antitumor efficacy of seventeen anticancer drugs in human breast cancer xenograft (MX-1) transplanted in nude mice. Cancer Chemother. Pharmacol. 10:182-186 (1983).

31. A. A. Epenetos, D. Snook, H. Durbin, P. M. Johnson and J. Taylor-Papadimitriou, Limitations of radiolabeled monoclonal antibodies for localization of human neoplasms. Cancer Res. 46:3183-3191 (1986).

32. M. H. Griffith, E. D. Yorke, B. W. Wessels, G. L. DeNardo and W. P. Neacy, Direct dose confirmation of quantitative autoradiography with micro-TLD measurement for radioimmunotherapy. J. Nucl. Med. 29:1795-1809 (1988).

THE USE OF HUMAN MONOCLONAL ANTIBODIES TO IDENTIFY AND ISOLATE BREAST TUMOR ASSOCIATED ANTIGENS

Anthony J. Strelkauskas and Paul H. Aldenderfer

Department of Pediatrics
Medical University of South Carolina
Charleston, SC 29425

INTRODUCTION

One of the greatest challenges in breast cancer research today involves the identification and isolation of breast cancer antigens. The study of antigens associated with these malignancies has been ongoing for years.

The use of monoclonal antibodies for cancer research has also gone on for several years. Several antigens have been identified in a variety of carcinomas using these probes. For example, the tumor associated antigens CA 19-9[1] and CA125[2] were identified using monoclonal antibodies derived from immunization of mice with colon and ovarian tumor cells. Similar studies have been done for pancarcinoma antigens[3], as well as melanoma antigens[4,5]. In fact, monoclonal antibodies are currently being used for radioimmunoguided surgery[6-8].

Breast cancer researchers have also used monoclonal antibodies for antigen identification[9-13], and the complexity of antigenic heterogeneity has been addressed[14-16]. Several laboratories have used monoclonal antibodies for detection of serum antigens[17-20]. The common bond associated with these studies is the use of murine monoclonal antibodies as probes. In many cases the antigens used to immunize these mice are prepared from either tumor cell lines or tumor tissue, using defined biochemical procedures. These procedures contain several steps which can destabilize and in some cases denature antigen molecules. Consequently, the animal is being immunized with molecules which are not only xenogeneic but also may not be in their natural configuration. This approach can lead to the generation of antibodies which are not specific or react with epitopes not necessarily associated with the natural antigen. This could dramatically amplify the degree of heterogeneity seen among tumors. Our approach decreases this amplification since it utilizes an allogeneic system (i.e., human monoclonal antibodies and human antigens) and an antigen found in serum. Although this serum component could be effected by enzyme activity in the serum, we feel it is in a more natural state than those obtained through biological procedures.

Our approach has been to utilize the most natural (i.e., least manipulated) system possible. Our earlier work in construction of stable human hybrid clones was very advantageous in this regard. We have produced over 50 stable human hybridomas using lymphocytes from breast

cancer patients who are producing high levels of antibody. Studies of
these monoclonals have been carried out and reported elsewhere[21]. In
studying these antibodies, we have found that they can efficiently and
reproducibly identify a serum antigen in breast cancer patients with
widespread disease. In addition, these monoclonals were reactive with
several human breast tumor cell lines while unreactive with normal
fibroblasts. Consequently, we had at our disposal, a sensitive and
specific probe with which to isolate putative antigen(s) as well as a
source of antigen (i.e., patients serum). Our hypothesis was simple.
First, human antibodies may be more selective for human antigens than
those produced in animals. Second, the antigens found in serum are in a
more natural and less denatured state than those obtained from tumor
cells by harsh and sometimes destructive biochemical methods. Therefore,
we should be able to isolate and purify these antigens from the serum
through specific fractionation and probing procedures.

The Antibodies Used

The monoclonal antibodies we used for these studies have been
described, as have the methods used for their construction[21]. The
monoclonal JDBl, produces both an IgM/kappa and IgG$_3$/kappa molecule. The
6052 monoclonal is a derivative of the JDBl clone which produces only
IgG$_3$ antibody. These antibodies react equally well with tumor tissue and
the breast cancer cell lines SW527, MCF-7, SKBr3, and T47D, while being
unreactive with normal fibroblasts. This positive reactivity can be seen
using both peroxidase and fluorescent staining as well as a quantitative
cellular elisa assay. Figure 1A shows the peroxidase staining of SW527

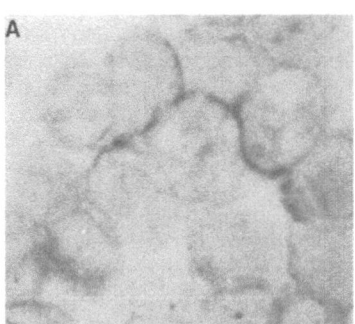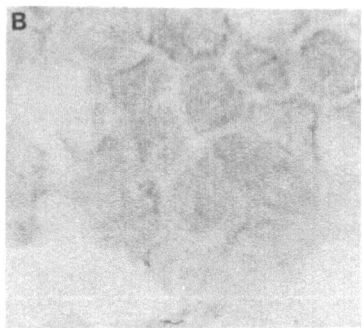

Figure 1. Peroxidase staining of SW527 human breast tumor cells. (A)
cells were sensitized with JDB1 antibody. (B) SW527 cells subjected to
peroxidase staining without prior sensitization by JDB1 antibody.

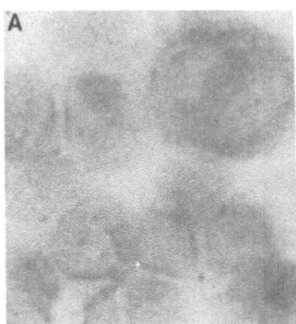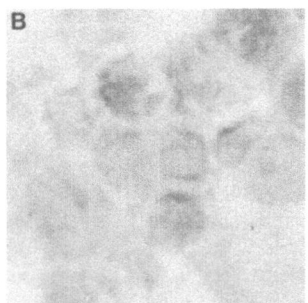

Figure 2. Peroxidase staining of MCF-7 breast tumor cells. (A) cells
were sensitized with the 6052 human monoclonal antibody. (B) Peroxidase
staining without prior sensitization by 6052 antibody.

with controls shown in Figure 1B. Peroxidase staining of MCF-7 cells using the 6052 monoclonal is shown in Figure 2A with control staining shown in Fig. 2B. Both antibodies also bind well to cells grown on coverslips (Fig. 3A JDB1, Fig. 3B 6052). Both are also capable of binding membrane antigens. Figure 4 shows an example of JDB1 binding as seen by indirect immunofluorescence.

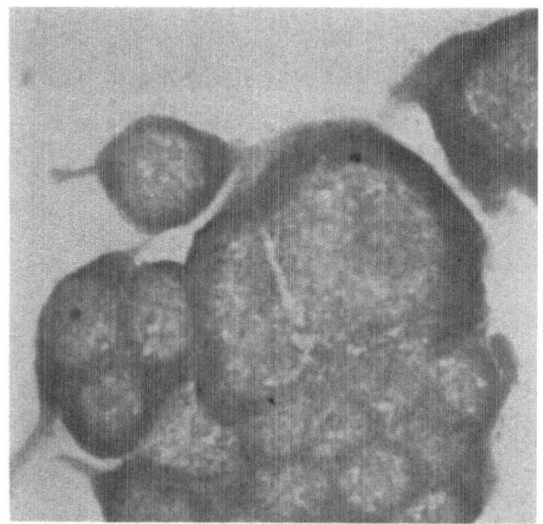

A

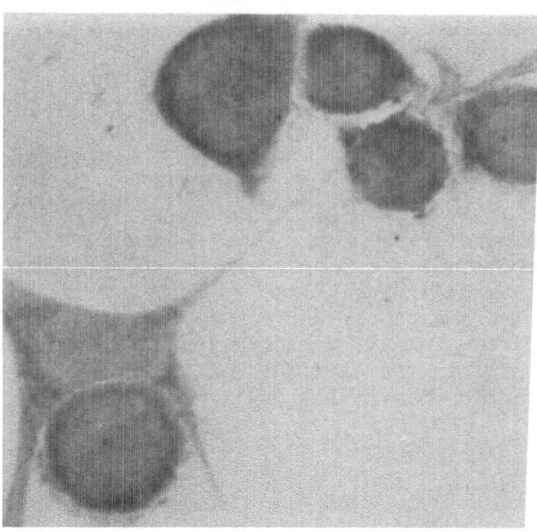

B

Figure 3. Peroxidase staining of cells grown onto sterile coverslips. (A) MCF-7 cells stained with JDB1 antibody. (B) SW527 cells stained with the 6052 antibody.

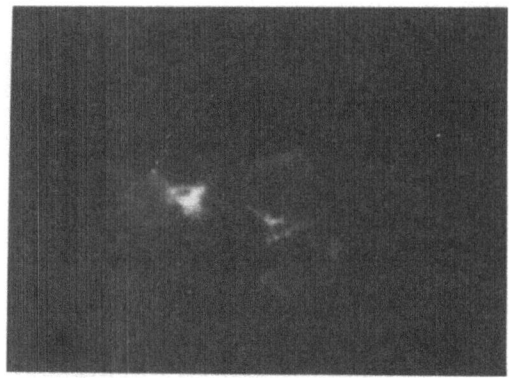

Figure 4.   Indirect immunofluorescence membrane staining of SW527 breast tumor cells using the JDB1 antibody.

Antigen Identification Tests

Utilizing JDB1 and 6052 monoclonal antibodies, serum antigen was initially detected in patients with ongoing disease with a latex agglutination test.   Though this test was rapid and inexpensive we could not use it to quantitate the antigen.   Therefore, we developed an antigen elisa assay described in Figure 5.   Using this system, we were able to identify and monitor levels of antigen in patients with breast cancer. To date, we have assayed over three thousand serum samples and have shown that the antigen identified by these antibodies may play a significant role in monitoring the progress of breast cancer patients especially as a predictive indicator of the onset of relapse.   In the interest of brevity and because this chapter concerns isolation of the antigen, we have not included these data.

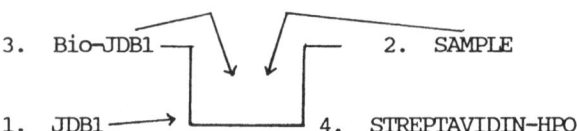

3.   Bio-JDB1   2.   SAMPLE

1.   JDB1   4.   STREPTAVIDIN-HPO

5.   SUBSTRATE

Figure 5.   Scheme for Antigen Elisa.   Immulon II plates (Nunc) were coated with monoclonal antibody overnight (1).   After washing, samples were added and incubated for 1 hour in a 37°C water bath (2), washed and incubated for an additional 60 minutes at 37°C with biotin labeled monoclonal antibody (3).   After washing streptavidin, HPO was added for 60 minutes at 37°C in the dark (4).   Substrate (ABTS) was added for 10 minutes (5) and color was read on a Dynatech 650 reader.

Presence of Antigen in Serum

Utilizing the elisa described above, we examined the serum of patient C.T. (Table 1).   It is clear that the antigen can be identified at dilutions of 1:40 and probably higher.   Several other important points are also illustrated in this table.   As can be seen, sera that are frozen and thawed are likely to show diminished reactivity.   Indeed, in studies not illustrated here, we have found that sera kept frozen for long periods will show a definite drop in our assay system.   We have also occasionally observed what appears to be a prozone affect when high

36

concentrations of serum are tested. This effect, though not extreme, is intermittently seen with some sera. The reasons for it are not understood, but may relate to the elisa system being used.

Table 1. Serum Antigen Titre
O.D. 410-490

EXP.1*		EXP. 2**		EXP. 3**	
1:2	.359	1:2	.309	1:5	.420
1:4	.231	1:4	.339	1:10	.460
1:8	.487	1:8	.401	1:20	.512
1:16	.236	1:16	.354	1:40	.446
1:32	.112	1:32	.270		

*FROZEN SERUM
**FRESH SERUM (NEVER FROZEN)

When whole serum is run over affinity columns coupled with JDB1, there is total loss of reactivity (Table 2). As can be seen in Table 2, serum from patient C.T. shows good reactivity of its antigen by elisa before passage through a sepharose 4B column coupled with JDB1 antibody. After passage, the reactivity is no longer detectable. In contrast, serum from SES, a normal control, shows no reactivity. Interestingly, a similar experiment utilizing an affinity column coupled with 6052 antibody does not remove all of the antigen activity (Table 3).

Table 2. Affinity Column Binding of Antigen

O.D. 410-490

	1:2	1:4	1:8	1:16	1:32	1:64
C.T. SERUM BEFORE JDB1 CHROMATOGRAPHY	.386	.337	.348	.280	.218	.110
C.T. SERUM AFTER JDB1 CHROMATOGRAPHY	.054	.022	.013	----	----	----
SES SERUM BEFORE JDB1 CHROMATOGRAPHY (CONTROL)	.065	.008	----	----	----	----

Table 3. Binding of JDB1 Compared to 6052

O.D. 410-490

	1:2	1:4	1:8	1:16	1:32
C.T. SERUM	.425	.458	.425	.347	.237
C.T. SERUM AFTER JDB1	.029	----	----	----	----
C.T. SERUM AFTER 6052	.321	.402	.369	.259	.166

These results indicate that the antigen found in patients sera can be removed by affinity chromatography using human monoclonal antibodies. Unfortunately, we have found this one step procedure can not be effectively used. In each of the experiments we found that polyacrylimide gel electrophoresis of putatively pure antigen gave three to four bands, only one of which was identified by our monoclonal antibodies. We therefore chose to utilize Sephadex G200 chromatography as a preliminary fractionation step.

Scheme for Isolation and Purification of Antigen

The steps used for purification of serum antigen are outlined in Figure 6. Basically, the scheme involves two steps. First, serum is chromatographed using Sephadex G200. Each of the fractions is then examined for antigen using our antigen elisa assay.

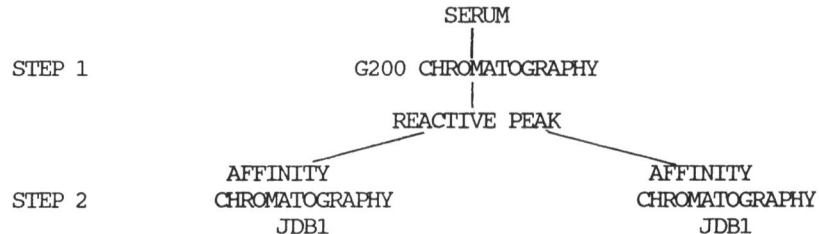

STEP 1

STEP 2

Figure 6. Isolation of Serum Antigen

The activity is always found on the front end of the second (gamma globulin) peak (Fig. 7). We have used this procedure multiple times on 4 different sera and the results are remarkably similar. Utilizing this two step procedure for antigen isolation, we have successfully isolated a serum component reactive with our monoclonal antibody. Table 4 shows the values obtained during two step purification with JDB1. As can be seen, the pooled G200 fraction contains over 90% of the antigen activity. After purification over a JDB1 antibody affinity column, the antigen activity was dramatically decreased. The bound antigen fraction eluted from the affinity column shows good reactivity in the antigen elisa. The difference in levels of reactivity between the G200 and purified antigen fractions is due primarily to the concentrations of each fraction as well as the possibility that some antigen may be lost during this purification process. Western blot analysis of G200 fractions using JDB1 monoclonal antibody shows the reactive band lies at about 35,000 M.W. (Fig. 8). Western blotting of affinity purified antigen using either 6052 or JDB1 antibody shows a single band of approximately 35,000 M.W. which can be identified by both 6052 and JDB1 (Fig. 9).

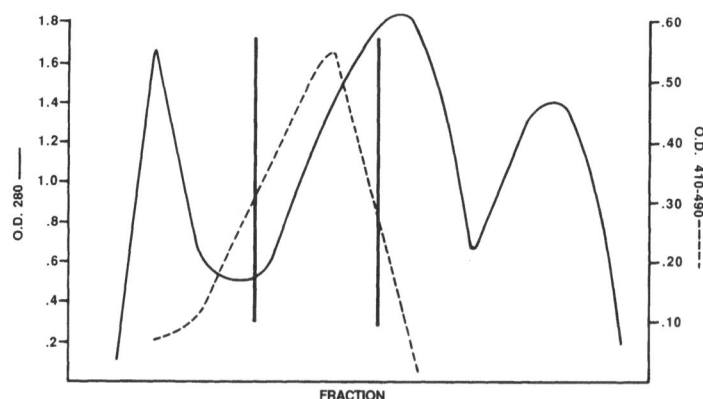

Figure 7. Sephadex G200 chromatography of patient C.T. serum. Dotted line indicates antigen reactivity.

Table 4. Eliza Analysis of Serum Fractions

	O.D. 410-490	
	1:2	1:4
C.T. G200	.736	.667
C.T. G200 POST JDB1	.141	.160
C.T. SERUM	.807	.780
PURIFIED AG	.423	.390

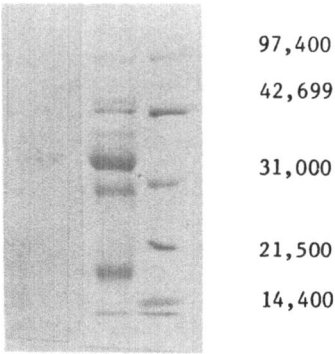

		97,400
		42,699
		31,000
		21,500
		14,400

A   B   C

Figure 8.   Western blot analysis of G200 fractions. Lane A, G200 fraction blotted with JDB1 antibody. Lane B, G200 fraction stained with Coomasie blue. Lane C, contains molecular weight standards.

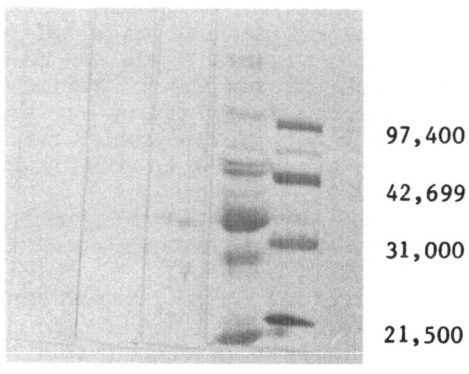

97,400

42,699

31,000

21,500

A   B   C   D   E

Figure 9.   Western blot of affinity purified antigen. Lane A contains purified antigen from patient C.T. blotted with JDB1 antibody, while Lane B contains the same antigen blotted with the 6052 antibody. Coomasie blue stain was used on the isolated antigen (Lane C), as well as the G200 fraction (Lane D). Molecular weight standards are shown in Lane E.

Perhaps of greater interest is the fact that purification of serum antigen from two patients give the same results. The same 35,000 molecular weight protein can be purified from sera of both patients (Fig. 10). Taken together with the fact that this antigen can be identified by our antigen assay in patients with a variety of different breast tumor types, we are led to believe it may be a common antigen. That is not to say a specific tumor antigen, but one which may be present in a variety of these patients. Further, large scale studies need to be done in order to confirm this possibility and antigens from a variety of women must be purified and sequenced in order to prove this hypothesis.

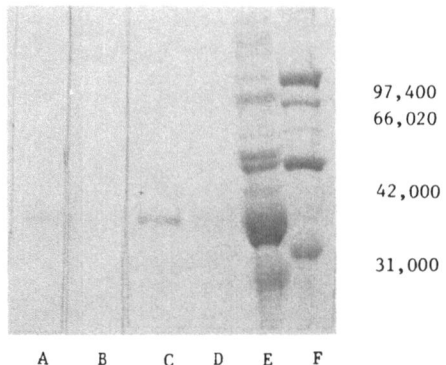

Figure 10. Western blot analysis of purified antigen. Lane A contains antigen isolated from patient C.T. blotted with JDB1 antibody, while Lane B contains purified antigen from patient V.F. Purified antigen from both patients, as well as the G200 fraction from patient V.F., are found in Lanes C, D, and E, stained with Coomassie blue. Lane F contains molecular weight standards.

Directions

There are almost more questions than answers in the studies shown above. We believe these isolated antigens can be useful in diagnostics as well as therapeutics. A variety of diagnostic questions which may be answered by the identification and quantitation of this serum antigen are outlined in Table 5. Provided adequate trials can be carried out, this antigen may be of tremendous use for the monitoring of patients with breast cancer and the possibility of improving treatments. More importantly, if a rise in this antigen can predict the onset of relapse, testing for this antigen may provide for an earlier and more effective response to recurrent disease.

Table 5. Utility in Diagnosis

1. Is this antigen present in all forms of breast cancer?

2. Does the titre of antigen rise and fall in relationship to changes in disease activity?

3. Can a rise in antigen levels predict the onset of relapse?

4. Can quantitative analysis of antigen levels be beneficial to the patients course of treatment?

A second and perhaps more important possibility for the use of these antigens is in therapy. Table 6 outlines some of these possibilities. With regard to the ability of this antigen to elicit an immunological response, we have begun preliminary experiments in which purified antigen was injected into rabbits. After boosting, the serum was tested for antibody to human breast cancer tumor cells with encouraging preliminary results indicating that the rabbit will produce antibodies which will bind to human breast tumor cells. After exposure to the purified antigen, serum from these same rabbits taken before exposure to antigen showed no reactivity with tumor cells.

Table 6. Utility in Therapy

1. Can this antigen be used therapeutically?

2. Can presentation of this antigen to animals lessen or eliminate the development of tumors after exposure to tumor cells?

3. If so, by what immunological mechanism?

4. Can the gene be cloned?

Should this antigen be capable of building or enhancing an immune response, it would be of great importance therapeutically. Unfortunately, there would be several problems to overcome, not the least of which would be supply. To this end, we have endeavored to clone the gene coding for this antigen. Once again, studies are very encouraging. Table 7 shows the results of experiments in which messenger RNA isolated from the human breast tumor cell line SW527 and translated in a commercially available rabbit reticulocyte system, will produce proteins identifiable in our antigen elisa. cDNA libraries have been constructed and screening awaits the protein sequencing of our purified antigen, which is currently underway.

Table 7. Antigen Elisa on Translational Products*

		O.D. 410-490
mRNA	Control (non-specific message)	---
mRNA	SW527	.659
mRNA	Duck globin	.009

*Messenger RNA isolated from the breast cancer cell line was used in a rabbit reticulocyte translational system. The translated products were tested in the standard antigen elisa using JDB1/Bio JDB1.

Conclusions and Discussion

Utilizing human monoclonal antibodies, we have isolated a glycoprotein antigen with a molecular weight of approximately 35-40,000 daltons. The isolation procedures employed 2 steps. The first was Sephadex G200 chromatography of serum from patients who test positive in our antigen elisa system. The positive fraction containing all of the antigen activity is located on the front end of the second peak. This location is identical for sera from several different patients, but no reactivity is seen in any fractions of G200 chromatography, of normal sera. The antigen can be easily identified in this G200 fraction by western blotting with either JDB1 or 6052 antibody. When the G200 fraction is passed over an affinity column coupled with either of these monoclonal antibodies the antigen can be purified. This purified antigen, which stains with both Coomasie and Alcyan blue indicating it is a glycoprotein, is very positive in our antigen elisa and can be easily seen by western blot analysis. We have injected this antigen into rabbits and obtained antibody which will react with human breast tumor cells.

The presence of this antigen may be important for the monitoring of patients with this disease in a fashion similar to earlier reports[18,19]. In our hands, over ninety percent of women with ongoing metastatic disease are positive for this serum antigen and longitudinal monitoring of its level can predict the onset of relapse up to 6 months before it is clinically obvious in some cases. Aside from the possible diagnostic importance of this antigen, there are obvious implications for its use therapeutically. Since we have shown in preliminary studies that immunization of rabbits with the purified glycoprotein can elicit an antibody response to human breast cancer cells, there is the possibility that it could help in potentiating the immune response of women with this disease. Obviously, a great deal remains to be done before any reliable comments on this possibility can be made. One of the major logistical problems for development of such information will be the supply of purified antigen. Purification steps as outlined, though effective, rely on the availability of patient sera, a component which is not available in sufficient quantity. To circumvent this problem, we have begun studies aimed at large scale production of the antigen through cloning of the gene coding for this antigen. Preliminary results are very encouraging, since we have isolated mRNA from the breast tumor cell lines SW527 which, when translated, produces a variety of proteins including the antigen identified by our antibodies. cDNA libraries have been constructed and probing awaits the sequencing of our purified antigen, which is currently underway. Successful cloning of the gene will allow for intensive study of the therapeutic potential of this antigen.

Unfortunately, the use of human monoclonal antibodies as probes for distinct tumor antigens has not progressed as rapidly as it should. There are several reasons for this, the most often cited is the difficulty in producing stable human clones. These problems have been examined,[22] and certainly, there are several technical approaches to hybridoma development which must be reexamined. We feel our construction techniques[23] are very dependable and can be effectively used for development of human monoclonal antibodies. We also feel that these antibodies may be more sensitive and specific for human antigens, and may alter and perhaps even change our understanding of tumor antigens and antigenic heterogeneity.

References

1. H. Koprowski, Z. Steplewski, and K. Mitchell, Colorectal carcinoma antigens detected by hybridoma antibodies, Somatic Cell Genet. 5:957-972 (1979).

2. R.C. Bast Jr., M. Ferney, L.M. Nadler, R.B. Colvin, and R.C. Knapp, Reactivity of monoclonal antibody with human ovarian carcinoma, J. Clin. Invest. 68:1331-1337 (1981).

3. T.L. Klug, M.A. Sattler, D. Colcher, and J. Schlom, Monoclonal antibody immunoradiometric assay for an antigenic determinant (CA72) on a novel pancarcinoma antigen (TAG-72), Int. J. Cancer 38:661-669 (1986).

4. A.C. Morgan, D.R. Galloway, and R.A. Reisfeld, Production and characterization of monoclonal antibody to a melanoma specific glycoprotein, Hybridoma 1:27-36 (1981).

5. S. DelVechio, J.C. Reynolds, R.C. Blasberg, R.D. Neumann, J.A. Carrasquilla, I. Hellstrom, and S.M. Larson, Measurement of local Mr 97,000 and 250,000 protein antigen concentration in sections of human melanoma tumor using in vitro quantitative autoradiography, Cancer Res. 48:5475-5481 (1988).

6. D. Colcher, J. Esteban, J.A. Carrasquillo, P. Sugarbaker, J.C. Reynolds, G. Bryant, S.M. Larson, and J. Schlom, Complementation

of intractivitary and intravenous administration of a monoclonal antibody (B72.3) in patients with carcinoma, Cancer Res. 57:4218-4224 (1987).

7.   E.W. Martin, C.M. Mojzisik, G.H. Hinkle, J. Sampsel, M.A. Siddiqi, S.E. Tuttle, B. Sickle-Santanello, D. Colcher, M.O. Thurston, J.G. Bell, W.B. Farrar, and J. Schlom, Radioimmunoguided surgery: a new approach to the intraoperative detection of tumor using monoclonal antibody B72.3, Am. J. Surg. In press (1988).

8.   B.J. Sickle-Santanello, P.J. O'Dwyer, C. Mojzisik, S.E. Tuttle, G.H. Hinkle, A. Sardi, J.P. Minton, E. W. Martin, Radioimmunoguided surgery using the monoclonal antibody B72.3 in colorectal tumors, Dis. Colon Rectum. 30:761-764 (1987).

9.   D. Colcher, P. Horan Hand, M. Nuti, and J. Schlom, A spectrum of monoclonal antibodies reactive with human mammary tumor cells, Proc. Natl. Acad. Sci. USA 78:3199-3203 (1981).

10.   M. Nuti, Y.A. Teramoto, R. Mariani-Costantini, P. Horan Hand, D. Colcher, and J. Schlom, A monoclonal antibody (B72.3) defines patterns of distribution of a novel tumor associated antigen in human mammary carcinoma cell populations, Int. J. Cancer 29:529-545 (1982).

11.   J. Hilkens, F. Buijs, J. Hilgers, P. Hageman, J. Calafar, A. Sonnenberg, and M. van der Valk, Monoclonal antibodies against human milk-fat globule membrane detecting differentiation antigens of the gland and its tumors, Int. J. Cancer 34:197-206 (1984).

12.   I.O. Ellis, C.P. Hinton, J. MacNay, C.W. Elston, A. Robbins, A.A. Owainati, R.W. Blamey, R.W. Baldwin, and B. Ferry, Immunocytochemical staining of breast carcinoma with the monoclonal antibody NCRC 11: a new prognostic indicator, Br. Med. J. 290:881-883 (1985).

13.   J. Burchell, H. Durbin, and J. Taylor-Papdimitriou, Complexity of expression of antigenic determinant recognized by monoclonal antibodies HMFG-1 and HMFG-2, in normal and malignant human mammary epithelial cells, J. Immunol. 131:508-513 (1983).

14.   M.S. Lan, R.C. Bast, M.I. Colnaghi, R.C. Knapp, D. Colcher, J. Schlom, and R.S. Metzghar, Co-expression of human cancer-associated epitopes on mucin molecules. Int. J. Cancer 39:68-72 (1987).

15.   P. Horan Hand, D. Colcher, D. Salomon, J. Ridge, P. Noguchi, and J. Schlom, Influence of spatial configuration of carcinoma cell populations in the expression of tumor associated glycoprotein, Cancer Res. 45:833-840 (1985).

16.   P. Horan Hand, M. Nuti, D. Colcher, J. Schlom, Definition of antigenic heterogeniety and modulation among human mammary carcinoma cell populations using monoclonal antibodies to tumor-associated antigens, Cancer Res. 43:728-735 (1985).

17.   D.F. Hayes, H. Sekine, T. Ohno, M. Abe, K. Keefe, and D.W. Kufe, Use of a murine monoclonal antibody for detection of circulating plasma DF3 antigen levels in breast cancer patients, J. Clin. Invest. 75:1671-1678 (1985).

18. J. Hilkens, V. Kroezen, J.M.G. Bonfrer, M. DeJong-Bakker, and P.F. Bruning, MAM-6 antigen, a new serum marker for breast cancer monitoring, Cancer Res. 46:2582-2587 (1986).

19. P.S. Linsley, V. Ochs, S. Laska, D. Horn, D.B. Ring, A.E. Frankel and J. Brown, Elevated levels of a high molecular weight antigen detected by antibody WI in sera from breast cancer patients, Cancer Res. 46:5444-5450 (1986).

20. J. Burchell, D. Wang, and J. Taylor-Papdimitriou, Detection of the tumor-associated antigens recognized by the monoclonal antibodies HMFG-1 and 2 in serum from patients with breast cancer. Int. J. Cancer 34:763-768 (1984).

21. A.J. Strelkauskas, C. Lofton, and P.H. Aldenderfer, Human monoclonal antibody: 2. Simultaneous expression of IgG and IgM with similar binding specificities by a human hybrid clone, Hybridoma 6:479-487 (1987).

22. A.J. Strelkauskas, "Human Hybridomas", Marcel Dekker, New York (1987).

23. A.J. Strelkauskas, and C.L. Taylor, Human monoclonal antibody. Construction of stable clones reactive with human breast cancer, Cancer Immunol. Immunother. 23:31-40 (1986).

CLINICAL AND MOLECULAR INVESTIGATIONS OF THE DF3 BREAST CANCER-ASSOCIATED ANTIGEN

Daniel F. Hayes, Miyako Abe, Javed Siddiqui, Carlo Tondini, and Donald W. Kufe

Laboratory of Clinical Pharmacology
Dana Farber Cancer Institute
Boston, MA 02115

GENERATION OF MAB DF3 AND IMMUNOPEROXIDASE STUDIES OF DF3 ANTIGEN DISTRIBUTION

The murine MAb DF3 is an IgG_1 which was generated against a membrane-enriched cell extract prepared from a human breast carcinoma metastatic to liver (1). Immunoperoxidase studies have demonstrated that MAb DF3 clearly distinguishes malignant and benign breast lesions. Whereas MAb DF3 produces a cytosolic staining pattern in 78% of breast carcinomas, such a pattern is observed in less than 10% of fibrocystic lesions or fibroadenomas (1). In contrast, reactivity of benign breast lesions with MAb DF3 is primarily on the apical borders of the ductules. MAb DF3 also reacts with a variety of non-mammary adenocarcinomas, but, of note, not with colon carcinomas (1). MAb DF3 does not react with tumors of mesenchymal origin. MAb DF3 also reacts with the apical surface of normal breast ductal epithelium, as well as the apical secretory surfaces of several other normal epithelial tissues such as liver, lung, kidney (distal collecting tubules), bladder, testis, uterus, ovary, and sebaceous and sweat glands (2). MAb DF3 does not react with normal adult spleen, colon, bone marrow, heart, stomach, duodenum, skin, or adrenal cortex (2).

BIOCHEMISTRY OF DF3 ANTIGEN

MAb DF3 recognizes a high molecular weight glycoprotein containing sialyl oligosaccharides present on a peptide backbone (3). Recognition of the binding site by MAb DF3 is altered but not abolished by treatment of the antigen with neuraminidase (4). Further characterization of the carbohydrate components of the DF3 antigen has revealed that the major oligosaccharides are the peanut agglutinin binding disaccharide (Galß1,3GalNAc, also designated as the Thomsen-Friedenreich antigen) and its mono- and di-sialylated derivatives (5). Comparison of these components with other sialomucin oligosaccharides from human and murine adenocarcinoma cell lines suggests considerable heterogeneity of expression of these complex carbohydrate epitopes.

45

The DF3 mucin-like glycoprotein belongs to a family of related but not identical high-molecular weight tumor-associated antigens. These antigens are identified by other MAbs generated against either breast carcinoma cell lines or human milk fat globule membranes and may be related to cellular differentiation (6). DF3 antigen expression by human breast cancers correlates with several markers of differentiation, such as nuclear grade (NG), histologic grade (HG), and estrogen receptors (ERP) (7). Furthermore, DF3 antigen production by cultured human breast carcinoma cells is enhanced by maturational agents such as butyric acid or phorbol esters (8,9).

DETECTION OF CIRCULATING DF3 AND RELATED ANTIGENS

We have developed a radioimmunoassay (RIA) and an enzyme linked immunoassay (EIA) with MAb DF3 to monitor circulating DF3 antigen levels in patients with breast cancer (10). While DF3 antigen can be detected at low levels in normal subjects, patients with breast cancer have very high levels. A separate MAb, designated 115D8, has been generated against human milk fat globule membranes by other investigators (11). MAb 115D8 identifies a high m.w. circulating antigen designated MAM-6 (12). While MAbs DF3 and 115D8 recognize the same family of mucin-like antigens, immunoperoxidase staining, solid phase immunoassays, and immunoblotting techniques have demonstrated that these MAbs react with distinct epitopes (6). An immunoradiometric assay (IRMA) has been developed with MAbs DF3 and 115D8 to determine levels of the circulating antigen, designated CA15-3 (13). While circulating CA15-3 levels are >22 U/ml in only 10% of normal control subjects, CA15-3 levels are >22 U/ml in more than 70% of patients with metastatic breast cancer.

CA15-3 levels have been compared with circulating CEA levels in the same population of patients with breast cancer. As listed in Table 1, significantly more patients with metastatic breast cancer have elevated CA15-3 antigen levels than elevated CEA levels. Only in those patients with liver metastases are the two assays comparably elevated.

To define the specificity of the CA15-3 assay, we have evaluated patients with a variety of benign conditions and non-breast malignancies. Approximately 20% of patients with benign breast abnormalities have CA15-3 levels > 22. CA15-3 levels are not elevated in pregnant or lactating women. However, CA15-3 levels are elevated in patients with acute hepatitis, chronic active hepatitis, or cirrhosis. Furthermore, certain patients with non-mammary, epithelial malignancies, such as colon, lung, and ovarian carcinomas, have elevated circulating CA15-3 antigen levels.

The CA15-3 assay has been shown to be reliable for monitoring patients with metastatic breast cancer (13,14) In a preliminary study, serial CA15-3 levels correlated with changes in clinical course in 42 of 57 patients (74%)(13). These results have been confirmed in a retrospective comparison of the value of CA15-3 and CEA in monitoring the clinical course of patients with metastatic breast cancer (14). In agreement with our previous studies, we observed that in patients with metastatic breast cancer CA15-3 levels are more commonly elevated than are CEA levels (McNemars test, p=0.01). Overall, serial changes in CA15-3 levels correlate with disease progression (PD), response (RD), or stability (SD) in a higher number of patients than do changes in CEA levels (60.3% vs 39.6%, p=.02). CA15-3 increases ≥25% more often than CEA in patients with PD (75% vs 58.3%) and decreases ≥25% more often than CEA in patients with RD. Moreover, specificity of CA15-3 is as good or better than for CEA. In a logistic regression model, changes in CA15-

Table 1. Comparison of CA15-3 and CEA Levels in Patients with Breast Cancer

PERCENT OF PATIENTS WITH

STAGE	CA15-3 >22.0 U/ML	CEA >3.0 NG/ML	P VAL	CA15-3 >30 U/ML	CEA >5.0 NG/ML	P VAL
NORMAL CONTROLS	9.4	9.4		1.3	1.3	
PRIMARY BREAST CANCER	29	7	.01<P<.02	19	0	.005<P<.01
METASTATIC BREAST CANCER	73	55	<0.001	63	41	<0.001
LOCAL ONLY	50	19	.01<P<.02	38	12	.02<P<.05
BONE ONLY	79	59	0.07	71	44	0.02
LIVER	83	88	NS	79	75	NS

From Ref. 13, with permission.

Table 2. SENSITIVITY OF CHANGES IN CA15-3 LEVELS TO MONITOR CLINICAL COURSE IN PATIENTS WITH METASTATIC BREAST CANCER

DISEASE COURSE	Nº PTS	Nº OF PATIENTS (%) WITH CHANGES IN ANTIGEN LEVEL THAT CORRELATE WITH CLINICAL COURSE							
		CA15-3		CEA		CA15-3 and CEA		CA15-3 or CEA	
		Nº	%	Nº	%	Nº	%	Nº	%
PROGRESSION	24	18	75.0	14	58.3	12	50.0	20	83.3
RESPONSE	21	8	38.1	5	23.8	3	16.6	10	47.6
STABLE	8	6	75.0	2	25.0	2	25.0	6	75.0
OVERALL*	53	32	60.3	21	39.6	17	32.0	36	67.9

**p=.02
From ref 14, with permission

3 levels correlate significantly with both PD (p=0.0004) and RD (p=0.02), while changes in CEA levels do not (PD, p=0.34; RD, p=0.92). Furthermore, correlations obtained when using both antigens together fail to improve the results obtained with CA15-3 alone (Table 2).

In summary, the CA15-3 IRMA is a new and potentially useful assay for the evaluation and monitoring of patients with breast cancer. The assay is more sensitive in this population than CEA, and more reliably reflects changes in the clinical course of patients with this disease. Prospective trials are underway to further evaluate the clinical utility of the CA15-3 assay in patients with metastatic disease and in patients with primary breast cancer.

POLYMORPHISM OF CIRCULATING DF3 ANTIGEN

Immunoblots used to determine the molecular weight of the circulating DF3 antigen have demonstrated that MAb DF3 reacts heterogeneously with one or more circulating antigens of molecular weight ranging from 300-450 Kd (10). This heterogeneity is observed in plasma from both patients and controls, although the extent of reactivity of MAb DF3 is clearly greater with plasmas obtained from breast cancer patients. Subsequently, we have examined the heterogeneity of DF3 antigen expression to determine whether certain patterns are detectable in different individuals (15). We have observed at least four distinct DF3 antigens, designated slow (S), intermediate (I), rapid (R), or very rapid (VR), based upon the electrophoretic mobility in 3-15% polyacrylamide gels (Figure 1).

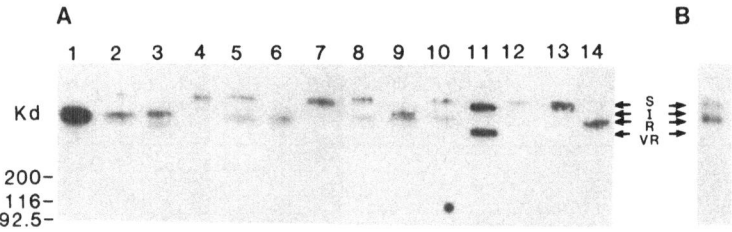

Figure 1.   Immunoblot analysis after 3-15% PAGE of plasmas from patients with metastatic breast cancer.   From ref. 15, with permission.

Moreover, the electrophoretic pattern of plasma DF3 antigen was comparable to that detected in a malignant pleural effusion from a patient with metastatic breast cancer. A similar but not identical pattern was observed in the urine of this patient. Likewise, the pattern of circulating DF3 antigen in plasma from a lactating woman was similar but not identical to that in her milk and urine. The patterns of DF3 antigen expression in a patient with metastatic breast cancer and ten of her family members suggest that the DF3 antigenic heterogeneity is a result of a genetically determined polymorphism which is expressed in an autosomal, codominant fashion (Figure 2).

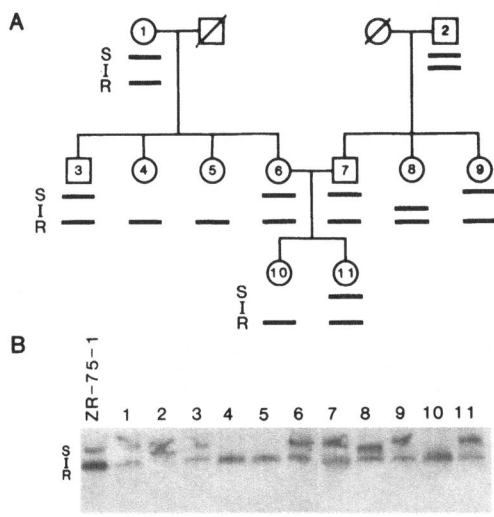

Figure 2. Relationship of DF3 electrophoretic mobilities among family members.
A. Family pedigree and schematic representaion of DF3 antigen mobilities for each
member. B. Immunoblot results obtained for plasma samples from the family members.
Electrophoretic mobilities are categorized as slow (S), intermediate (I), and rapid (R).
Lane numbers correspond to subject designation in family pedigree. Subject six is a
patient with metastatic breast cancer. From ref. 15, with permission.

These findings have been confirmed by Western blot analysis of serum
from members of 17 additional caucasian families. Although several other
plasma proteins exhibit electrophoretic polymorphisms (16), DF3 antigen
appears distinct on the basis of: 1) electrophoretic migration; 2) presence in
human milk (3); 3) expression on the surface of epithelial cells (1); and 4)
absence on erythrocytes and granulocytes (unpublished data). Thus, DF3
antigen appears to represent a previously undescribed circulating
polymorphism.

ISOLATION AND SEQUENCING OF A cDNA CODING FOR THE PROTEIN CORE OF THE
DF3 ANTIGEN.

In relation to the observation of an electrophoretic polymorphism of the
DF3 antigen, we have isolated a 309 bp partial cDNA clone from a lambda gt11
library of the breast cancer cell line, MCF-7. This clone, designated pDF9.3,
identifies a segment of the gene which codes for the core protein of the DF3
antigen (17). Southern blot analyses of EcoRI digested DNAs from several
human tumor cell lines with the pDF9.3 probe reveals restriction fragment
length polymorphisms (RFLPs) (Figure 3).

Northern blot analysis with the pDF9.3 clone of total cellular RNA from
the same human cancer cell lines demonstrates a polymorphism of transcript
size between 4.1 and 7.1 Kb. The different sized transcripts detected by pDF9.3
correspond with the DF3 antigen polymorphisms as monitored by
immunoblotting analysis (Figure 4).

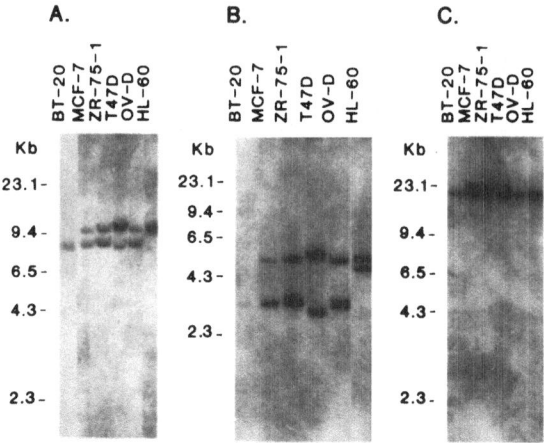

Figure 3. Southern blot analysis of genomic DNA with the pDF9.3 probe. DNAs (20μg) from human tumor cell lines were digested to completion with EcoRI (A), PstI (B), and HindIII (C) and electrophoresed in 0.6% agarose gels. The gels were denatured and the DNA fragments were transferred to nylon filters. The filters were hybridized with the ^{32}P-labeled pDF9.3 cDNA insert. The filters were then washed and exposed to x-ray film. From ref. 17, with permission.

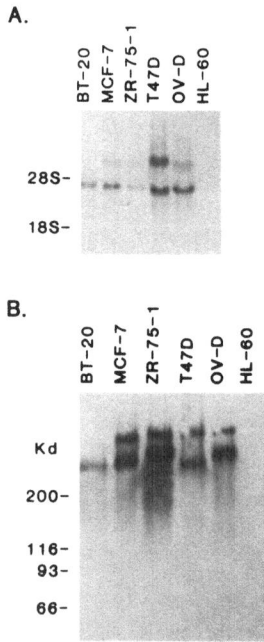

Figure 4. RNA transfer blot analysis with pDF9.3 and immunoblotting with MAb DF3. (A) Total cellular RNA (20μg) from human tumor cell lines was electrophoresed in a 1.1% agarose/formaldehyde gel, transferred to nitrocellulose, and hybridized with the ^{32}P-labeled pDF9.3 cDNA insert. (B) Extracts of the human tumor cells were analyzed by 3-15% SDS PAGE, immunoblotted with MAb DF3, and then allowed to react with rabbit anti-mouse immunoglobulin and ^{125}I-labeled protein A. From ref. 17, with permission.

These data suggest that the transcripts detected by Northern analysis code for the DF3 core protein and that the size of these transcripts determines the relative size of the MAb DF3 reactive glycoproteins.

The reactivity of MAb DF3 with a ß-galactosidase/pDF9.3 fusion protein indicates that the cDNA insert contains an open reading frame that codes for the DF3 epitope. Sequencing of the pDF9.3 segment demonstrates tandem repeats of approximately 60 bp (Figure 5).

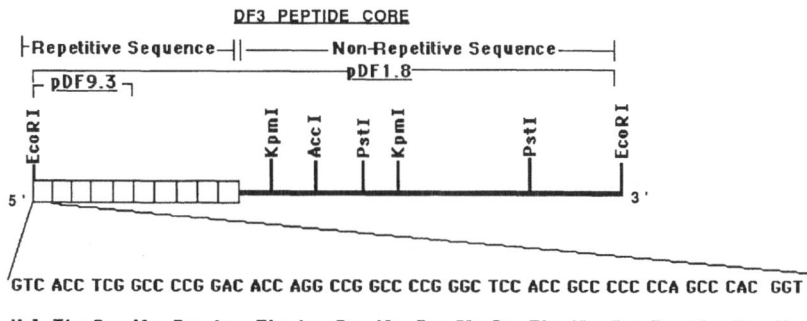

Figure 5. Schematic representation of gene coding for DF3 antigen peptide core

These repeats are nearly identical, with the exception of an occasional transversion, and they are highly rich (85%) in G+C base pairs. The deduced amino acid sequence demonstrates that the tandems are relatively proline rich and that they contain several potential sites for O carbohydrate linkage. Comparison of the pDF9.3 sequences with that of all genes with known sequences fails to reveal any significant homology.

We have suggested that variations in the size of the DF3 alleles could be due to differences in the number of these repeats and might occur as a result of unequal crossing-over events (17). Such a mechanism has recently been described to account for the allelic size difference of the complement receptor 1 (CR1)(18). We have also proposed that the presence of closely related repeats could explain the observation that MAb DF3 binds to two or more epitopes on the same DF3 molecule (17). To further investigate these and other questions related to the DF3 gene, we have isolated a larger cDNA clone (pDF1.8) (Figure 5) which is currently being evaluated.

The data generated with the DF3 gene probes provide further support for the concept that a family of related, but not identical, high-molecular weight, mucin-like polymorphic antigens is produced by human secretory epithelial cells and their malignant counterparts. The DF3 glycoprotein is also detected by another MAb, designated Ca1, that reacts with a wide range of human tumors (6). The binding site for MAb Ca1 on the DF3 glycoprotein is distinct from that defined by MAb DF3. Recent studies have described a genetic polymorphism of the Ca1 antigen in human urine (19). The locus coding for these urinary mucins (designated PUM, "peanut lectin binding urinary mucins," or, more recently designated PEM, "polymorphic epithelial mucin") is a hypervariable minisatellite of human DNA (20). A partial cDNA clone (pMUC10) which codes in part for PEM has been identified from a lambda gt11 MCF-7 breast cancer cell line cDNA library (20,21). The pMUC10 probe identifies a gene with a similar, if not identical, RFLP pattern to that observed with the DF3 gene probes. Partial sequence analysis has demonstrated that PEM, like DF3 antigen, contains several highly conserved 60bp-tandem repeats

(22). The nucleotide sequence of these repeats is identical to that of the pDF9.3. More extensive sequence analyses of these genes are currently ongoing which will allow further comparison of the moieties within this family of antigens.

In summary, DF3 antigen is a member of a highly polymorphic family of mucin glycoproteins. Detection of these proteins in human plasma has led to the development of a clinically useful serologic assay for the evaluation and monitoring of patients with metastatic breast cancer. Biochemical and genetic analyses are providing insights into the molecular nature of these antigens, and may allow generation of even more valuable clinical tools. The widespread tissue distribution and the presence in secretory fluids of these mucins imply an important, but yet unidentified, biologic role.

REFERENCES

1. D. Kufe, G. Inghirami, M. Abe, D. Hayes, H. Justi-Wheeler, and J. Schlom: Differential reactivity of a novel monoclonal antibody (DF3) with human malignant versus benign breast tumors. Hybridoma 3, 223-232, 1984.

2. D. Hayes, E. Friedman, D. Kufe: Radioimmunoscintigraphy of human carcinoma: Characterization of monoclonal antibodies; in Antibodies in Radiodiagnosis and Therapy; Zalutsky, MR (ed), CRC Press, (in press).

3. H. Sekine, T. Ohno, and D. Kufe: Purification and characterization of a high molecular weight glycoprotein detectable in human milk and breast carcinomas. J. Immunol. 135:3610-3615, 1985.

4. M. Abe, D. Kufe: Effects of maturational agents on expression and secretion of two partially characterized high molecular weight milk-related glycoproteins in MCF-7 breast carcinoma cells. J. Cell. Phys. 126:126-132, 1986.

5. S. Hull, A. Bright, M. Abe, D. Kufe, and L. Carraway: Oligosaccharides of the DF3 antigen of the BT-20 human breast carcinoma cell line. J. Cell. Biochem. Supp. 12E:130-133, 1988

6. M. Abe, and D. Kufe: Identification of a family of high molecular weight tumor-associated glycoproteins. J. Immunol. 139:257-261, 1987.

7. J. Lundy, A. Thor, R. Maenza, J. Schlom, F. Forouhar, M. Testa and D. Kufe: Monoclonal antibody DF3 correlates with tumor differentiation and hormone receptor status in breast cancer patients. Breast Cancer Res. Treat. 5:269-276, 1985.

8. M. Abe, D. Kufe: Sodium butyrate induction of milk-related antigens in human MCF-7 breast carcinoma cells. Cancer Res. 44:4574-4577, 1984.

9. M. Abe, D. Kufe: Effect of sodium butyrate on human breast carcinoma (MCF-7) cellular proliferation, morphology, and CEA production. Breast Cancer Research and Treatment 4:269-274, 1984.

10. D. Hayes, T. Ohno, M. Abe., H. Sekine, and D. Kufe: Detection of elevated plasma DF3 antigen levels in breast cancer patients. J. Clin. Invest. 75:1671-1678, 1985.

11. J. Hilkens, F. Buijs, J. Hilgers, P. Hageman, J. Calafat, A. Sonnenberg, and M. Van der Valk: Monoclonal antibodies against human milk fat globule membranes detecting differentiation antigens of the mammary gland and its tumors. Int. J. Cancer 34:197-206, 1984.

12. J. Hilkens, V. Kroezen, H. Bonfrer, M. De Jong-Bakker, and P. Bruning: MAM-6 antigen, a new serum marker for breast cancer monitoring. Cancer Res. 46:2582-2587, 1986.

13. D. Hayes, V. Zurawski, and D. Kufe: Comparison of circulating CA15-3 and carcinoembryonic antigen in patients with breast cancer. J. Clin. Oncol. 4:1542-1550, 1986.

14. C. Tondini, D. Hayes, R. Gelman, I. Henderson, and D. Kufe: Comparison of CA15-3 and carcinoembryonic antigen in monitoring the clinical course of patients with metastatic breast cancer. Cancer Res. 48:4107-4112, 1988.

15. D. Hayes, H. Sekine, D. Marcus, C. Alper, and D. Kufe: Genetically determined polymorphism of the circulating human breast cancer-associated DF3 antigen. Blood 71:436-440, 1988.

16. C. Alper, and D. Nathan: Serum proteins and other genetic markers of the blood; in Hematology of Infancy and Childhood (ed III); Nathan GD , Oski F (eds.) WB Saunders, pp 345-360 (1988).

17. J. Siddiqui, M. Abe, D. Hayes, E. Shani, E. Yunis, and D. Kufe: Isolation and sequencing of a cDNA coding for the human DF3 breast carcinoma-associated antigen. Proc. Natl. Acad. Sci. USA 85:2320-2323, 1988.

18. V. Holers, D. Chaplin, J. Leykam, B. Gruner, V. Kumar, and J. Atkinson: Human complement C3b/C4b receptor (CR1) mRNA polymorphism that correlates with the CR1 allelic molecular weight polymorphism. Proc. Natl. Acad. Sci. (USA) 84:2459-2463, 1987.

19. D. Swallow, B. Griffiths, M. Bramwell, G. Wiseman, J. Burchell: Detection of the urinary PUM polymorphism by the tumour-binding monoclonal antibodies Ca1, Ca2, Ca3, HMFG1, and HMFG2. Dis. Markers 4:247, 1986.

20. D. Swallow, S. Gendler, B. Griffiths, G. Corney, J. Taylor-Papadimitriou, and M. Bramwell: The human tumour-associated epithelial mucins are coded by an expressed hypervariable gene locus PUM. Nature (London) 328:82-84, 1987.

21. S. Gendler, J. Burchell, T. Duhig, D. Lamport, R. White, M. Parker, and J. Taylor-Papadimitriou: Cloning of partial cDNA encoding differentiation and tumor-associated mucin glycoproteins by human mammary epithelium. Proc. Natl. Acad. Sci. (USA). 84:6060-6064, 1987.

22. S. Gendler, J. Taylor-Papadimitriou, T. Duhig, J. Rothbard, and J. Burchell: A highly immunogenic region of a human polymorphic epithelial mucin expressed by carcinomas is made up of tandem repeats. J. Biol. Chem. 263:12820-12823, 1988.

This work was supported by Public Health Service Grants No. CA38869, CA10141, and by grants from Associazione Italiana per la Ricerca sul Cancro and the European Organization for Research on Treatment of Cancer, and by a Burroughs Wellcome Award in Clinical Pharmacology.

AN ASSAY FOR CRYPTIC TUMOR ANTIGENS

IN SERA OF WOMEN WITH BREAST CANCER

R. Kinders, J. Slota, J. Patrick, C. Plate, I. Kafer,
W. Caminiti, H. Rittenhouse and G. Manderino

Abbott Laboratories
Department 90C, R1B
North Chicago, IL   60064

The utility of circulating mucins as breast cancer markers was first proposed by Ceriani, et al. (1) and was rapidly confirmed and expanded by many other laboratories, including those of Chu, Taylor-Papadimitriou, Hilgers and Kufe (2-5). The antibodies used in mucin assays measure epitopes expressed on or cross-reactive with the human milk-fat globule membrane (HMFG) antigens. Assays using antibodies developed in many of the above mentioned laboratories are now commercially available, and have been used with some success in monitoring breast cancer patients.

Immunoassays for these markers measure epitopes at least partly composed of oligosaccharides, which are linked to the protein core through serine or threonine in O-glycosidic linkages (6). The oligosaccharide chains are expressed in multiple copies per glycoprotein molecule (7), and recent evidence indicates that the peptide core to which the carbohydrate chains are attached also has a repetitive structure (8). Immunoassays for these molecules can be problematic because of the high epitope density which may be present on some but not all molecules, and the variability of carbohydrate chain synthesis from individual to individual. In addition, the high negative charge and water of hydration of these molecules, properties associated with the presence of sialic acid on many, but not all of the carbohydrate chains (6-8), may affect assay performance. In some cases, the sialic acid is an important part of the epitope recognized by tumor specific antibodies (9), and in other cases it is not (10,11).

We have constructed an assay for a mucin-like glycoprotein which we believe has utility in monitoring breast cancer patients' response to therapy. In addition, we have devised a method of modifying the behavior of these glycoproteins in the assay system, resulting in improved assay performance and specificity without adding steps to the assay. The assay utilizes sialidase (C. Perfringens) to expose tumor-associated antigens that are cryptic in some, but not all, patients' sera because of sialylation of the epitopes. The presence of cryptic cell surface antigens, some of them tumor-associated, has been reported by several laboratories, notably of Burger, Springer and Feizi (12-14).

We present here some data on a cryptic tumor antigen assay for HMFG associated epitopes generated in our laboratories. A mouse monoclonal to the paragloboside family of oligosaccharides, M85/34, is used as the catcher and the peroxidase conjugated probe is the breast cancer MAb (F36/22) generated in T.M. Chu's laboratory at Roswell Park Memorial Institute (11,20).

MATERIALS

Defatted human milk fat globule membrane preparations were provided by R. Ceriani, John Muir Cancer and Aging Research Institute, Walnut Creek, CA. Sera from women judged to be normals by personal histories and physical examination by Dr. K. McCarty, Jr., were used to establish the normal cutoff for the assay. Other sera were from various sources and were acquired by the Abbott Laboratories serum bank. NCI blind panel specimens were obtained from Dr. R. Aamodt, Biological Markers Program, National Cancer Institute, Bethesda, MD. Glycolipid preparations were provided by Samar Kundu, Abbott Laboratories. Anti-sera to paragloboside was obtained from Dainabot, Ltd.

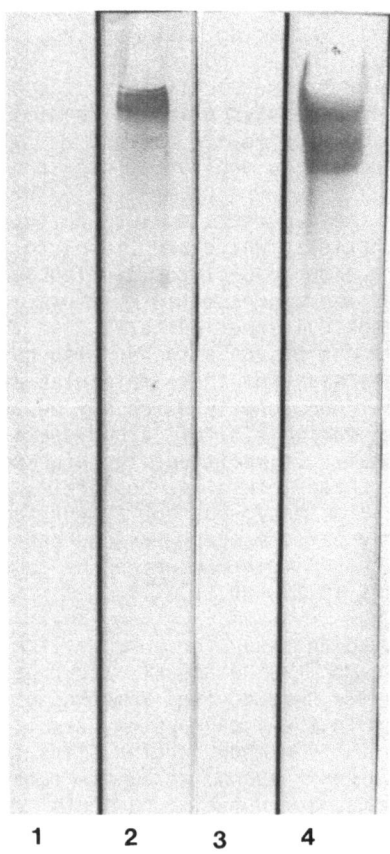

1   2   3   4

Fig. 1. Western blot of HMFG, developed with MAb MA85/34 (Lane 2) or control mouse IgM (Lane 1), or with MAb F36/22 (Lane 4) or control mouse IgG (Lane 3).

METHODS

NCI panel analyses were performed by the Breast Cancer Biomarkers Data Center, Information Management Services, Inc., Silver Spring, MD.

Monoclonal antibody M85/34, A mouse IgM, was generated by immunization of BALB/c mice with a high molecular mass fraction purified from an ovarian cancer patient's ascites fluid. Fusions of spleens and SP2/0 mouse myeloma cells were performed by conventional methods. Hybridomas were selected based on screening of antibody reactivity with immunogen, immunohistochemical analysis of tumor tissue sections, erythrocyte and lymphocyte reactivities, and with other normal tissues.

M85/34 was used to coat microtitre plates or 1/4 inch polystyrene beads. The reaction wells or beads were incubated with either standards containing extracts of the human breast tumor cell line T47D, control sera and/or ascites fluids from breast cancer patients, or test sera diluted 1/22 in the reaction well. Each reaction also contained neuraminidase (type X, Sigma). The beads, neuraminidase and specimens were incubated for 2 hours at $37^{\circ}C$. Conjugated F36/22 was then added to each well and incubated for 1 hr at $37^{\circ}C$. After a final wash, O-phenylenediamine/peroxide (Abbott) was added and reacted for 30 min. The reaction was stopped by the addition of an equal volume of 1 N sulfuric acid and read at 492 nM using either a Biotek Autoreader or the Abbott Quantum Automated Spectrophotometer, which used an internal program to convert the absorbance to arbitrary units/mL for each specimen assayed.

RESULTS

Monoclonal antibody F36/22 recognizes a repetitive epitope present on a mucin-like glycoprotein found on ductal epithelia, mammary carcinoma tissue, and circulating in the blood of women with breast cancer (4). The antigen, ductal carcinoma antigen (DCA) has been affinity purified, biochemically and immunochemically characterized (10). The antibody is a murine IgG3.

Monoclonal antibody (MAb) M85/34 was raised to mucin purified from a cancer patient ascites and recognizes a repetitive epitope on a high molecular mass antigen present in HMFG membrane, T47D and MCF-7 extracts (Fig.1) with a similar tissue distribution to F36/22 (immunocytochemical data to be published elsewhere).

The M85/34 epitope is predominantly, if not exclusively carbohydrate in nature, expressed on meconium glycolipids, and minimally composed of N-acetyllactosamine attached to a GalNac moiety in an O-glycosidic linkage to peptide (11) (Fig.2). M85/34 does not recognize the LacNac structure when it is attached to GlcNac in an N-glycosidic linkage. The epitope does not require sialic acid and is putatively identified as the I/i blood group substances. The MAb is a murine IgM and, consistent with its specificity, it is a cold agglutinin. It has been suggested that the i blood group can be viewed as an oncofetal antigen (16).

CRYPTICITY OF THE EPITOPES

Data generated during the characterization of the MAbs suggested that the presence of sialic acid on oligosaccharide chains bearing the F36/22 or M85/34 epitopes interfered with MAb binding. This was true for antigen preparations from cell extracts (MCF-7, T47D), human serum specimens, human ascites fluids, and meconium glycolipid extracts.

I   II

1   2   3   4   5   6   1   2   3   4   5   6

Fig 2. High performance TLC binding of anti-paragloboside and M85/34.
Lane 1:250 nG sialosyl (a2-3) lacto-n-isooctasylceramide (SA-I).
Lane 2: 250 nG neuraminidase treated SA-I. Lane 3: 250 nG
sialosyl (a2-3) lacto-n-norhexaosylceramide (SA-i). Lane 4: 250
nG neuraminidase treated SA-i. Lane 5: 500 nG paragloboside.
Lane 6: neutral glycolipids from meconium.

We examined a number of serum specimens from normal women, women
with benign breast disease, and breast cancer patients to determine if
crypticity of epitopes was a factor in circulating mucins. The assays
were performed as two step EIAs, with or without neuraminidase treatment
of each of the serum specimens. There was a substantial increase in the
reactivity of a number of the cancer patient specimens in the assay,
without a concurrent increase in the reactivity of the control specimens
(Table 1).

NCI BLIND PANEL RESULTS

We tested a prototype plate EIA with an NCI blind panel, performing
the actual assay at Roswell Park Memorial Institute. The panel consisted
of 36 controls, 36 Stage I or II breast cancers, 36 Stage IV breast cancers and 36 benign breast disease patients. Human milk fat globule membrane extract, kindly provided by R. Ceriani, was used as the standard
antigen (Fig. 3).

The patient scores for the cryptic tumor antigen (CTA) prototype
assay, Abbott CEA, and Centocor CA 15-3 are shown in Table 2.

The panel contained 24 duplicate specimens. Correlation of
duplicates run blind are shown in Fig. 4. The correlation of the blind
duplicates was 0.987, and the p value (=0.00000) indicated a very high
degree of reproducibility of even the prototype assay.

TABLE 1. Effects of Neuraminidase Digestion on Specimen Reactivity in the M85/34-F36/22 Assay.

SPECIMEN	CATEGORY	NATIVE	NEURAMINIDASE TREATED O.D. 490	NASE/NATIVE
333	Adv.BrCa	0.550**	1.484**	2.7
332	"	0.078	0.208	2.7
331	"	0.082	0.484*	5.9
280	"	0.056	0.170	3.0
279	"	0.090	0.419*	4.7
281	"	0.106 B	0.245	2.3
319	"	0.049	0.110	2.2
320	"	0.084	1.887*	22.5
269	"	0.419**	0.704**	1.7
270	"	0.074	0.445*	6.0
91	Early BrCa	0.062	0.180	2.9
49	"	0.074	0.232	3.1
51	"	0.052	0.166	3.2
21	"	0.060	0.486*	8.1
33	"	0.055	0.236	4.3
26	"	0.055	0.342*	6.2
119	N. Male	0.056	0.154	2.8
361	"	0.058	0.207	3.6
12	N. Fem.	0.113 B	0.296	2.6
79	"	0.060	0.280	4.7
15	"	0.071	0.268	3.8
51	"	0.050	0.130	2.6
369	"	0.054	0.144	2.7

** Specimens with elevated values without neuraminidase treatment.

* Specimens with elevated values only after neuraminidase treatment.

B Specimens with values within 5% of the cutoff value for normal vs. elevated values.

TABLE 2. NCI Blind Panel Results

Group	N	Number Assayed Positive (and percent)		
		CA 15-3 (30 U/mL)	CEA (5 nG/mL)	CTA (30 U/mL)
Controls	36	3 (8.3)	0	3 (8.3)
Benign Breast	36	4 (11.6)	0	2 (5.6)
Breast Ca.				
Stage I	18	1 (5.6)	3 (16.7)	6 (33.3)
Stage II	18	6 (33.3)	1 (5.6)	3 (16.7)
Stage IV	36	18 (50.0)	7 (19.4)	20 (55.6)
Sensitivity		35%	15%	40%
Specificity		90%	100%	93%

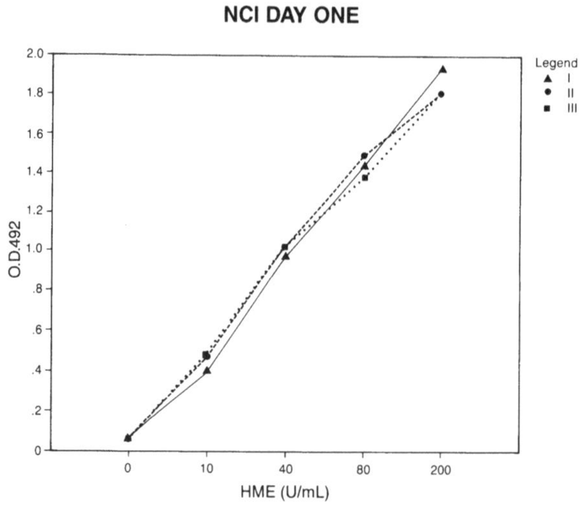

NCI DAY ONE

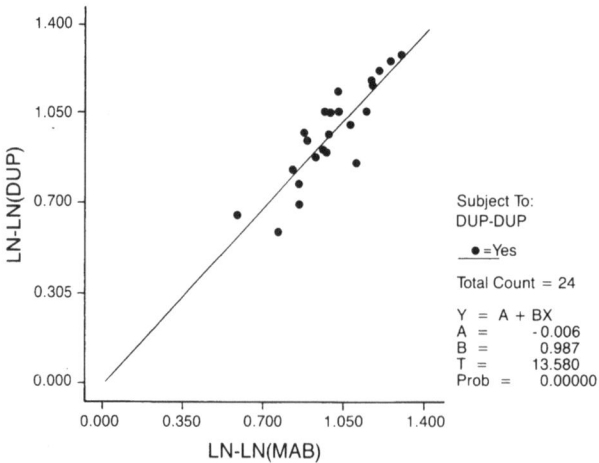

Fig 3. HMFG (HME) standard curves from three different 96-well plates (I,II,III), plotted as U/mL vs A492.

FIG. 4 Correlation of values obtained on independent assay of duplicate blind panel members, graphed and calculated by IMS, Inc. (See methods).

RESEARCH USE BCM (BREAST CANCER MUCIN) ASSAY, IN-HOUSE CLINICAL DATA

The prototype assay was converted into a 1/4" polystyrene bead EIA format for further clinical studies. This was done using the standard Abbott quarter-inch bead format, with M85/34 as the solid phase antibody, and F36/22 HRPO conjugate as the probe. A number of materials were available for use as standards. Cell extracts from the human breast cancer line MCF-7 served as primary standard. The kit configuration uses a four point standard curve, and two control specimens are provided. Standards and controls are diluted in parallel with the patient specimens to be assayed. The final specimen dilution is 1:21. The results are reported as arbitrary units and the units are calculated on the Abbott Quantum spectrophotometer.

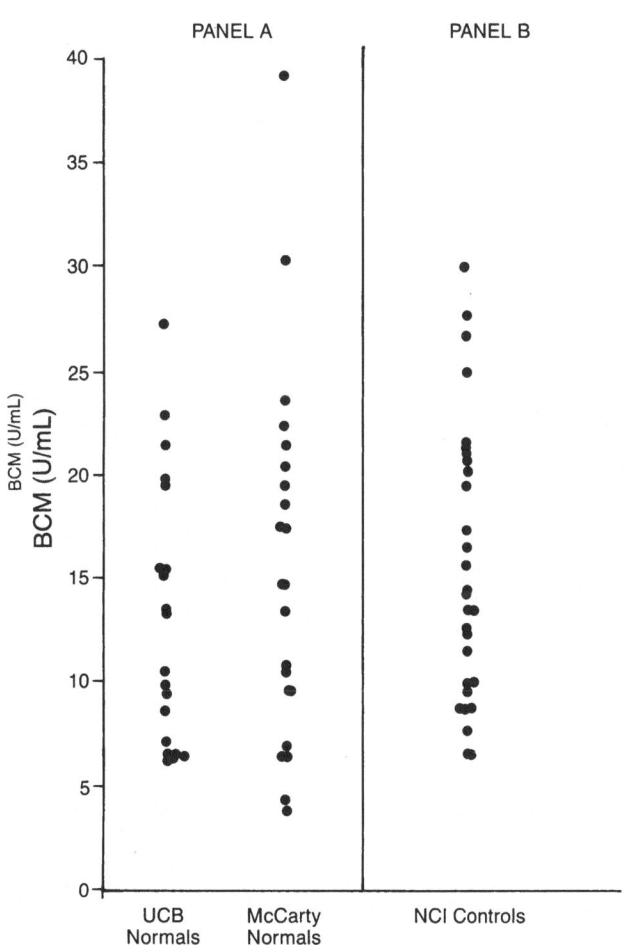

Fig. 5   Scatter diagram of BCM-EIA values for normal women (Panel A) and NED controls provided by NCI biological markers program.

We established the normal specimen range and a cutoff to separate normal from elevated specimens in the bead EIA using two groups of healthy women: Women with normal histories and no evidence of benign breast disease by physical exams were identified by Dr. K. McCarty (N=22), and a group of rand m normal controls provided by the Abbott serum bank (N=20). Scatter diagrams of the specimens are shown in Fig. 5A. The mean U/mL was 13.75. with a Std. Dev. of 6.8 U, resulting in a 3 Std. Dev. cutoff of 34.13 U/mL. One specimen from a woman judged normal repeatedly assayed at a value of about 39 U/mL. The proposed cutoff was

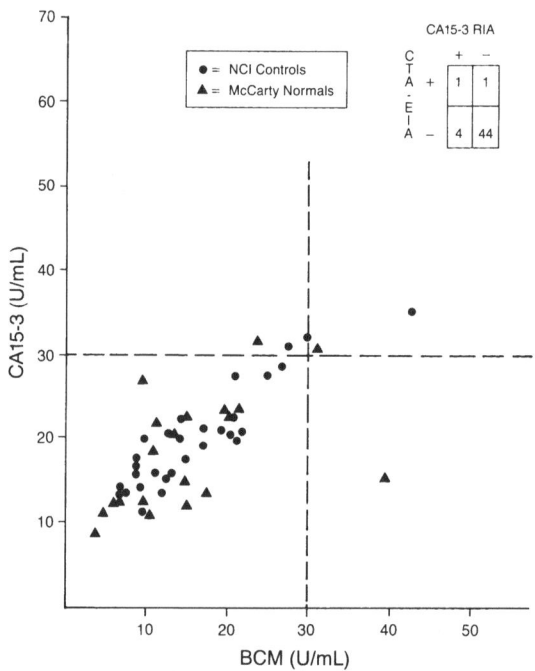

Fig. 6 Comparison of assay values of normals and controls for the BCM EIA and CA 15-3 RIA.

used to evaluate the controls (which were age-matched to the cancer patients) from the NCI panel (N=30), again in a double-blinded manner. For this group the mean was 15.56 U/mL with a Std. Dev. of 6.67 U/mL. As shown in panel 5B, 29 specimens from this group fell below the 35 U/mL predicted 3 standard deviation cutoff (range 6.5 to 30 U/mL). One specimen reproducibly assayed at 43 U/mL, well beyond the 3 Std. Dev. cutoff for either the control or the normals population, and was elevated regardless of whether the 43 value was included in the calculation of the Mean and Std. Dev.

Although CTA and CA 15-3 assays were found to be strongly correlated differences between the assays, often striking, were observed probably due to the different epitopes recognized by the two assays, and the effects of the neuraminidase treatment of specimens in CTA. An interesting point is that the scores on normal women and women with benign breast disease were strikingly similar for the two assays (r≳.94). (Fig. 6).

Not surprisingly, the arbitrary units and cutoff are similar to those used for the Centocor CA 15-3 assay, since both assays are measuring circulating HMFG mucin glycoproteins (r=0.9).

The BCM bead EIA and the CA 15-3 RIA were then tested on a panel of 528 specimens, in a double blinded fashion, in a head to head comparison with the CA 15-3 RIA. The results are shown as the percent of specimens from each of 3 groups reading within an assay range (Table 3). For ease of comparison, we used the CA 15-3 assay ranges and cutoffs to compare assay performances. The results of this panel suggested that the BCM-EIA had a significantly better sensitivity for breast cancer than did the CA 15-3 assay, while maintaining at least equivalent specificity.

TABLE 3. NUMBER OF SPECIMENS ASSAYED IN EACH RANGE (U/mL)

Patient Group	Percent			
	CTA Bead EIA			
	0-30	30.1-38	38.1-200	200
Normals/benign Breast/controls N=154	95.5	4.5	0	0
Stages I & II Breast Cancer N=49	83.7	4.1	12.2	0
Stage IV Breast Cancer N=325	22.8	12.0	51.0	14.2
	Centocor CA 15-3 RIA			
Normals/benign Breast/controls N=154	93.5	6.5	0	0
Stages I & II Breast cancer N=49	89.8	10.2	0	0
Stage IV Breast cancer N=325	43.0	13.2	29.5	14.2

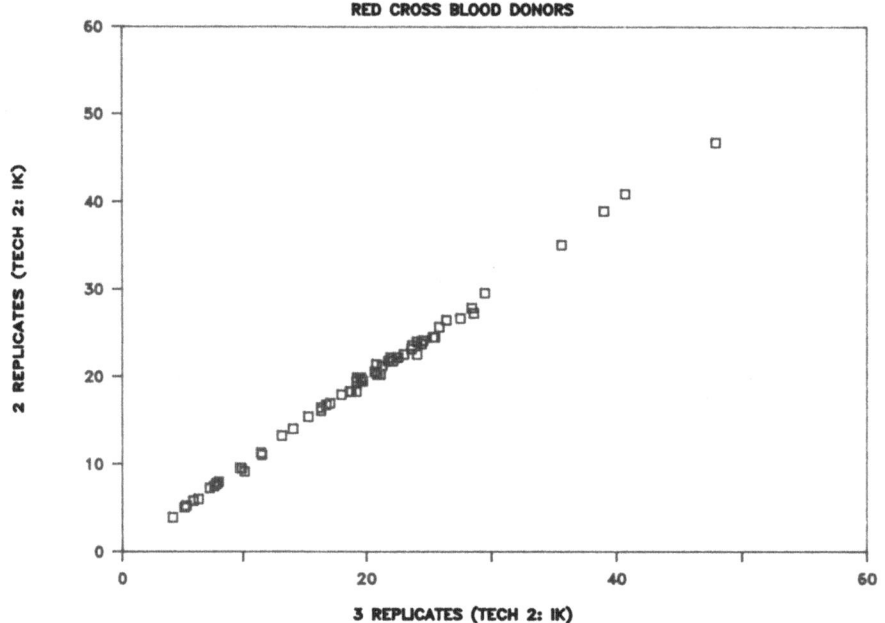

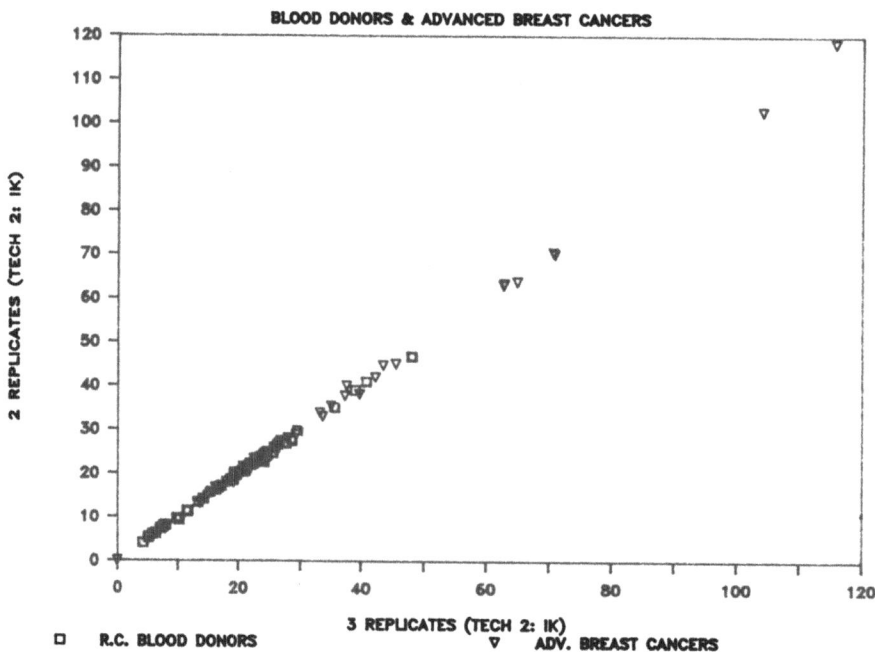

Fig. 7   BCM assay performance.   60 Red Cross blood donors and 48 breast
cancer patients were assayed in triplicate on the BCM EIA.   The
mean of the first two tubes (2 replicates) was then plotted
against the mean of all three tubes (3 replicates).

Assay reproducibility was comparable to CEA, with typical CVs of 4% (range 1-12%). Higher CVs were not clustered or associated with any particular sample group, as shown in Fig. 7, which compares the means of duplicates with the means of triplicate determinations over the low range or entire range of the assay.

PATIENT TRACKING SERIES

Tracking series from 38 patients, of a minimum of 4 time points, were examined by BCM EIA (Fig. 8). The retrospective results suggested that the assay correlated with clinical outcomes for 27 of the patients. Abbott CEA one-step was performed on the same group of patients, with apparent clinical correlation for 18 of these. The use of both assays resulted in agreement with clinical status for 31 of the 38. Centocor CA 15-3 appeared to track 23 of the 31 patients, adding one additional patient to BCM alone, but none to BCM plus CEA.

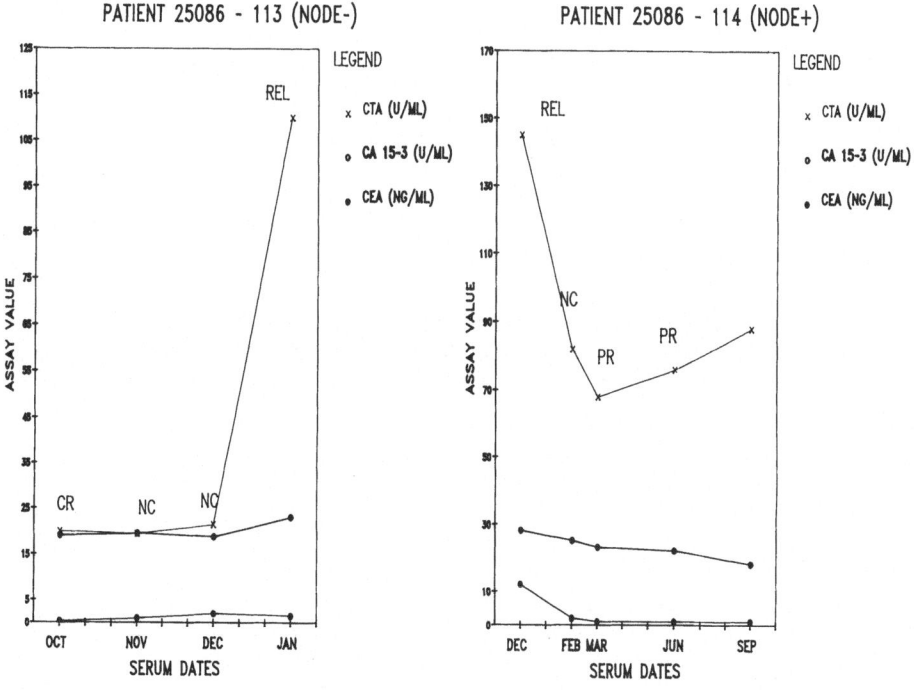

Fig. 8   Retrospective tracking series of a node negative (113) and a node positive (114) breast cancer patient. The patients were reported to have active advanced disease at the last time point in each series. The sera were assayed with Abbott CEA one-step EIA, Centocor CA 15-3 RIA, and Abbott BCM EIA. CR: Complete response to therapy; NC: no change; Rel: relapse; PR: partial response.

DISCUSSION

The clinical utility of circulating mucin markers has been the subject of intense research over the last decade. While no antigens have been identified which are useful as serum markers for patient screening, considerable data supporting a potential role for these markers in monitoring disease status of the patient. Our early data on the BCM assay suggest that mucin molecules bearing the DCA and I/i epitopes (10,14,16) can be effectively used in disease monitoring, providing good sensitivity for advanced breast cancer (76%) and acceptable specificity (95%). In addition, the cryptic tumor antigen assay format allowed the positive detection of 16% of Stage I and II breast cancer patients tested.

The use of neuraminidase in the assay proved to be entirely beneficial. No control or benign disease patients' sera which had been negative without neuraminidase treatment became positive after treatment, while some marginally elevated sera from this group fell below the cutoff after neuraminidase treatment, presumably due to reduction in non-specific interactions. Furthermore, the use of neuraminidase increased overall assay sensitivity by more than 30%. We attribute the beneficial effect to the well known heterogeneity of both the human cancer patient population as a whole, and to that of the individual tumor cells. The removal of sialic acid to allow MAb access to the oligosaccharide core structure substantially increases the ability to measure mucin in some sera, while having no effect on others. The neuraminidase treatment step has been incorporated into the assay kit, and requires no additional specimen handling compared to standard bead format EIAs or RIAs.

The BCM assay is currently being tested in independent clinical laboratories in Europe and the U.S. These data will identify clinical utility of the assay for disease detection and patient monitoring.

ACKNOWLEDGEMENTS

We would like to thank Dr. T. M. Chu, Roswell Park Memorial Institute, and Dr. Ken McCarty, Jr., Duke University Medical Center, for their assistance which were key ingredients in the success of this project. We also would like to thank Drs. Joyce Taylor-Papadimitriou, Roberto Ceriani and Byron Anderson for their advice and comments. Finally, we would like to thank Ms. Carol Dostalek without whom we would not have had a manuscript.

REFERENCES

1. R. L. Ceriani, M. Sasaki, H. Sussman, W. M. Wara, and E. W. Blank, Circulating human mammary epithelial antigens in breast cancer, Proc. Natl. Acad. Sci. U.S.A. 79:5420-5424 (1982).
2. J. Burchell, D. Wang, and J. Taylor-Papadimitriou, Detection of tumor-associated antigens recognized by the monoclonal antibodies HMFG-1 and 2 in serum from patients with breast cancer, Int. J. Cancer 34:763-768 (1984).
3. J. Hilkens, F. Buijs, J. Hilgers, P. Hageman, J. Calafat, A. Sonnenberg, and M. van der Valk, Monoclonal antibodies against human milk-fat globule membranes detecting differentiation antigens of the mammary gland and its tumors, Int. J. Cancer 34:197-206 (1984).

4. L. D. Papsidero, T. Nemoto, G. A. Croghan, and T. M. Chu, Expression of ductal carcinoma antigen in breast cancer sera as defined using monoclonal antibody F36/22, Cancer Res. 44:4653-4657 (1984).
5. D. F. Hayes, T. Ohno, M. Abe, H. Sekine, and D. W. Kufe, Detection of elevated plasma DF3 levels in breast cancer patients, J. Clin. Invest. 75:1671-1678 (1985).
6. S.-I. Hakamori, Tumor-associated carbohydrate antigens, Ann. Rev. Immunol. 2:103-126 (1984).
7. H. G. Rittenhouse, G. L. Manderino, and G. M. Hass, Mucin-type glycoproteins as tumor markers, Lab. Med. 16:556-560 (1985).
8. D. M. Swallow, B. Griffiths, M. Bramwell, G. Wiseman, and J. Burchell, Detection of the urinary PUM polymophism by the tumor-binding monoclonal antibodies Ca1, Ca2, Ca3, HMFG1 and HMFG2, Disease Markers 4:247-254 (1986).
9. J. L. Magnani, Z. Steplewski, H. Koprowski, and V. Ginsburg, Identification of the gastrointestinal and pancreatic cancer-associated antigen detected by monoclonal antibody 19-9 in the sera of patients as a mucin, Cancer Res. 43:5489-5492 (1983).
10. L. D. Papsidero, G. A. Croghan, E. A. Johnson, and T. M. Chu, Immunoaffinity isolation of ductal carcinoma antigen using mono-clonal antibody F36/22, Molec. Immunol. 21:955-960 (1984).
11. B. Anderson, J. Slota, S. Kundu, J. Patrick, G. Manderino, H. Rittenhouse, and J. Tomita, Characterization of monoclonal anti-bodies to paragloboside and sialosyl-PG, and an improved chroma-togram binding assay for rapidly identifying antibodies to tumor antigens, J. Cell Biochem. Suppl. 110:157 (1987).
12. M. M. Burger, A difference in the architecture of the surface membrane of normal and virally transformed cells, Proc. Natl. Acad. Sci. U.S.A., 62:994-1001 (1969).
13. G. F. Springer, T and Tn, general carcinoma antigens, Science 224:1198-1206 (1984).
14. H. C. Gooi, K.-I. Uemura, P. Edwards, C. S. Foster, N. Pickering, and T. Feizi, Two mouse hybridoma antibodies against human milk-fat globules recognize the I(MA) antigenic determinant, Carbohy-drate Res. 120:293-302 (1983).
15. L. D. Papsidero, G. A. Croghan, M. J. O'Connell, L. A. Valenzuela, T. Nemoto, and T. M. Chu, Monoclonal antibodies (F36/22 and M7/105) to human breast carcinoma, Cancer Res. 43:1742-1747 (1983).
16. T. Feizi and R. A. Childs, Carbohydrates as antigenic determinants of glycoproteins, Biochem. J. 245:1-11 (1987).

SESSION II

BIOSYNTHESIS OF THE CELL SURFACE SIALOMUCIN FROM ASCITES 13762 RAT MAMMARY ADENOCARCINOMA CELLS: INTRACELLULAR MATURATION

Steven R. Hull, Julie Spielman and Kermit L. Carraway

Department of Anatomy and Cell Biology
University of Miami School of Medicine
Miami, FL 33101

INTRODUCTION

Considerable attention has been directed in recent years toward tumor cell surface sialomucins (Carraway and Spielman, 1986). The presence of these O-glycosylated glycoproteins has been correlated with metastasis in the 13762NF rat mammary adenocarcinoma (Steck and Nicolson, 1983), and they are proposed to protect carcinomas from immune destruction by "masking" cell surface antigens, including histocompatibility antigens (Codington, 1981). Monoclonal antibodies prepared against whole tumor cells (Lan et al., 1985), tumor cell membranes (Kufe et al., 1984) or human milk fat globule membranes (Taylor-Papadimitriou, 1981) in many cases react specifically with carcinoma cell sialomucins and are being investigated for their potential in diagnosis and therapy (Schlom, 1986). Why should these mucin-like molecules, which are also products of normal tissues (Ceriani et al., 1983), be recognized as "carcinoma-associated antigens"? One possibility is that changes in the glycosylation of these glycoproteins in carcinomas yields epitopes which are absent or uncommon in normal tissues or other tumors (Hull and Carraway, 1988). An example of this phenomenon is the presence of "incomplete" oligosaccharides on many carcinomas, including the Thomsen-Friedenreich (T) and Tn antigens (Springer, 1984), whose carbohydrate components are the disaccharide Galβ1,3GalNAc and monosaccharide GalNAc, respectively. Examination of the general sialomucin biosynthesis pathway (Fig. 1) shows that the saccharides of these antigens are biosynthetic precursors (Carraway and Hull, 1989).

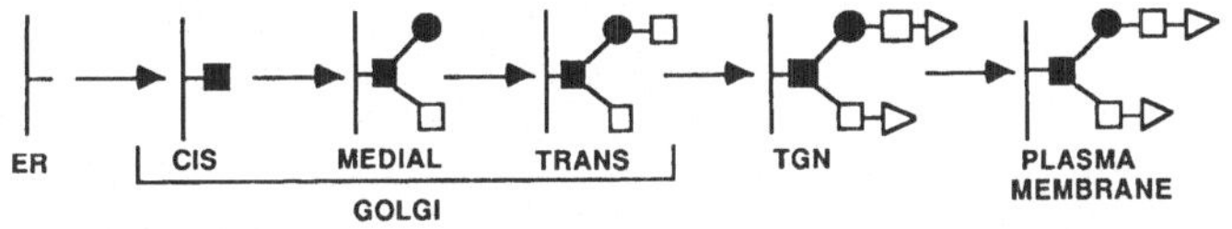

Fig. 1 Proposed general pathway for O-glycosylation (Carraway and Hull 1989). GalNAc, (■); GlcNAc(●); Gal, (□); sialic acid, (▷). TGN, Trans-Golgi network.

An understanding of the expression of these antigens requires knowledge of the biosynthesis of the sialomucins. Toward this goal we have been investigating the biosynthetic pathway for the cell surface sialomucin ASGP-1 of ascites sublines of the 13762 rat mammary adenocarcinoma (Carraway and Spielman, 1986; Spielman et al., 1987). These cells are an appropriate model because of the abundance of the sialomucin on the ascites cells (about 0.5% of the **total** cell protein) (Sherblom et al., 1980) and the presence of "incomplete" oligosaccharides on the cell surface, including T antigen disaccharide detected by staining with fluorescent peanut agglutinin (PNA) (Helm and Carraway, 1981), which is specific for the disaccharide. Pulse-chase studies of the transit of ASGP-1 through the cells show that 60-80 min is required from the time of polypeptide synthesis to its appearance at the cell surface (Spielman et al., 1987). In contrast, less than 10 min was required from the time of addition of carbohydrate to appearance at the cell surface. Analyses of the individual sugars of the cell surface ASGP-1 oligosaccharides showed that

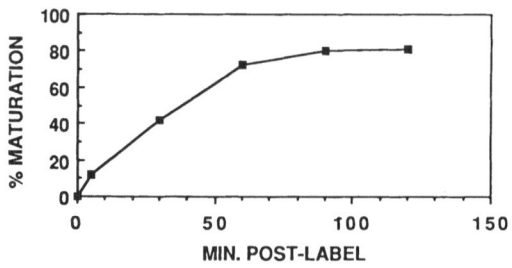

Fig. 2. Conversion of immature to pre-mature form of ASGP-1.

initiation of oligosaccharide synthesis was occurring within 10 min of appearance at the cell surface. Thus, a fraction of the ASGP-1 oligosaccharides are being synthesized late in the transit pathway (Spielman et al., 1987).

MATURATION OF ASGP-1

To investigate this transit pathway, pulse-chase labeled intermediates of ASGP-1 were analyzed by gel filtration chromatography in sodium dodecyl sulfate (SDS). Three discrete forms of ASGP-1 were identified (Spielman et al., 1988). A poorly glycosylated immature form was detected by PNA precipitation and gel filtration in less than 5 min after labeling with threonine (Spielman et al., 1987,1988). This form was chased into a larger, more heavily glycosylated pre-mature form with a half-time of about 30 min (Fig. 2). The rapid appearance of the immature form of ASGP-1 suggests that it is being produced in the endoplasmic reticulum. Moreover, the half-time for the immature to pre-mature transition and the resulting "burst" of glycosylation are consistent with a transfer from the endoplasmic reticulum to the Golgi.

Table 1. Major oligosaccharides synthesized by 13762 MAT-B1 ascites cells in the presence and absence of monensin (Spielman et al., 1988).

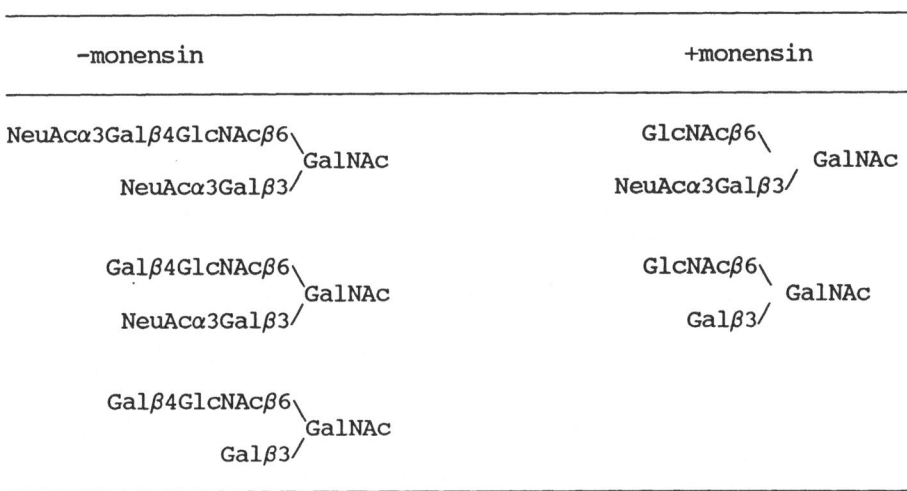

−monensin	+monensin
NeuAcα3Galβ4GlcNAcβ6\ GalNAc / NeuAcα3Galβ3	GlcNAcβ6\ GalNAc / NeuAcα3Galβ3
Galβ4GlcNAcβ6\ GalNAc / NeuAcα3Galβ3	GlcNAcβ6\ GalNAc / Galβ3
Galβ4GlcNAcβ6\ GalNAc / Galβ3	

This transfer has been shown to be a rate-limiting step in glycoprotein maturation in other cell systems (Lodish, 1988). Finally, the pre-mature form was converted to a mature form with a half-time of greater than 4 hr.

To investigate the individual steps in the maturation of ASGP-1, we examined the effects of monensin, a perturbant of Golgi functions and glycoprotein biosynthesis (Tartakoff, 1983). In the absence of monensin the major oligosaccharides synthesized by 13762 MAT-B1 ascites cells are the tetrasaccharide and its monosialo and disialo derivatives (Table 1). In the presence of monensin the tetrasaccharide and its derivatives are greatly reduced, leading to a substantial reduction in size of the ASGP-1 produced. In their place are synthesized a trisaccharide and its monosialo derivative (Spielman et al., 1988). From these structures it is apparent that monensin has specifically prevented the addition of β1,4-galactose to the 1,6-arm of the oligosaccharide without inhibiting the addition of sialic acid to the 1,3-arm. Since monensin also inhibits the addition of sulfate to glucosamine of the 1,6-arm, we have proposed that the mechanism of monensin action in these cells involves specific disruption of the Golgi compartment containing β1,4-galactosyltransferase and sulfate transferase without significantly affecting prior or subsequent compartments involved in the ASGP-1 biosynthesis pathway (Fig. 3) (Spielman et al., 1988). These results also indicate that the β1,4-galactosyltransferase is predominantly in a separate compartment from sialyltransferase.

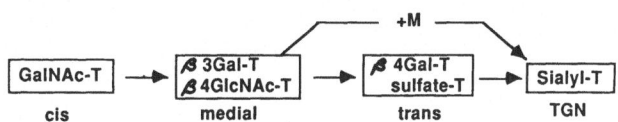

Fig. 3. Proposed enzyme locations during glycoprotein transit through Golgi compartments and monensin (M) effect.

Table 2. Major sulfated oligosaccharides of MAT-B1 cells.

S-1	^-O_4S-GlcNAcβ6\ Galβ3/ GalNAc		S-2	^-O_4S-GlcNAcβ6\ NeuAcGalβ3/ GalNAc	

TERMINAL MATURATION STEP

What is the nature of the conversion from pre-mature to mature ASGP-1? Since sialic acid is the final sugar added to the oligosaccharides, one might expect that the pre-mature to mature conversion simply involves sialylation of pre-existing neutral oligosaccharides, primarily tetrasaccharide. However, the fact that we have observed late initiation of oligosaccharides suggests a second possible mechanism, i.e., complete synthesis of new oligosaccharides in a late compartment of the transit pathway. To distinguish between these two mechanisms, we have asked two questions. How does the rate of sialylation compare to the rate of conversion from pre-mature to mature ASGP-1? Are sialylated oligosaccharides completely synthesized in a late compartment in the transit pathway?

To simplify the determination of the kinetics of sialylation, we examined the sialylation of sulfated oligosaccharide. MAT-B1 cells have only two major sulfated oligosaccharides on ASGP-1 (Hull and Carraway, 1989), as shown in Table II. Thus the sialylation kinetics for the sulfated oligosaccharide involves only one conversion, compared to several conversions among several products of nonsulfated oligosaccharides. Pulse-chase analyses of sulfate-labeled MAT-B1 cells showed that sulfated trisaccharide S-1 was rapidly chased into sialylated, sulfated trisaccharide with a half-time of less than 5 min (Fig. 4). Thus, the rate of sialylation of sulfated oligosaccharide is much faster than the rate of conversion of pre-mature to mature ASGP-1 (half-time >4 hr).

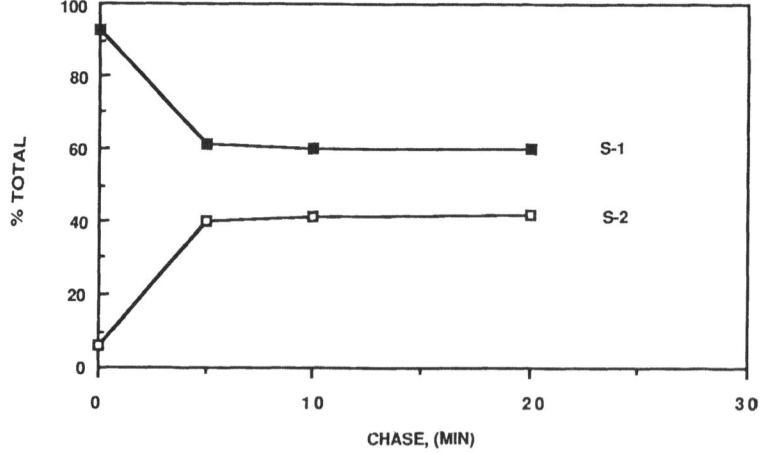

Fig. 4. Pulse chase sulfate labeling of S-1 and S-2. Analyses were performed as previously described (Hull and Carraway, 1989).

We have previously shown that the T antigen disaccharide Galβ1,3GalNAc, which appears at the cell surface of MAT-B1 cells, is synthesized in a late compartment of the transit pathway (Hull and Carraway, 1988). Disaccharide synthesized earlier is elongated and does not appear at the cell surface in this precursor form. We have proposed that this late synthesis of disaccharide is due to aberrant localization of the enzymes synthesizing the disaccharide to a late compartment (Hull and Carraway, 1988). These results raise the question of whether this late compartment is capable of synthesizing all of the ASGP-1 oligosaccharides as part of the process of maturation from the pre-mature to mature form of the glycoprotein.

To investigate the synthesis of sialylated oligosaccharides late in the transit pathway, we pulse-labeled MAT-B1 cells for 5

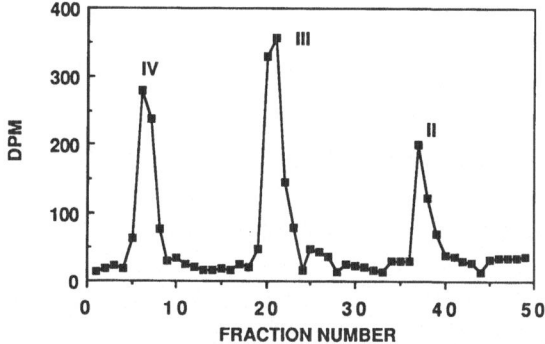

Fig. 5. Isolation of neutral, monosialo and disialo oligosaccharides from pulse-chase labeled, cell surface ASGP-1. Cells were pulse labeled 5 min with glucosamine, chased with unlabeled glucosamine for 10 min and treated with trypsin to release labeled ASGP-1 glycopeptides (Hull and Carraway, 1988; Spielman et al., 1987). Oligosaccharitols were released from the glycopeptides with alkaline borohydride and fractionated by anion exchange HPLC (Hull and Carraway, 1989).

min with ^{3}H-glucosamine and chased for 10 min with unlabeled glucosamine. The cells were treated with trypsin to release cell surface ASGP-1 glycopeptides (Hull and Carraway, 1988; Spielman et al., 1987), which were precipitated with PNA (Hull and Carraway, 1988). The carbohydrates were released from the glycopeptides with alkaline borohydride as oligosaccharitols, which were separated into neutral, mono-anionic and di-anionic fractions by anion exchange HPLC (Fig. 5). The anionic species were hydrolyzed with mild acid to release sialic acid, which was separated from the neutral oligosaccharitol core by HPLC, as shown in Fig. 6 for the monosialotetrasaccharide. Analysis of the radioactivity profiles showed that the oligosaccharitol core was heavily labeled, but that the sialic acid contained almost no label.

To examine the label distribution in the oligosaccharitol core, the neutral oligosaccharitol was hydrolyzed to its constituent sugars and fractionated by HPLC (Fig. 7). Quantitation of the label in glucosamine and galactosamine indicated label was incorporated in similar amounts into the two amino sugars in neutral, monosialo and disialo derivatives of the tetrasaccharide. Since the ratio of label in the two sugars is also similar to the ratio found in mature ASGP-1 (Spielman et al., 1987), incorporation of both sugars appears to be occurring in the late compartment for all of the oligosaccharides.

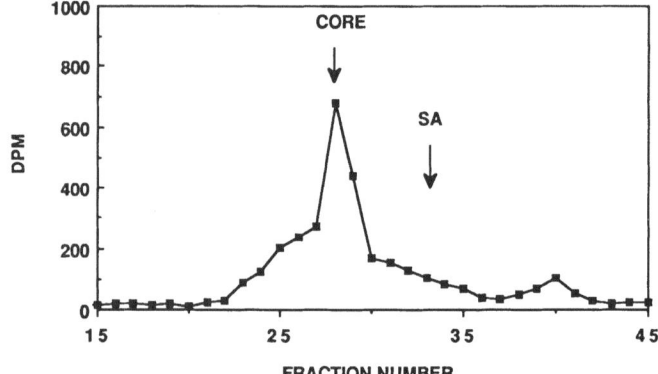

Fig. 6. Analysis of label in neutral core and sialic acid from mono-sialylated tetrasaccharide oligosaccharitol of cell surface ASGP-1. Mono-sialylated oligosaccharitol, isolated as in Fig. 5, was hydrolyzed with 0.05 N sulfuric acid at 80°C for 1 hr to release sialic acid. The products were fractionated by HPLC to separate the neutral core from sialic acid.

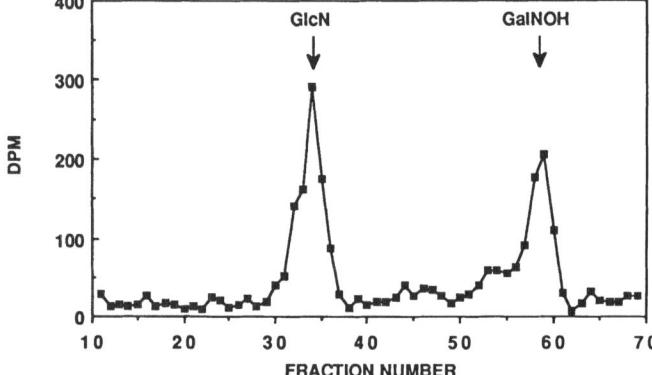

Fig. 7. Analysis of label in glucosamine and galactosamine from mono-sialylated tetrasaccharide oligosaccharitol of cell surface ASGP-1. Mono-sialylated oligosaccharitol was hydrolyzed in 4 N HCl at 105°C for 6 hr to release all monosaccharides, and glucosamine and galactosaminitol were separated by HPLC.

These results indicate that sialylated as well as neutral oligosaccharides are being completely synthesized in the late compartment of the ascites 13762 cells. Interestingly, these studies show glucosamine label appearing in galactosamine, but not sialic acid, in the cell surface ASGP-1 oligosaccharides. This observation is not due to a failure to label the sialic acid pool, because a chase of 60 min results in the appearance of label in the sialic acid. The simplest explanation is that the sialo-oligosaccharides are being synthesized and their glycoprotein molecules transported to the cell surface faster than the glucosamine is able to equilibrate with the CMP-sialic acid pool in the late compartment.

CONCLUSIONS

The results of our studies can best be explained by the model presented in Fig. 8. ASGP-1 is synthesized in the endoplasmic reticulum and glycosylated on a fraction of its serine and threonine residues. In a rate-determining step, the ASGP-1 is transferred to the Golgi, where it undergoes rapid and extensive glycosylation and transfers through a series of three compartments, each of which adds one or two sugars. The final transit in these rapid transfers is into the <u>trans</u>-Golgi network (TGN), in which the nascent oligosaccharides are rapidly sialylated. The final rate-determining step is the transfer to the plasma membrane. While the glycoprotein is residing in the last compartment before this transfer, it is additionally glycosylated by "filling in" the unoccupied glycosylation sites and elongating and terminating the monosaccharides produced. This slow process constitutes the final maturation step in the biosynthesis and may even involve recycling between the cell surface and the late biosynthesis compartment.

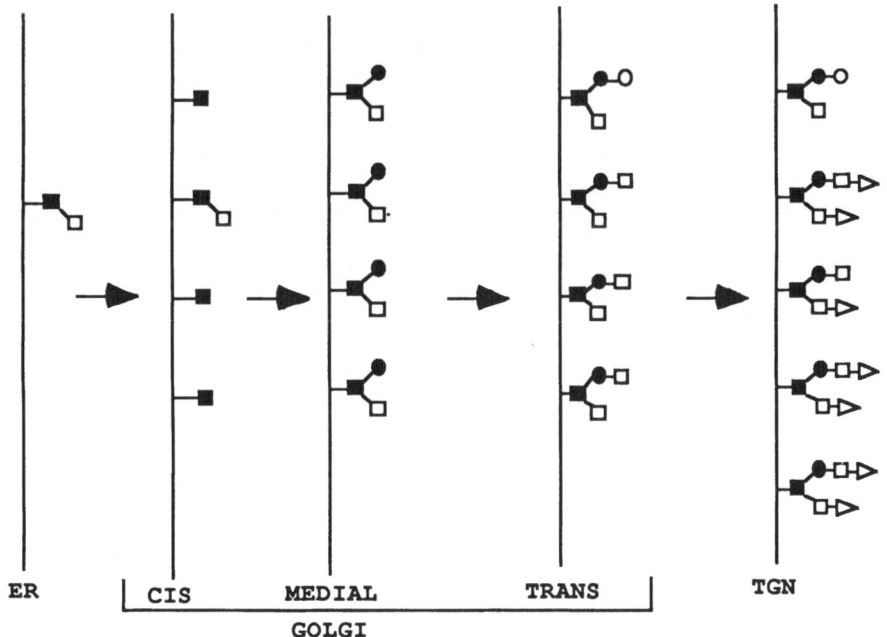

Fig. 8. Proposed model for ASGP-1 biosynthesis. GalNAc, [■]; GlcNAc, [●]; Gal, [□]; sialic acid, [▷]; sulfate, [○]. TGN, <u>Trans</u>-Golgi network.

ACKNOWLEDGMENTS

This work was supported by National Institutes of Health Grant CA 31695 and the Papanicolaou Comprehensive Cancer Center of the University of Miami (National Institutes of Health Grant CA 14395).

REFERENCES

Carraway, K. L. and Hull, S. R., 1989, O-Glycosylation pathway for mucin-type glycoproteins, BioEssays, in press.

Carraway, K. L., and Spielman, J., 1986, Structural and functional aspects of tumor cell sialomucins, Molec. Cell. Biochem., 72:109-120.

Ceriani, R. L., Peterson, J. A., Lee, J. Y., Moncada, R., and Blank, E. W., 1983, Characterization of cell surface antigens of human mammary epithelial cells with monoclonal antibodies prepared against human milk fat globule, Somatic Cell Genetics, 9:415-427.

Codington, J. F., 1981, Masking of cancer cell surface antigens, Handbook of Cancer Immunol., 8:171-203.

Helm, R. M., and Carraway, K.L., 1981, Evidence for the association of two cell surface glycoproteins of 13762 mammary ascites tumor cells, Exp. Cell Res., 135:418-424.

Hull, S. R., and Carraway, K. L., 1988, Mechanism of expression of Thomsen-Friedenreich (T) antigen at the cell surface of a mammary adenocarcinoma, FASEB J., 2:2380-2384.

Hull, S. R., and Carraway, K. L., 1989, Sulfation of the tumor cell surface sialomucin of the 13762 rat mammary adenocarcinoma, J. Cell. Biochem., in press.

Kufe, D., Inghirami, G., Abe, M., Hayes, D., Justi-Wheeler, H., and Schlom, J., 1984, Differential reactivity of a novel monoclonal antibody (DF3) with human malignant versus benign breast tumors, Hybridoma, 3:223-232.

Lan, M. S., Finn, O. J., Fernstein, P. D., and Metzgar, R.S., 1985, Isolation and properties of a human pancreatic adenocarcinoma-associated antigen, Cancer Res., 45: 305-310.

Lodish, H. F., 1988, Transport of secretory and membrane glycoproteins from the rough endoplasmic reticulum to the Golgi. A rate-limiting step in protein maturation and secretion, J. Biol. Chem., 263:2107-2110.

Schlom, J., 1986, Basic principles and applications of monoclonal antibodies in the management of carcinomas, Cancer Res., 46:3235-3238.

Sherblom, A. P., Buck, R. L., and Carraway, K.L., 1980, Purification of the major sialoglycoproteins of 13762 MAT-B1 and MAT-C1 rat mammary adenocarcinoma cells by density gradient centrifugation in cesium chloride and guanidine hydrochloride, J. Biol. Chem., 255:783-790.

Spielman, J., Rockley, N. L., and Carraway, K. L., 1987, Temporal aspects of O-glycosylation and cell surface expression of ascites sialoglycoprotein-1, the major cell surface sialomucin of 13762 mammary ascites tumor cells, J. Biol. Chem., 262:269-275.

Spielman, J., Hull, S. R., Sheng, Z., Kanterman, R., Bright, A., and Carraway, K. L., 1988, Biosynthesis of a tumor cell surface sialomucin. Maturation and effects of monensin, J. Biol. Chem., 263:9621-9629.

Springer, G. F., 1984, T and Tn, general carcinoma autoantigens, Science, 224:1198-1206.

Steck, P. A., and Nicolson, G. L., 1983, Cell surface glycoproteins of 13762NF mammary adenocarcinoma clones of differing metastatic potentials, Exp. Cell Res., 147:255-267.

Tartakoff, A. M., 1983, Perturbation of vesicular traffic with the carboxylic ionophore monensin, Cell, 32:1026-1028.

Taylor-Papadimitriou, J., Peterson, J. A., Arklie, J., Burchell, J., Ceriani, R. L., and Bodmer, W.F., 1981, Monoclonal antibodies to epithelial-specific components of the human milk globule membrane: Production and reaction with cells in culture, Int. J. Cancer, 28:17-21.

EPITHELIAL MUCIN ANTIBODIES AND THEIR EPITOPES: CORE PROTEIN EPITOPES

OF A POLYMORPHIC EPITHELIAL MUCIN (PEM)

Joyce Taylor-Papadimitriou, Joy Burchell, Sandra Gendler,
Martina Boshell and Trevor Duhig

Imperial Cancer Research Fund
P O Box 123
Lincoln's Inn Fields
London WC2A 3PX, U.K.

INTRODUCTION

Largely because of their complexity, the detailed structure of the
mucins has been difficult to analyze. This group of compounds is
categorized mainly by the fact that they contain a high level of
carbohydrate which is attached in O-linkage to serine and/or threonine via
the linkage sugar N-acetylgalactosamine. The mucous secretions produced by
some epithelial cells, particularly those lining the gastro-intestinal
tract and the lungs, contain mucins along with other products and these
components have been studied for some time at the biochemical level.
However, other glandular epithelial cells, such as the salivary gland,
breast, ovary, endometrium, and sweat glands, also produce mucins, and some
of these simpler mucins have recently received much attention. This is
because many antibodies selected for epithelial or tumor specificity have
been found to react with high molecular weight glycoproteins which are
produced by simple epithelial cells and have the properties of mucins.[1-9]

Analysis of the primary structure of mucins from various animal
species suggests that there is great variety in the structure of the carbohydrate side chains which may be composed of only one type of disaccharide,
as in ovine submaxillary mucin, or may be complex, containing several
sugars and branched chains as in most gastric mucins. However, the same
sugars are used to build up the side chains and similar epitopes may be
present on more than one mucin and even on other glycoproteins or
glycolipids. When an antibody reacts with several epithelial tissues and

carcinomas or with more than one component on Western blots, it is
therefore possible that glycoproteins with different core proteins but
similar oligosaccharide side chains are being detected.

Little is known about the detailed structure of the core protein of
mucins, and how variable these are within the same animal species. To
differentiate between mucins with different core proteins, it is necessary
to work with antibodies directed to the core proteins and, where these are
heavily glycosylated, with the deglycosylated material. Moreover, to
determine how many different genes there are within a species which code
for mucin core proteins, it is necessary to obtain some biochemical or
sequence data to define the protein(s), or to do this indirectly via gene
cloning. We have recently obtained such data for a human mucin which is
expressed by several simple epithelial cell types and abundantly by the
lactating mammary gland and by many carcinomas. This mucin, which we have
called the PEM mucin (polymorphic epithelial mucin) because of the high
degree of polymorphism seen at the DNA and protein level,[1,10,11] is highly
immunogenic and many antibodies raised against normal and malignant
epithelial cells or their membranes are directed to it. Interestingly,
core protein epitopes can be exposed in the mucin expressed by carcinomas,
which are masked in the normal mucin, suggesting that differences in
glycosylation occur in the normal and malignant cells.[2] Because the amino
acid sequence of the immunogenic region of the core protein is now known,[12]
it has been possible to map these epitopes in some detail, thus opening up
the possibility of a directed approach to the production of tumour specific
antibodies.

THE PEM MUCIN CORE PROTEIN

The component we refer to as the PEM mucin was originally purified by
Shimizu and Yamauchi and characterized by them as having the properties of
a mucin.[13] Antibodies to this component have been raised by several groups
(for review see ref. 14) using a variety of immunogens and accordingly it
has been given different names (epitectin,[15] PASO,[13] NPGP,[8] MAM6,[5] EMA[16]).
While it may seem to add to the confusion by giving it yet another name, a
salient feature, namely its polymorphism is implied from the new
nomenclature. As other mucins become characterized, it will be important

to agree on a general nomenclature which should take into account features of the mucin and not only the name of the tissue of origin.

Gendler et al. obtained partial cDNA clones coding for an immunogenic domain of the PEM mucin[10] and found it to be composed of 60bp tandem repeats coding for a 20 amino acid repeating unit.[12] The sequence contains potential glycosylation sites, and is shown in Figure 1. The polymorphism in the mucin which was originally noted at the protein level[1,11] has now

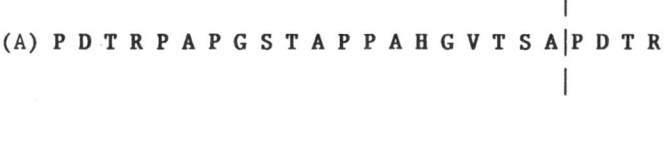

(A) P D T R P A P G S T A P P A H G V T S A|P D T R

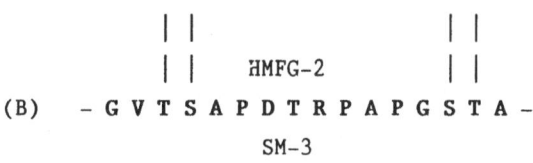

(B) – G V T S A P D T R P A P G S T A –

SM-3

Fig. 1. Sequence of tandem repeat element found in the PEM mucin (A) 24 amino acid peptide PDTR used to demonstrate binding of antibodies HMFG-1, HMFG-2 and SM-3. The last 4 amino acids are the first 4 of the next repeat unit. (B) Position of epitopes recognised by SM-3 and HMFG-2, between potential glycosylation sites.

been shown to be at the DNA level[10,12,17] and is due at least in part to the presence of differing numbers of tandem repeats.[12] The polymorphism in the gene coding for the PEM mucin is proving to be an extremely useful feature in analyzing changes which occur around this locus in cancer. The gene has been mapped to chromosome 1 in the region of 21q.[18] There are several reports of chromosomal breaks in this region observed in metaphase spreads of cells from breast cancers and eight oncogenes have been localized on this chromosome.[19-21] Preliminary results indicate that greater than 30% of informative breast tumors show an alteration at the PEM locus when DNA made from breast carcinomas is compared with constitutional DNA from the same patient (S. Gendler, personal communication). It is therefore important to extend the examination of this region, particularly in view of the repetitive sequences contained in the gene which could lead to an increase in recombination events.

GENERAL FEATURES OF MUCINS

The cDNA clones coding for the PEM mucin were selected from a λgt11 expression library made from MCF-7 mRNA[22] using antibodies directed to epitopes on the core protein.[2,10] Using a similar strategy and antibody DF3[4] Siddiqui and colleagues have also isolated partial cDNA clones of the PEM mucin and the 60bp repeat sequence has been confirmed.[23] Interestingly the sequence of the core protein of the porcine submaxillary mucin has recently been defined by Timpte et al.[24] and found to be composed of tandem repeats consisting of 81 amino acids. Also preliminary data suggest that the human colonic mucin also contains a domain made up of tandem repeats containing a high proportion of threonines (Kim, Y., pers. commun.).

Much of the work which has been done in the past on attempting to define the structure of mucins has been done using mucins isolated from mucus and has been concerned mainly with colonic, cervical, lung or ovarian cyst mucins. A model has been proposed for the structure of these mucins where heavily glycosylated domains are separated by stretches of naked peptide containing cysteines.[25-27] The PEM mucin and the submaxillary mucins contain low amounts of sulphur containing amino acids and would not fit such a model. Indeed the domain of the core protein of the PEM mucin which contains the tandem repeats appears to be glycosylated, but core protein epitopes are exposed between oligosaccharide side chains[12] (see Figure 1). The possibility however that mucin subunits are linked together by cysteine rich link proteins[25] cannot be excluded.

There are several examples of genes, many in lower organisms, coding for extracellular or surface antigens, which have a large domain in the coding sequence made up of tandem repeats (see Table 1). Some of these proteins, like the mucin described here, may be required to resist degradation, and the repetitive structure may lead to such a function even if the amino acid sequences are quite different. In the fibroin, Plasmodium and glue protein genes, allelic variations in length have also been described suggesting that the actual number of tandem repeats may not be critical for function. Of great interest is the observation that the repetitive elements in the exposed mucin core protein, like the repetitive region in Plasmodium circumsporozoite protein, form an immunogenic domain of the molecule.[32]   In thinking of the function of the mucin core protein to act as a scaffold for oligosaccharide attachment, a repetitive amino acid sequence should lead to a repetitive final structure, which in turn could lead to strong associations in oligomerization. Most mucins are found as aggregates and it may be that the property of self association is related to the ability to form many similar, possibly weak, attachments. If this is so we might expect to find that a repetitive structure is a key feature of most mucin core proteins, even though the individual sequences may show great divergence.

Table 1. Proteins with Tandem Repeats

Protein	Comments
Drosophila Glue Protein[28]	21bp repeat
Silk Fibroin[29]	Different organization of repeat units within the gene
DIF Induced Protein of Dictyostelium[30]	Extracellular structural protein (cysteine rich)
Circumsporozite Protein of Plasmodium[31]	Tandem repeat domain very immunogenic[32]
Involucrin[33]	Produced by differentiated keratinocytes

ANTIBODIES REACTIVE WITH CORE PROTEIN EPITOPES OF THE PEM MUCIN

The coding strand of the 60bp tandem repeat was established using synthetic oligonucleotides, deduced from each strand of the DNA, to probe Northern blots of MCF-7 total RNA.[12] There were two possible open reading frames and the correct one, shown in Figure 1, was determined by showing a positive reaction of three mucin-reactive antibodies (HMFG-1, HMFG-2, SM-3) with a synthetic peptide with sequence predicted from the nucleotide sequence. In this peptide the first four amino acids are repeated at the end to avoid missing an epitope, and it is referred to as the PDTR peptide.

The three monoclonal antibodies mentioned above were used to select the cDNA clones from the MCF-7 cDNA library and their spectrum of reactivity is indicated in Table 2. Two of these antibodies, HMFG-1 and -2 were developed and characterized several years ago[1,34] using the immunogens shown in the Table 2 and were, surprisingly, found to react with the deglycosylated mucin.[2,10] The third antibody, SM-3, was developed more recently against the deglycosylated component and shows a marked selectivity in its reaction with breast and other carcinomas.[2] All three antibodies were found to react with the β-galactosidase cDNA encoded fusion proteins produced by all of the clones including the smallest which contained only 73bp.[10]

Table 2. Reactivity of Antibodies Used to Select cDNA
Clones Coding for PEM

Antibody	Immunogen	Reactivity
HMFG-1 (1,34)	Extract of human milk fat globule (HMFG)	Reacts well with fully glycosylated mucin (FGM) in lactating gland. Less strong reaction with deglycosylated mucin (DGM) and breast cancers
HMFG-2 (1,34)	HMFG and cultured milk epithelial cells	Reacts strongly with DGM and breast cancers. Positive reaction but fewer epitopes on FGM
SM-3 (2)	Deglycosylated milk mucin	Reacts strongly with breast cancers and DGM. No reaction with FGM in lactating gland

The positive reactions of antibodies HMFG-1, HMFG-2 and SM-3 with the PDTR peptide were demonstrated using a solid phase ELISA assay and the specificity of the reaction was established by showing that the peptide competed effectively with the deglycosylated milk mucin for binding to the antibodies.[12] A range of antibodies developed in other laboratories were tested for their reaction with the PDTR peptide and several showed positive reactions including antibodies DF3,[4] M8[6] and Ca2.[9]

The amino acid sequence and composition of the repeat unit exhibit features which would be expected for the core protein of a mucin. There are five potential 0 glycosylation sites represented by serines and threonines separated by proline-rich stretches of 3,5 and 7 amino acids (see Figure 1A). The prolines would keep the molecule extended, so that even in the glycosylated molecule some epitopes on the core protein could be exposed, and these could be different depending on the pattern of glycosylation. The amino acid sequence suggests a linear structure with minimal conformation, and we have therefore attempted to identify more precisely the reactive epitopes by testing the reaction of the antibodies with overlapping octamers. The SM-3 and HMFG-2 epitopes are similar; both appear to contain a threonine, but the SM-3 epitope requires more amino acids around this for reactivity than does the HMFG-2. The antibody HMFG-1 did not react positively with any of the octamers, but does react with a truncated peptide missing the first three amino acids of the peptide shown in Figure 1A.

GLYCOSYLATION OF THE PEM MUCIN BY THE NORMAL MAMMARY GLAND AND BY BREAST CANCER

Since the first antibodies to the PEM mucin were developed, it became clear that the profile of epitopes expressed on the mucin produced by the normal mammary gland at lactation was different from the profile of epitopes expressed on the cancer associated mucin.[1] The enhanced tumour specificity of the antibody SM-3 directed to the deglycosylated PEM,[2] indicates that epitopes of the core protein which are normally masked can be exposed in the cancer associated mucin. This suggests that at least some of the differences between the normally processed mucin and the mucin expressed in breast cancers are due to differences in glycosylation patterns. The exposure of core protein epitopes in the cancer mucin could be due to underglycosylation of potential glycosylation sites, or to a reduction in the length of the added oligosaccharide side chains. The mapping of the SM-3 and HMFG-2 epitopes to amino acids around a threonine residue in the tandem repeat sequence (Figure 1B), indicates that this is probably unglycosylated in the cancer associated mucin. The presence of the HMFG-2 epitope (albeit in lower numbers)[1] on the normally processed mucin suggests however, that at least some of these sites are also not glycosylated in the normally processed mucin. Indirect evidence for shorter oligosaccharide side chains on the cancer-associated mucin is provided by the observation that the SM-3 epitope which is only exposed in this form of the mucin, contains extra amino acids flanking the HMFG-2 epitope, some of which are apparently masked in the normally processed component. Direct evidence from the analysis of oligosaccharide side chains on the various mucins is now becoming available to support the idea that the oligosaccharide side chains on cancer associated mucins are shorter than those on the normal component. Hanisch and colleagues[35] have analyzed in detail some of the oligosaccharides of a mucin isolated from milk. Analysis of the total sugars in this component shows it to be somewhat different to the PAS-0 component first studied by Shimizu and Yamauchi although both are clearly mucin glycoproteins (see Table 3). Although sialic acid is present in the mucin isolated by Hanisch,[35] only the neutral oligosaccharide side chains were analyzed in detail. These were found to contain between 4 and 14 sugars, and made up of polylactosamine chains containing an unusual β(1-6) linkage; some of the longer chains are branched. At least some of the mucin molecules analyzed by Hanisch et al. carry epitopes recognized by antibodies HMFG-1 and 2 (Burchell, J., Taylor-Papadimitriou, J., Hanisch, F.G. MS in preparation).

Table 3. Sugar Composition of Mucin Isolated from Human Milk

Sugar	Hanisch et al.[35] µg/mg	Shimizu & Yamauchi[13] µg/ml
Fucose	93.2	70
Mannose	Trace	–
Galactose	350.2	380
GalNAc	51.0	159
GlcNAc	146.5	210
NeuAc	35.5	169

These extended side chains may be compared to the very short sugar chains found in the DF-3 reactive component produced by BT20 cells,[37] which consist of Galβ1-3GalNAc or the mono or disialylated derivaties of the disaccharide.

Further evidence for the presence of short oligosaccharide side chains on cancer-associated mucins comes from work with the antibody B72.3 which has recently been reported to be directed towards sialosyl-Tn(NeuAcα2→6GalNAcα1→OSer or Thr).[39] This is the disaccharide found on ovine submaxillary mucin and in fact this mucin has been used to immunize mice to produce monoclonal antibodies reacting with sialylated Tn.[39] These antibodies together with B72.3 show considerable tumour specificity. Preferential staining of tumours with antibodies or lectins directed to the Tn antigen itself has also been reported.[40,41]

Thus it appears that the oligosaccharide side chains on cancer associated mucins may be terminated early, in some cases due to premature sialylation, with the effect of unmasking core protein epitopes and introducing new carbohydrate epitopes, many of which contain sialic acid.[39,42-44] Antibodies to these epitopes will then show a high degree of specificity in their reaction with tumour tissue. In this context it is interesting to note that antibody OC125, which is widely used in monitoring ovarian cancer[45] is also directed to a large glycoprotein and appears to be directed to a sialic acid containing epitope.[36]

Evidence that changes in the sialylation pattern are occurring in the tumour associated PEM also comes from the reactivity of the monoclonal antibody M18.[6] M18, which recognises an oligosaccharide determinant, reacts strongly with PEM produced by normal breast epithelium but shows very little staining on breast carcinomas. However when the sections are treated with neuraminadase, 86% of breast carcinomas stain although no change is observed in the lactating breast.[46] Thus sialic acid masks the M18 epitope in PEM produced by carcinomas but not in the normal PEM.

APPLICATIONS OF ANTIBODIES TO THE PEM MUCIN

Monoclonal antibodies to the PEM mucin have been used for some time in in vitro and in vivo tumour diagnosis and to a limited extent have been tested in tumour therapy (for review see Ref. 14). Now that the molecular basis for a differential reaction with the tumour associated mucin is being elucidated, the development, characterization and application of these antibodies should be possible in a more directed way. The tumour specific core protein epitopes typified by that recognized by antibody SM-3 can be defined at the peptide level, and consequently it should be possible to develop a range of antibodies of different classes and affinities to such an epitope. These antibodies should be useful in histological diagnosis, in in vivo diagnosis and, because of their very limited reaction with normal tissues, possibly in therapy based on drug or toxin targeting. Our investigations to date however of the SM-3 antibody in serum diagnostic tests suggest that the epitope may be found on the circulating mucin found in some normal subjects (4-6%) as well as in the majority of breast and ovarian cancer patients. This suggests that oligosaccharide side chains of the mucin shed by normal tissues may be degraded to some extent before appearing in serum (in fact the molecular weight of the serum component appears to be slightly lower than the corresponding tissue mucin). It may be therefore that antibodies to the new carbohydrate epitopes appearing on the cancer associated mucin will play an important role in effective tumour specific detection of the mucin in serum. Interestingly, the Ca15.3 test uses a core protein antibody and an antibody directed to a non-selective carbohydrate epitope for mucin detection. Also, antibodies to sialyated oligosaccharide epitopes on mucins other than the PEM mucin have been used in serum diagnostic tests.[44,45,47]

In view of the immunogenic nature of the repeat domains of the mucins and of the fact that some of the newly expressed epitopes on the cancer associated mucins may be considered non-self, one further application of anti-mucin antibodies which must now be considered is their possible use in active immunisation against cancers.

REFERENCES

1. J. Burchell, H. Durbin and J. Taylor-Papadimitriou, Complexity of expression of antigenic determinants recognised by monoclonal antibodies HMFG-1 and HMFG-2, in normal and malignant human mammary epithelial cells, J. Immunol. 131:508 (1983).
2. J. Burchell, S. Gendler, J. Taylor-Papadimitriou, A. Girling, A. Lewis, R. Millis and D. Lamport, Development and characterization of breast cancer reactive monoclonal antibodies directed to the core protein of the human milk mucin, Cancer Res. 47:5476 (1987).

3. A. B. Griffiths, J. Burchell, J. Taylor-Papadimitriou, S. Gendler, A. Lewis, K. Blight and R. Tilly, Immunological analysis of mucin molecules expressed by normal and malignant mammary epithelial cells, Int. J. Cancer 40:319 (1987).
4. H. Sekine, T. Ohno and D. Kufe, Purification and characterization of a high molecular weight glycoprotein detectable in human milk and breast carcinomas, J. Immunol. 135:3610 (1985).
5. J. Hilkens, F. Buijs, J. Hilgers, P. Hagemann, J. Calafat, A. Sonnenberg, and M. Van der Valk, Monoclonal antibodies against human milk fat globule membranes detecting differentiation antigens of the mammary gland and its tumour, Int. J. Cancer 34:197 (1984).
6. C. Foster, P.A. Edwards, E.A. Dinsdale and A.M. Neville, Monoclonal antibodies to the human mammary gland. I. Distribution of determinants in non-neoplastic mammary and extra mammary tissues, Virchows Arch. (Path. Anat.) 394:279 (1982).
7. M. Price, S. Edwards, A. Owainati, J.E. Bullock, B. Ferry, R.A. Robins and R.W. Baldwin, Multiple epitopes on a human breast carcinoma associated antigen, Int. J. Cancer 36:567 (1985).
8. R. L. Ceriani, J. A. Peterson, J. Y. Lee, R. Moncada and E. W. Blank, Characterisation of cell surface antigens of human mammary epithelial cells with monoclonal antibodies prepared against human milk fat globule, Som. Cell Genet. 9:415 (1983).
9. M.E. Bramwell, V.P. Bhavanandan, G. Wiseman, and H. Harris, Structure and function of the Ca antigen, Br. J. Cancer 48:177 (1983).
10. S. J. Gendler, J. M Burchell, T. Duhig, D. Lamport, R. White, M. Parker and J. Taylor-Papadimitriou, Cloning of partial cDNA encoding differentiation and tumor-associated mucin glycoproteins expressed by human mammary epithelium, Proc. Natl. Acad. Sci. USA. 84:6060 (1987).
11. B. Griffiths, A. Gordon, J. Burchell, M. Bramwell, A. Griffiths, M. Price, J. Taylor-Papadimitriou, D. Zanin, and D.M. Swallow, The breast tumour-associated epithelial mucins and the peanut lectin binding urinary mucins are coded by a single highly polymorhpic gene locus 'PUM', Dis. Markers 6:185 (1988).
12. S. Gendler, J. Taylor-Papadimitriou, T. Duhig, J. Rothbard, and J. Burchell, A highly immunogenic region of a human polymorphic epithelial mucin expressed by carcinomas is made up of tandem repeats, J. Biol. Chem. 263:12820 (1988).
13. M. Shimizu and K. Yamauchi, Isolation and characterisation of mucin-like glycoproteins in human milk fat globule membranes. J. Biochem. 91:515 (1982).
14. J. Burchell, and J. Taylor-Papadimitriou, Antibodies to human milk fat globule molecules, Cancer Invest. (in press).
15. S.A. Bader and H. Harris, Regulation of epitectin production in a malignant cell line, J. Cell Sci. 87:375 (1987).
16. E. Heyderman, K. Steele, and M.G. Ormerod, A new antigen on the epithelial membrane: Its immunoperoxidase localization in normal and neoplastic tissues, J. Clin. Pathol. 32:35 (1979).
17. D.M. Swallow, S. Gendler, B. Griffiths, G. Corney, J. Taylor-Papadimitriou, and M.E. Bramwell, The human tumour-associated epithelial mucins are coded by an expressed hypervariable gene locus PUM, Nature 328:82 (1987).
18. D. Swallow, S. Gendler, B. Griffiths, A. Kearney, S. Povey, D. Sheer, R. Palmer and J. Taylor-Papadimitriou, The hypervariable gene locus PUM, which codes for the tumour associated epithelial mucins, is located on chromosome 1, within the region 1q21-24, Ann. Hum. Genet. 51:289 (1987).

19. J.M. Trent, Cytogenetic and molecular biologic alterations in human breast cancer: a review, Breast Can. Res. & Treatment 5:221 (1985).

20. N.B. Atkins, Chromosome 1 aberrations in cancer, Cancer Genet. Cytogenet. 21:279 (1986).

21. E. Gebhart, S. Bruderlein, M. Augustus, E. Siebert, J. Feldner, and W. Schmidt, Cytogenetic studies on human breast carcinomas. Br. J. Cancer Res. & Treatment 8:125 (1986).

22. P. Walter, S. Green, G., Greene, A. Krust, J.-M. Bornert, J.-M. Heltsch, A. Staub, E. Jensen, G. Scrace, M. Waterfield and P. Chambon, Cloning of the human estrogen receptor cDNA. Proc. Natl. Acad. Sci. USA. 82:7889 (1985).

23. J. Siddiqui, M. Abe, D. Hayes, E. Shani, E. Yunis, and D. Kufe, Isolation and sequencing of a cDNA coding for the human DF3 breast carcinoma-associated antigen, Proc. Natl. Acad. Sci. USA. 85:2320 (1988).

24. C.S. Timpte, A.E. Eckhardt, J.L. Abernethy, and R.L. Hill, Porcine submaxillary gland apomucin contains tandemly repeated, identical sequences of 81 residues, J. Biol. Chem. 263:1081 (1988).

25. A. Wesley, M. Mantle, D. Man, R. Quereshi, G. Forstner and J. Forstner, Neutral and acidic species of human intestinal mucin, J. Biol. Chem. 260:7955 (1985).

26. J.R. Clamp, A. Allen, R.A. Gibbons and G.P. Roberts, Chemical aspects of mucins, Br. Med. Bull. 34:25 (1978).

27. R.L. Shogrun, A.M. Jamieson, J. Blackwell and N. Jentoft, The thermal depolymerisation of porcine submaxillary mucin, J. Biol. Chem. 259:14657, 1984.

28. M.A.T. Muskavitch, and D.S. Hogness, An expandable gene that encodes a drosophila glue protein is not expressed in variants lacking remote upstream sequences, Cell 29:1041 (1982).

29. R.F. Manning and I.P. Gage, Internal structure of the silk fibroin gene of bombyx mori. II. Remarkable polymorphism of the organization of crystalline and amorphous coding sequences. J. Biol. Chem. 255:9451 (1980).

30. J.G. Williams, A. Ceccarelli, S. McRobbie, H. Mahbubani, R.R. Kay, A. Early, M. Berks, and K.A. Jermyn, Direct induction of dictyostelium prestalk gene expression by DIF provides evidence that DIF is a morphogen, Cell 49:185 (1987).

31. L.S Ozaki, P. Svec, R.S. Nussenzweig, V. Nussenzweig, and G.N. Godson, Structure of the plasmodium knowlesi gene coding for the circumsporozoite protein, Cell 39:815 (1983).

32. G.N. Godson, J. Ellis, P. Svec, D.H. Schlesinger, and V. Nussenzweig, Identification and chemical synthesis of a tandemly repeated immuogenic region of Plasmodium knowlesi circumsporozoite protein. Nature 305:29 (1983).

33. R.L. Eckert, and H. Green, Structure and evolution of the human involucrin gene, Cell 46:583 (1986).

34. J. Taylor-Papadimitriou, J.A. Peterson, J. Arklie, J. Burchell, R.L. Ceriani, and W.F. Bodmer, Monoclonal antibodies to epithelium-specific components of the human milk fat globule membrane: production and reaction with cells in culture, Int. J. Cancer 28:17 (1981).

35. F.-G. Hanisch, G. Uhlenbruck, J. Peter-Katalinic, H. Egge, J. Dabrowski, and U. Dabrowski, Structures of neutral O-linked polylactosaminoglycans on human skim milk mucins, J. Biol. Chem. (in press).

36. F.-G. Hanisch, G. Uhlenbruck, C. Dienst, M. Stottrop and E. Hippauf, Ca125 and Ca19-9: two cancer-associated sialylsaccharide antigens on a mucus glycoprotein from human milk, Eur. J. Biochem. 149:323 (1985).

37. S.R. Hull, A. Bright, K.L. Carraway, M. Abe, and D. Kufe, Oligosaccharides of the DF-3 antigen of the BT20 human breast carcinoma cell line, J. Cell. Biochem. Suppl. 12E:130 (1988).

38. D. Colcher, P. Horan Hand, M. Nuti and J. Schlom, Production of monoclonal antibodies reactive with human mammary carcinomas, Proc. Natl. Acad. Sci. USA. 78:3199 (1981).

39. T. Kjeldsen, H. Clausen, S. Hirohashi, T. Ogawa, H. Iijima and S. Hakomori, Preparation and characterization of monoclonal antibodies directed to the tumour associated O-linked sialosyl-2→6α-N-acetylgalactosaminyl (Sialosyl-Tn) epitope, Cancer Res. 48:2214 (1988).

40. H.K. Takahashi, R. Metoki and S. Hakomori, Immunoglobulin G3 monoclonal antibody directed to Tn antigen (tumor-associated α-N-acetylgalactosaminyl epitope) that does not cross-react with blood group A antigen, Cancer Res. 48:4361 (1988).

41. A.J. Leathem and S.A. Brooks, Predictive value of lectin binding on breast-cancer recurrence and survival, The Lancet May 9:1054 (1987).

42. A. Kurosaka, S. Fukui, H. Kitagawa, H. Nakada, Y. Numata, I. Funakoshi, T. Kawasaki and I. Yamashina, Mucin-carbohydrate directed monoclonal antibody, FEBS Lett. 215:137 (1987).

43. J. Magnani, B. Nilsson, M. Brockhaus, D. Zopf, Z. Steplewski, H. Koprowski and V. Ginsburg, A monoclonal antibody-defined antigen associated with gastrointestinal cancer is a ganglioside containing sialylated lacto-N-fucopentaose II, J. Biol. Chem. 257:14365 (1982).

44. D. Chia, P.I. Terasaki, N. Suyama, J. Galton, M. Hirota and S. Katz, Use of monoclonal antibodies to sialylated Lewis[x] and sialylated Lewis[a] for serological tests of cancer, Cancer Res. 45:435 (1985).

45. R.C. Bast Jr., T.L. Klug, E. St. John, E. Jenison, J.M. Niloff, H. Lazarus, R.S. Berkowitz, T. Leavitt, C.T. Griffiths, L. parker, V.R. Zurawski and R.C. Knapp, A radioimmunoassay using a monoclonal antibody to monitor the course of epithelial ovarian cancer, N. Eng. J. Med. 309:883 (1983).

46. C. Foster, and A.M. Neville, Monoclonal antibodies to the human mammary gland. III. Monoclonal antibody LICR-LON-M18 identifies impaired expression and excess sialylation of the 1(Ma) cell surface antigen by primary breast carcinoma cells, Hum. Pathol. 15:82 (1984).

47. J.L. Magnani, Z. Steplewski, H. Koprowski and V. Ginsburg, Identification of the gastrointestinal and pancreatic cancer-associated antigen detected by monoclonal antibody 19.9 in the sera of patients as a mucin, Cancer Res. 43:5489 (1983).

CELL HETEROGENEITY AND COMPLEXITY OF BREAST EPITHELIAL SURFACE ANTIGENS EXPRESSION AND MOAB THERAPY

Jerry A. Peterson, Edward Blank, Cindy Zoellner, Sean Enloe, Garrett Walkup and Roberto L. Ceriani

John Muir Cancer and Aging Research Institute, 2055 North Broadway, Walnut Creek, CA 94596

INTRODUCTION

The advent of monoclonal antibodies has opened a new area of breast cancer therapy, and because of unique aspects compared to conventional therapy new approaches have to be defined, and new problems addressed. Monoclonal antibodies have to be selected specifically for therapy, ideal characteristics have to be defined, conjugates must be selected, conjugation methods must be evaluated, and appropriate target antigens have to be identified. One aspect of the latter that must be taken into consideration is the complexity and cell heterogeneity in expression of most antigens that have an appropriate tissue or tumor cell specificity for therapy. This paper will address the question of antigenic heterogeneity in approaching the use of monoclonal antibodies for therapy of breast cancer.

Because of the difficulty of obtaining truly tumor specific antibodies, in fact there is a question that truly tumor specific antigens really exist, our approach has been to select monoclonal antibodies against normal breast epithelial cells that either have a tissue or cell-type specificity (1). Normal breast epithelial antigens, although they are expressed on normal gland are present on most breast tumors and their metastases and are often expressed at greater levels in breast tumors, both from the fact that the tumor has an enormous epithelial component compared to the normal gland and also are often present in higher concentrations even at a single-cell level.

In this paper we will address the methods by which we will evaluate both the monoclonal antibodies and target antigens considering the complexity and heterogeneity of antigenic expression in breast tumors. With regard to the monoclonal antibodies, those will be selected that have the greatest specificity for breast carcinomas and are most prevalent both on an individual cell basis in individual tumors and are expressed in most breast carcinomas in different breast cancer patients. With regard to antigenic heterogeneity there are two basic levels of heterogeneity, (1) heterogeneity among patients, and cell-to-cell heterogeneity among the tumor cells of any given tumor. Since each patient may have unique characteristics, the tumor of each patient should be examined with regard to the percentage positive cells and the level of antigen expression. We have shown already that the level of expression of the antigens under study is different in different patients (2). Also, the percentage of positive cells differs among patients. Furthermore, we have previously shown that the tumors of some patients are more variable than others, expressed as rate of phenotypic variability (2).

In order to establish criteria for evaluating results of therapy, effectiveness of treatment, and why some patients respond and others do not, we have conducted preclinical studies to evaluate quantitatively the antigen expression in tumors using flow cytometry. We hope that if we know the characteristics of the tumor antigen expression that are associated with better response to therapy, we will be better able to select patients for therapy.

RESULTS AND DISCUSSION

The MoAbs that we have selected for the preclinical studies and for the first clinical trials in patients are all prepared against delipidated human milk fat globule membranes (HMFG) and were selected for specificity for breast epithelial cells (3). Five monoclonal antibodies will be discussed, Mc3, Mc8, Mc5, BrE1, and BrE2. Mc3 and Mc8 which have been described previously (3), react with a 46K glycoprotein, while Mc1, Mc5, BrE1 and BrE2 identify a large molecular weight mucin-like glycoprotein complex, which when prepared from HMFG has an apparent molecular weight of approximately 400K (3). The two monoclonal antibodies against the 46K antigen stain normal breast and breast carcinomas in a weak diffuse manner histologically, but do not stain any other normal tissues nor tumors. Mc5 and BrE2 stain almost 100% of breast carcinomas examined, and also stain normal breast tissue on the apical region of the epithelial component. Each stain selected areas of a few other normal tissue besides breast, which include lung, kidney, pancreas, sweat gland, and some epithelial tumors of non-breast origin. The rationale for using them for therapy is that the amount of antigen in breast tumors is vastly greater than in normal tissues, due both the greater epithelial component of the tumor compared to normal breast and other tissue, and that the single cell content in tumor cells is often much greater than in normal. Also, a similar MoAb (Mc1, i.e., HMFG2) labeled with I-131 has been injected into patients without significant toxicity (4). The MoAb BrE1 binds strongly to breast tumors but does not bind normal breast tissue, in spite of the fact that it was prepared using normal breast epithelial membranes, namely HMFG membranes. The only normal tissues it binds are lung and kidney.

Each of the three MoAbs against the breast mucin complex binds a different epitope as shown by competition studies. Moreover, they also bind to the polypeptide portion of this highly glycosylated glycoprotein. This latter is demonstrated unequivically by the fact that they all bind to fusion proteins we have synthesized in bacteria using lambda gt11 clones containing cDNA inserts we have selected from a lambda gt11 library of MCF7 breast carcinoma cells. The library has been screened with each of the above-mentioned MoAbs and cDNA clones have been selected that bind to each. For example, the clone NP4-3 was found to produce a fusion protein that was bound strongly by BrE2, but not by the other MoAbs against the breast mucin complex, such as Mc1, Mc5 or BrE1, nor to Mc3 or Mc8 against the 46K glycoprotein (Table 1). Since Mc1 (also called HMFG-2) does not bind this fusion protein, NP4-3 is a cDNA clone either for a different polypeptide or a different region of the same polypeptide of the breast mucin that was cloned by others (5). A single band of approximately 120,000 molecular weight was stained in a western blot of the Y1089 lysate of NP4-3 with BrE2.

Table 1. Radioimmunobinding analysis of fusion proteins from the λ phage clone NP4-3 with MoAb against breast epithelial mucin (Mc1, Mc5, BrE1, BrE2) and 46K glycoprotein (Mc3, Mc8).

	cpm bound[a]	
Monoclonal Antibody	NP4-3 lysate	λgt11 lysate
Mc1 (>400K)[b]	851	827
Mc5 (>400K)	535	663
BrE1 (>400K)	742	
BrE2 (>400K)	5,403	610
Mc3 (46K)	373	433
Mc8 (46K)	729	1,718

[a] Bacterial lysates were prepared from E. culi strain λ1089 infected with either λNP4-3 clone or λgt11, as a control, and bound to wells of microtiter plates. Specific binding was determined by incubations with the different MoAbs followed by ^{125}I-labeled goat anti-mouse Ig.

[b] Numbers in parentheses indicates the molecular weight of the antigens identified by the different MoAbs.

At this point I would like to bring up the subject of so-called tumor associate antigens. I feel that this term is a misnomer and its use stems from wishful thinking on our part that there are unique characteristic of tumors. Tumor specific antigens have been searched for decades and except for viral antigens, have usually turned out to be normal antigens expressed in an aberrant manner, in some cases giving rise to the term oncofetal antigens. This misconception is exemplified by our MoAb BrE1, which was prepared using normal HMFG membranes as the immunogen, which are in fact derived from the plasma membrane of the breast epithelial cell (1). If one tested only breast epithelial cells it could be termed breast tumor specific since it binds breast tumors but does not bind to normal breast. On the other hand, it binds normal lung epithelial cells and lung tumors. I feel that a more appropriate term could be something like frequently-occurring tumor-associated phenotypic alterations.

In initial experiments to establish quantitative methods using the flow cytometer to assess antigen content in different breast tumors and evaluate the heterogeneity of antigen expression, we have examined a number of breast carcinoma cell lines for the expression of the large molecular weight breast mucin complex using the three different MoAbs discussed above, Mc5, BrE1, and BrE2. Since in breast carcinoma cells this antigen is expressed sometimes both on the cell surface and in the cytoplasm, we stained both live cells and cells fixed in 70% ethanol using fluoresceinated MoAbs. The staining of the live cells represents surface staining and the fixed cells the total antigen content per cell. The cells were run on an EPICS 753 flow cytometer. Histograms were analyzed using the IMMUNO program on the EASY 88 system, using fluoresceinated nonspecific IgG1 as a control. Data was collected both on a logrithmic and linear mode. The former allowed better separation and evaluation of the entire population of stained cells, permitting the comparison of relative antigen content and percentage of positive cells. The latter allowed calculation of the coefficient of variation on the positive staining population which gives a quantitative estimate of the heterogeneity of the antigen expression at the single cell level.

From the analysis of a dozen different breast carcinoma cell lines, it became apparent that the epitope identified by the MoAb Mc5 was most often expressed on the cell surface, while the epitopes identified by BrE1 and BrE2 was more often found in the cytoplasm. For example, as shown in Figure 1 for two different cell lines, MDA-MB-331 and SKBR3, almost all the MDA-MB-331 cells (98%) stained on the cell surface with Mc5, this represented most of the epitope since there was only a slight increase in percentage positive and average intensity of staining when fixed cells are stained for total antigen. In contrast, the epitopes identified by BrE1 and BrE2 are primarily in the cytoplasm (Figure 1). SKBR3 cells stained less intensely with all 3 MoAbs, but the same general pattern was maintained although it had a larger proportion of cytoplasmic

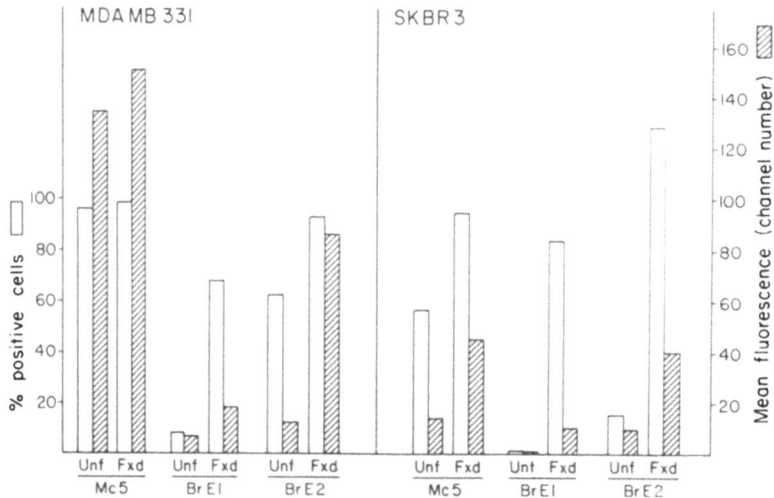

Fig. 1. Flow cytometry analysis of surface and total antigen content in two breast carcinoma cell lines with MoAbs against different epitopes of a breast mucin-like glycoprotein. Staining of unfixed cells (Unf) represents surface antigen and of fixed cells (fxd) represents total antigen content (surface and cytoplasm).

staining with Mc5. The relative surface-cytoplasmic distribution of the epitopes for the different breast carcinoma cell lines was maintained when these tumors are grown as transplanted tumors in nude mice as shown in Figures 2 and 3, for Mc5 and BrE2, respectively, where the IMMUNO program analysis of the flow cytometric histograms are presented. There appears to be somewhat more antigen expressed in the cultured cells than in the tumors, however this may be due to the different ways in which the cells are prepared for analysis. The cell from tumors are mechanically dispersed while the cultured cells are removed from the culture vessels with trypsin and then grown suspended in methyl cellulose culture medium for 48 hours before analysis (6).

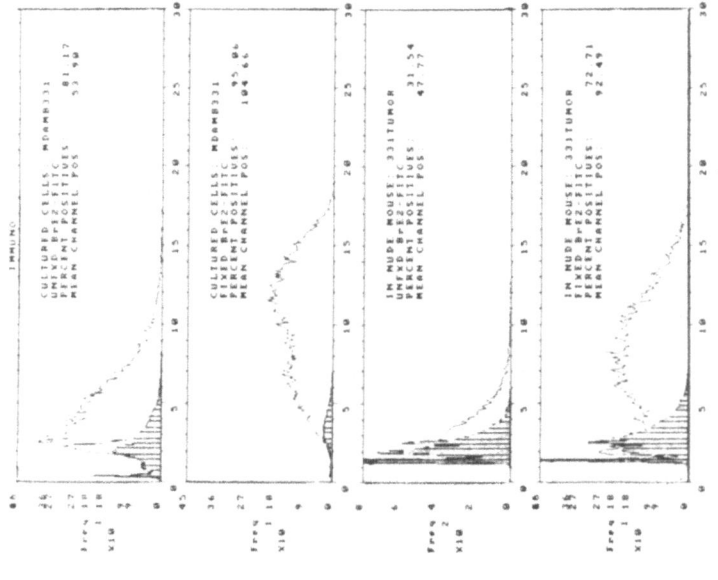
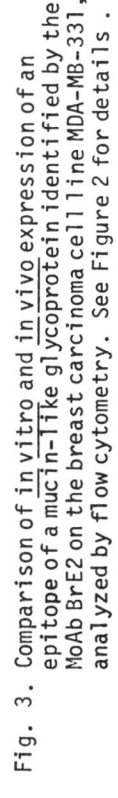

Fig. 2. Comparison of in vitro and in vivo expression of an epitope of mucin-like glycoprotein identified by the MoAb Mc5 on the breast carcinoma cell line MDA-MB-331, analyzed by flow cytometry. Staining of unfixed cells (unfxd) represents surface staining profile and of fixed cells represent total antigen content. Shaded histogram represents cells stained with a nonspecific fluoresceinated IgG_1 used as a control.

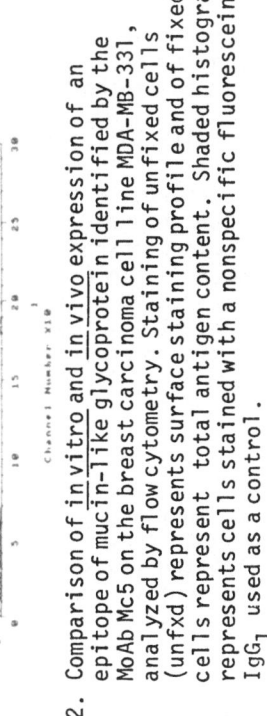

Fig. 3. Comparison of in vitro and in vivo expression of an epitope of a mucin-like glycoprotein identified by the MoAb BrE2 on the breast carcinoma cell line MDA-MB-331, analyzed by flow cytometry. See Figure 2 for details .

With regard to quantitative differences among the cell lines, there is as much as a 20 fold variation among the different breast cell lines with regard to the mean antigen content. The single cell heterogeneity within each cell line is also enormous, being as much as 100 fold. In fact, each cell line has a unique distribution of the different epitopes of the large molecular weight mucin. Furthermore, the relative antigen content determined by flow cytometry correlates with the intensity of staining seen when sections of the different tumors are stained histologically using immunoperoxidase methods (data not shown).

The structure of the breast mucin complex has not been yet determined in detail, nor has its method of synthesis in the cell been elucidated. However, there is speculation that the detection of this antigen in the cytoplasm of tumor cells compared to the exclusive surface location in normal cells, suggests that some breast tumor cells may be deficient in the processing of this molecule. The difference among the MoAbs described here may indicate that they are identifying molecular species of the mucin at different stages of maturation. If this is the case, they will provide useful tools for isolating molecules in different stages of maturation and help elucidate these stages and characterizing the alterations that are occurring in the tumor cells. The fact that each tumor has a unique profile of staining with these three MoAbs, demonstrates the heterogeneity of the breast tumors and that different tumor may have a different altered expression of the enzymes that are responsible for the processing of this molecule.

Quantitative analysis with flow cytometry, such as the above, of tumor target antigen content and cell heterogeneity for patients considered for MoAb therapy will be useful in the clinical trials to evaluate the relationship between antigen content and heterogeneity and response to therapy and in future selection of patients and predicting response. Since there is a correlation between flow cytometry antigen profile and immunohistochemical analysis, in the cases where there is not enough tumor tissue for flow cytometry these studies can permit a more rational means to obtain a prediction of response from immunohistochemistry which will always be available with every patient.

With regard to MoAb therapy and target antigen content and heterogeneity, we have demonstrated, in previous studies, that when nude mice carrying transplanted breast tumor MX1 are treated with a cocktail of unconjugated MoAbs (Mc1, Mc5, Mc3, and Mc8) there was an inhibition of growth compared with similar tumor-bearing mice treated with nonspecific immunoglobin (7). When the antigen content of the tumor that did grow in the treated mice, albeit, at a reduced rate, were compared to the control mice, it was found that there was a greatly diminished level of antigen in the treated tumors compared to the control tumors. This indicates that there can be a selection of antigen deficient tumor cells as a result of the treatment.

Since we have found that radiolabeled MoAbs are much more effective at killing established breast tumors in nude mice (7), we felt it would be important to quantitate the effect of this latter treatment on the antigen content in the tumor cells that survive the treatment. This is important to know, since we have also shown in the nude mouse system that consecutive treatments with ^{131}I-labeled MoAbs is more effective in reducing the growth rate of transplanted tumors and controlling it for a longer period of time, than a single injection (7). In a series of experiments with nude mice transplanted with MX1 breast tumors, we have compared quantitatively the total antigen content by flow cytometry in tumors of treated and untreated mice. Since there may be considerable variation between different mice, we did a series of experiments where a large group of mice were transplanted with fragments of tumor taken from a single mouse. Some were treated and some were not. For the flow cytometric analysis, tumors from two mice from each group were prepared, stained, and analyzed the same day using the same batch of fluorescent MoAbs. Contrary to the studies with treatment with the unconjugated MoAbs, in the tumors from the mice treated with a single dose of ^{131}I-labeled MoAbs there was never a reduction in antigen content. Four separate experiments are presented in Figure 4. Surprisingly, in some mice there was an actual and significant increase in mean antigen content as a result of the treatment. In other experiments, the increase in antigen content was more than two fold, and in addition, there appears to be a change in the single cell distribution of the antigen in the tumor cell population and in the coefficient of variation (Figure 5). The significance of the latter result is that it would permit sequential treatments with radiolabeled MoAbs.

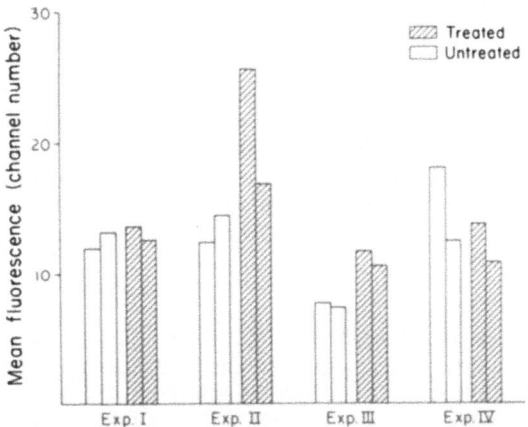

Fig. 4. Effect of ^{131}I-labeled MoAb therapy on target antigen content in breast carcinomas (MX-1) in nude mice, analyzed by flow cytometry. In each experiment tumors from 2 treated and 2 untreated nude mice were analyzed and mean total antigen content determined within the positive cell population by the IMMUNO program of EASY88 program for the EPICS flow cytometer. Mice were treated with a cocktail of MoAbs Mc1, Mc3, Mc5, and Mc8.

At the moment we can only speculate on the mechanism of this increase in antigen content as a result of in vivo treatment with radiolabeled MoAbs. It must be considered that the killing effect of the radiolabeled MoAb is not necessarily related to the level of antigen content of the individual cells, since the range of the isotope is great enough to kill surrounding cells. Also, the antibody can bind to the halo of antigen that most likely surrounds the tumor mass and still kill. Since the radiation would primarily kill cells that are more rapidly growing and synthesizing DNA, there could be a selection of the slower growing

cells. In fact, repeatedly we have found that the tumors that eventually
grow in the treated mice are slower growing when compared to untreated
control mice (8).

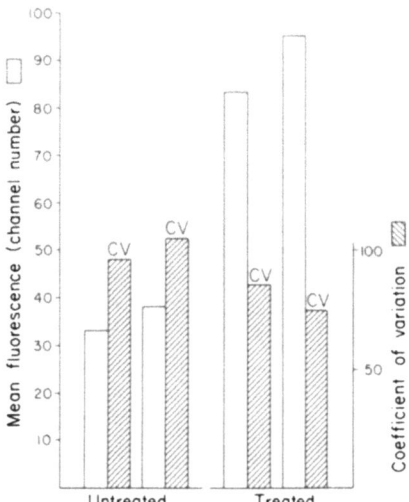

Fig. 5. Therapy with ^{131}I-labeled MoAbs of breast carcinomas
(MX-1) transplanted in nude mice results in a
significant increase in target antigen content and a
decrease in coefficient of variation. Tumors stained
with fluoresceinated MoAb Mc5 were analyzed by flow
cytometry.

An important aspect of MoAb therapy that can be evaluated with flow
cytometry is the relationship between the level and distribution of
target antigen content and the effectiveness of therapy. In the case of
the MX1 tumor in nude mice, a considerable percentage of the antigen is
expressed in the cytoplasm and the radiolabeled MoAb therapy is still
effective. It will be possible to obtain minimal levels of tumor antigen
that are necessary for effective therapy, and therefore be able to
include patients that may otherwise be excluded from therapy. Also,
these studies exemplify the uniqueness of each tumor and justifies the
careful evaluation of each patient being considered for therapy.

ACKNOWLEDGEMENTS

This work is supported by NIH Grants CA39936, 39932, 42767, and BRSG
RR05929.

REFERENCES

1. R. L. Ceriani, K. E. Thompson, J. A. Peterson and S. Abraham, Surface
    differentiation antigens of human mammary epithelial cells
    carried on the human milk fat globule. Proc. Natl. Acad. Sci.
    USA 74:582-586 (1977).
2. R. L. Ceriani, J. A. Peterson and E. W. Blank, Variability in surface
    antigen expression of human breast epithelial cells cultured
    from normal breast, normal tissue peripheral to breast
    carcinoma, and breast carcinomas. Cancer Res. 44:3033-3039
    (1984).

3. R. L. Ceriani, J. A. Peterson, J. Y. Lee, R. Moncada and E. W. Blank, Characterization of cell surface antigens of human mammary epithelial cells with monoclonal antibodies prepared against human milk fat globule. Somat. Cell Genetics 9:415-427 (1983).

4. H. P. Kalofonos and A. A. Epenetos, Antibody guided diagnosis and therapy of patients with breast cancer, in: "Immunological Approaches to the Diagnosis and Therapy of Breast Cancer," R. L. Ceriani, ed., Plenum Press, New York, p. 245-257 (1987).

5. S. J. Gendler, J. M. Burchell, T. Duhig, D. Lamport, R. White, M. Parker and J. Taylor-Papadimitriou, Cloning of partial cDNA enciding differentiation and tumor-associated mucin glycoproteins expressed by human mammary epithelium, Proc. Natl. Acad. Sci. USA 84:6060-6064 (1987).

6. J. A. Peterson, J. C. Bartholomew, M. Stampfer and R. L. Ceriani, Analysis of expression of human mammary epithelial antigens in normal and malignant breast cells at the single cell level by flow cytofluorimetry, Exp. Cell Biol. 49:1-14 (1981).

7. R. L. Ceriani, E. W. Blank and J. A. Peterson, Experimental immunotherapy of human breast carcinomas implanted in nude mice with a mixture of monoclonal antibodies against human milk fat globule components, Cancer Res. 47:532-540 (1987).

8. R. L. Ceriani and E. W. Blank, Experimental therapy of human breast tumors with ^{131}I-labeled monoclonal antibodies prepared against the human milk fat globule, Cancer Res. 48:4664-4672 (1988).

THE ONCOGENIC POTENTIAL OF MEMBRANE RECEPTOR PROTEINS

ENCODED BY MEMBERS OF THE HUMAN erbB PROTO-ONCOGENE FAMILY

Matthias H. Kraus

Laboratory of Cellular and Molecular Biology
National Cancer Institute
Bethesda, Maryland

INTRODUCTION

Investigations of genetic alterations associated with neoplasia have identified a limited set of cellular genes, termed proto-oncogenes, which are highly conserved in vertebrate evolution. Acute transforming retroviruses have substituted viral genes essential for replication with these discrete segments of host genetic information. When incorporated within the retroviral genome, such transduced sequences acquire the ability to induce neoplastic transformation (1,2). Analysis of products of viral oncogenes has revealed important insights concerning the physiological roles of their normal cellular counterparts, designated proto-oncogenes. In particular, recent evidence has established a direct link between oncogene products and growth factor receptors. The v-*erbB* oncogene was identified as a structurally altered version of the epidermal growth factor (EGF) receptor (3), while v-*fms* shares homology with colony stimulating factor-1 (CSF-1) receptor (4).

More recently, we and others have identified a second human homologue of v-*erbB*, designated *erbB*-2, whose coding sequence encompasses structural features of a tyrosine kinase receptor with close homology to the EGF receptor protein (5-8). An important consequence of these findings has been the ability to test with specific model systems the role of altered growth factor receptor expression in the neoplastic process. We have investigated the transforming properties of the EGF receptor and *erbB*-2 in vitro and have identified aberrations of these genes associated with naturally occurring malignancies, in particular human mammary neoplasia. Our findings have implications concerning the conditions under which the altered expression of growth factor receptor molecules of the *erbB* proto-oncogene family may exert a role in tumor initiation or progression.

RESULTS

Identification of a novel EGF receptor-related gene, erbB-2, amplified in a human mammary adenocarcinoma

As an approach to identify activated oncogenes which encode receptor-related proteins, we subjected DNAs of mammary tumor tissues and cell lines to Southern blot analysis utilizing v-erbB as a probe (5). In an effort to identify genes that might be candidates for new receptor coding sequences of this gene family, we employed hybridization conditions of moderate stringency under which protooncogenes related to other viral oncogenes of the tyrosine kinase family did not hybridize (data not shown). Thus, any gene detected might be expected to have a closer relationship to v-erbB than to other members of the tyrosine kinase family. DNA prepared from a human mammary carcinoma, MAC117, showed a pattern of hybridization differing both from that observed with DNA of normal human placenta and the A431 squamous-cell carcinoma line. In A431 DNA, we observed four EcoR I fragments that had increased signal intensities compared to those of corresponding fragments in placenta DNA. In contrast, MAC117 DNA contained a 6-kilobase pair (kbp) fragment, which appeared to be amplified compared to corresponding fragments observed in both A431 and placenta DNAs. These findings were consistent with the possibility that the MAC117 tumor contained an amplified DNA sequence related to, but distinct from the EGF receptor (5).

To define its structure, we undertook the molecular cloning of the 6-kbp EcoRI fragment and we determined its nucleotide sequence in the region most homologous to v-erbB. This sequence contained two regions of nucleotide sequence homology to v-erbB separated by 122 nucleotides. By comparison of the predicted amino acid sequence of the clones designated pMAC117 with corresponding sequences of several members of the tyrosine kinase family, the most striking homology of 85% was observed with the human EGF receptor and v-erbB (5).

The availability of cloned probes of the gene made it possible to investigate its expression in a variety of cell types. The probe detected a single 5-kb transcript in A431 cells (5). Under the stringent conditions of hybridization utilized, this probe did not detect any of the three RNA species recognized by EGF receptor complementary DNA. Thus, the gene, designated erbB-2, represented a new functional gene within the tyrosine kinase family, closely related to, but distinct from the gene encoding the EGF receptor (5). The complete coding structure of erbB-2 was determined by isolation of the entire coding sequence as complementary DNA to the mRNA (8,9,10). The predicted amino acid sequence identified overall structural homology to the EGF receptor protein including a cysteine-rich extracellular domain, a transmembrane region, and a highly conserved tyrosine kinase domain.

Mechanisms activating receptor-like proto-oncogenes of the erbB gene family in human mammary neoplasia

The initial identification of erbB-2 gene amplification in tissue from a primary mammary adenocarcinoma suggested the possibility that erbB-2 overexpression might contribute to neoplastic growth in this tumor type (5). To assess the role of erbB-2 in human mammary neoplasia, we compared mRNAs of 16 mammary tumor cell lines to normal human fibroblasts, M413, and a human mammary epithelial derived cell line, HBL100 (10). Increased expression of an apparently normal size 5 kb transcript was detected in 8 of 16 tumor cell lines, when total cellular RNA was subjected to Northern blot analysis (data not shown). An aberrantly sized erbB-2 mRNA was not detected in any of the cell lines analyzed. The amount of erbB-2 transcript in the 8 cell lines overexpressing erbB-2 was measured by dot blot analysis (Table 1).

To investigate alterations of the *erb*B-2 gene associated with its overexpression, we examined the gene locus by Southern blot analysis in these same cell lines (10). The normal restriction pattern was detected in all DNA samples tested, indicating that gross rearrangements in the proximity of the *erb*B-2 coding region had not occurred. When compared with normal human DNA, the *erb*B-2 specific restriction fragments appeared amplified in several cell lines including SK-BR-3, BT474, and MDA-MB361. Quantitation of *erb*B-2 gene copy number was accomplished using DNA dot blot analysis. These studies revealed a 4 to 8 fold *erb*B-2 gene amplification in SK-BR-3 and BT474 relative to diploid human DNA and a 2 to 4 fold *erb*B-2 gene amplification in the MDA-MB453 and MDA-MB361 cell lines. Thus, gene amplification was associated with overexpression in the four cell lines with the highest levels of *erb*B-2 mRNA (Table 1). In contrast gene amplification could not be detected by Southern blot analysis or DNA dot blot analysis in four tumor cell lines in which the *erb*B-2 transcript was increased to intermediate levels (10).

Table 1. Gene amplification and overexpression of EGF-R or *erb*B-2 in mammary tumor cell lines

| | EGF-R | | *erb*B-2 | |
	gene copies[a]	mRNA[b]	gene copies	mRNA
M413	2	1	2	1
HBL100	2	1	2	1
MCF-7	2	<1	2	1
BT20	8-16	16	2	1
MDA-MB468	64	32	-	1
SK-BR-3	2	1	8-16	128
BT474	2	1	8-16	128
MDA-MB361	2	1	4-8	64
MDA-MB453	2	<1	4	64
ZR-75-1	2	1	2	8
ZR-75-30	2	<1	<2	4
MDA-MB175	2	<1	2	8
BT483	2	<1	<2	8

[a] gene copy number in comparison to normal diploid DNA
[b] mRNA level relative to HBL100 and normal fibroblasts

In chemically induced rat neuroblastomas, a point mutation within the transmembrane region activates *neu* (11), the rat homologue of *erb*B-2, to acquire transforming activity in the NIH3T3 transfection assay. We have reported a lack of transforming activity of a large group of human mammary tumors and tumor cell lines in this assay (10,12). These included those which exhibited *erb*B-2 gene amplification and/or overexpression in the absence of aberrant transcript sizes. Thus, our studies suggested that a structurally normal *erb*B-2 coding sequence was overexpressed in these mammary tumor cell lines.

We also analyzed total cellular RNA of the same mammary tumor cell lines for evidence of EGF receptor mRNA overexpression. Increased amounts of apparently normal size EGF receptor mRNA were observed in BT20 and MDA-MB468 (10). These two cell lines have been shown to contain amplified EGF receptor genes. EGF receptor transcripts were elevated 16-fold in BT20 and 32-fold in MDA-MB468 above the level seen in normal human fibroblasts as determined by RNA dot-blot analysis (Table 1).

EGF receptor or erbB-2 overexpression detected at all tumor stages of mammary cancer is maintained during tumor progression in vivo

Our findings in mammary tumor cell lines are paralleled by similar observations using primary mammary tumors (Table 2) (13). Among 57 mammary tumor patients analyzed we detected erbB-2 gene amplification with high levels of protein product, comparable to the level detected in SK-BR-3 in 11 tumors (19%). In contrast, EGF receptor gene amplification with overexpression of its encoded protein was observed in 2 tumors (4%). In addition, 14 of 53 (26%) mammary tumor patients exhibited moderately increased erbB-2 protein levels in the absence of gene amplification. Similar alterations resulting in overexpression of the EGF receptor without detectable gene amplification were associated with 2 (4%) mammary tumors among 47 patients analyzed (13).

Table 2. Overexpression of EGF-receptor and erbB-2 at different stages of mammary cancer

	CLINICAL STAGE				TOTAL
	I	II	III	IV	(% POSITIVE)
EGF-R overexpression:					
a) with gene amplification	0/12[a]	1/23	1/7	0/15	2/57 (4%)
b) without gene amplification	0/8	1/22	0/5	1/12	2/47 (4%)
erbB-2 overexpression:					
a) with gene amplification	3/12	1/23	1/7	6/15	11/57 (19%)
b) without gene amplification	3/9	7/23	1/6	3/15	14/53 (26%)

[a] positive patients/patients analyzed

Increased expression of the erbB-2 protein, which occurred in a total of 47% of the mammary tumor patients analyzed, was detected in all tumor stages of mammary neoplasia. Overexpression of the EGF receptor was observed at lower frequency with 4 mammary tumors (9%) of stages II-IV exhibiting elevated protein levels among 47 patients analyzed. In 7 cases, it was possible to investigate such alterations in primary and metastatic lesions derived from the same patient. Two patients at stage II and 1 patient at stage III had moderately elevated erbB-2 expression levels in the absence of gene amplification. In 2 patients at stage IV, a high level of erbB-2 expression was associated with gene amplification. Similarly, the EGF receptor was overexpressed at intermediate levels in 1 patient at stage IV in the absence of gene amplification and at high level in 1 patient of stage II who harbored a 16 fold gene amplification of the EGF receptor. In these 7 patients, the levels of expression and gene copy numbers of erbB-2 or EGF receptor were found to be similar in the primary tumor and metastatic lesion of the same patient (13). Moreover, in one patient (#7) we detected EGF receptor overexpression without gene amplification at similar levels in the primary tumor and in 3 separate lymph node metastasis. Concordance of elevated membrane protein levels of erbB-2 or EGF receptor in matched primary and metastatic lesions combined with the observation that such alterations are detectable as early as stage I and II mammary tumors, indicate that membrane receptor overexpression can develop at a relatively early stage in the pathway of human mammary cancer and is maintained during tumor progression (13).

The erbB-2 gene is a potent oncogene when overexpressed in NIH/3T3 cells

To directly assess the effects of erbB-2 overexpression on cell growth properties, expression vectors based on the transcriptional initiation sequences of either the Moloney murine leukemia virus long terminal repeat (MLV-LTR) or the SV40 early promoter were constructed in an attempt to express the erbB-2 cDNA at different levels in NIH/3T3 cells (14). To assess the biologic activity of our human erbB-2 vectors, we transfected NIH/3T3 cells with serial dilutions of each DNA. As shown in Table 3, a LTR-based erbB-2 expression vector, LTR-1/erbB-2, induced

Table 3.   Transformed phenotype induced by overexpression of erbB-2

DNA[a]	Transforming activity (FFU/pmol)[b]	Colony-forming efficiency in agar (%)[c]	Cell number for 50% tumor incidence[d]
LTR-1/erbB-2	4.1×10^4	45	10^3
SV40/erbB-2	$< 10^0$	< 0.01	$> 10^6$
LTR/erbB	5.0×10^2	20	5×10^4
LTR/ras	3.6×10^4	35	10^3
pSV2/gpt	$< 10^0$	< 0.01	$> 10^6$

a   NIH3T3 cells transfected with 1 µg/plate were selected by their ability to grow in the presence of killer HAT medium.
b   Focus-forming units (FFU)/pmol of cloned DNA added
c   Cells were plated at 10-fold serial dilutions in 0.33% soft agar medium containing 10% calf serum. Visible colonies comprising >100 cells were scored after 14 days.
d   NFR nude mice were subcutaneously inoculated with each cell line. Ten mice were tested at cell concentrations ranging from 10^3 to 10^6 cells/mouse. Tumor formation was monitored twice weekly for up to 30 days.

transformed foci at high efficiencies of 4.1×10^4 focus-forming units per picomole of DNA (ffu/pmol). In striking contrast, the SV40/erbB-2 construct failed to induce any detectable morphological alteration of NIH/3T3 cells transfected under identical assay conditions (Table 3). Since the SV40/erbB-2 construct lacked transforming activity, these results demonstrated that the higher levels of erbB-2 expression under LTR influence correlated with its ability to exert transforming activity (14).

To compare the growth properties of NIH/3T3 cells transfected by these genes, we analyzed the transfectants for anchorage-independent growth in culture, a property of many transformed cells (15). The colony-forming efficiency of the LTR-1/erbB-2 transformant was very high and comparable to that of cells transformed by LTR-driven v-H-*ras* and v-*erbB* (Table 3). Moreover, the LTR/erbB-2 transfectants were as malignant *in vivo* as cells transformed by the highly potent v-H-*ras* oncogene and 50-fold more tumorigenic than cells transfected with v-*erbB*. In contrast, SV40/erbB-2 transfectants failed to display anchorage-independent growth *in vitro* and did not grow as tumors in nude mice even when 10^6 cells were injected (Table 3) (14).

While the predicted erbB-2 protein bears structural similarity to the EGF receptor, there is evidence that EGF is not the ligand for the erbB-2 product (16,17). In fact, the normal ligand for this receptor-like protein has yet to be identified. If

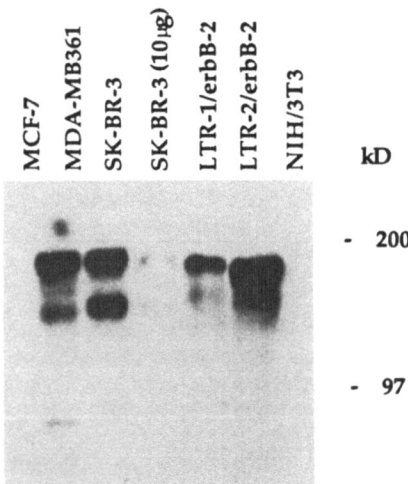

Fig.1.   Immunoblot analysis of erbB-2 proteins in
         LTR/erbB-2 transformed NIH3T3 cells and
         human mammary tumor cell lines

present in serum, this ligand might be responsible for stimulating the overexpressed erbB-2 product and triggering its transforming ability. To address this possibility, we investigated whether erbB-2 transformed cells maintained their altered phenotype when cultured in medium lacking serum (14). NIH/3T3 cells grow in a chemically defined medium which contains EGF, PDGF, or FGF, and high concentrations of insulin (W. Taylor, 0. Segatto, S.A. Aaronson, unpublished). These growth factors were excluded as possible exogenous ligands for the erbB-2 gene product (16,17). In medium lacking EGF, PDGF or FGF, LTR-1/erbB-2-transfected cells continued to exhibit a stable transformed phenotype by growing as foci of densely packed cells (14). These findings demonstrate that neither EGF nor any factors present in serum are required for maintaining the transformed phenotype of NIH/3T3 cells overexpressing erbB-2.

Human mammary tumors with amplified erbB-2 genes express the erbB-2 protein at high levels comparable to LTR/erbB-2 NIH/3T3 transformants

In order to assess the relevance of erbB-2 protein levels inducing *in vitro* transformation for erbB-2 overexpression in mammary neoplasia, we sought to compare the level of overexpression of the erbB-2-encoded 185 kd protein in human mammary tumor cell lines possessing amplified erbB-2 genes with that of NIH/3T3 cells transformed by the erbB-2 coding sequence (14). An anti-erbB-2 peptide serum detected several discrete protein species ranging in size from 150 to 185 kd in extracts of MDA-MB361 and SK-BR-3 mammary tumor cell lines, as well as LTR/erbB-2 NIH/3T3 transformants (Fig. 1). The relative levels of the 185-kd erbB-2 product were similar in each of the cell lines and markedly elevated over that expressed by MCF-7 cells, where the 185 kd erbB-2 protein was not detectable under these assay conditions. Thus, human mammary tumor cells which overexpressed the erbB-2 gene demonstrated levels of the erbB-2 gene product capable of inducing malignant transformation in a model system.

Overexpression of the EGF receptor confers a conditional growth advantage to NIH/3T3 cells

In an effort to comparatively assess whether overexpression of the normal EGF receptor could alter cell growth properties, we engineered an eukaryotic expression vector in which the EGF-R cDNA was put under the transcriptional control of the Mo-MLV LTR (18). This vector (LTR/EGF-R) was transfected onto NIH/3T3 cells which normally express a low number of functional EGF receptors (approximately 3×10^3 receptors per cell). As shown in Table 4, the LTR/EGF-R DNA construct failed to induce morphologically altered foci in NIH/3T3 cells in repeated experiments. In contrast, LTR/v-erbB, which encodes an oncogenically activated form of the avian EGF receptor (19) engineered in an identical expression vector, induced transformed foci with efficiencies of 3×10^2 focus-forming units per picomole of DNA (Table 4). We reasoned that if increased numbers of EGF receptors were to confer a selective growth advantage to NIH/3T3 cells, this advantage might be unmasked by the addition of EGF to the medium. Indeed, when the transfection assay was performed in medium supplemented with 20 ng/ml EGF, the same LTR/EGF-R construct displayed readily detectable transforming activity of around 2×10^2 focus-forming units per picomole of DNA (Table 4). The conditional nature of the transforming activity associated with LTR/EGF-R transfection strongly argues that the normal EGF-R gene was responsible for transforming activity observed in the presence of EGF. The specificity of the EGF effect was further demonstrated by the lack of a detectable increase in the transforming potential of the LTR/v-erbB DNAs upon EGF addition to the culture medium (Table 4) (18).

As an independent approach towards assessing the conditional nature of the growth alterations induced by the LTR/EGF-R construct, we investigated the ability of transfected NIH/3T3 cells to display anchorage-independent growth, a property known to correlate well with the malignant phenotype (15). Following transfection and marker selection, a mass population, designated NIH-EGF-R cells, was suspended in semisolid medium. In the absence of EGF supplement, the cells displayed only a low colony-forming ability of around 9.4%. However, upon addition of EGF to the agar medium, we observed a dramatic increase in colony formation (Table 4) with a shift towards large, progressively growing colonies (> 0.20 mm in diameter). The optimal EGF concentration for induction of this effect was 20 ng/ml (data not shown). In comparison, NIH/3T3 cells transfected with the v-*erbB* gene displayed a high clonogenic capability in semisolid medium that was not enhanced by EGF addition (Table 4) (18).

Table 4. Overexpression of the EGF receptor confers conditional growth advantage to NIH3T3 cells

DNA	Transforming activity[a] (FFU/pmol)		Growth in agar[b] (%)	
	- EGF	+ EGF	- EGF	+ EGF
LTR/EGF-R	< 10^0	2 x 10^2	0.4	19.7
LTR/v-*erbB*	3 x 10^2	3 x 10^2	12.7	15.4
pSV2/gpt	< 10^0	< 10^0	< 0.01	< 0.01

[a] 18 days after transfection using calcium phosphate precipitation EGF was added at 20ng/ml medium as indicated and focus formation was scored 8 days after EGF addition to duplicate plates. Specific transforming activity was assessed as focus-forming units (FFU) per pmol of cloned DNA added.

[b] Single cell suspensions were plated at 10-fold serial dilutions in 0.45% sea plaque agarose medium containing 10% calf serum. Colonies were scored at 14 days. The results represent the mean values of 3 independent experiments.

Human mammary tumor cells overexpress the EGF receptor at protein levels that confer conditional growth advantage to NIH/3T3 cells

The EGF receptor gene has been shown amplified and/or overexpressed in a wide array of human malignancies including mammary tumors and tumor cell lines (10,13,20-22). Hence, we sought to compare the levels of overexpression of the EGF-R protein in human tumor cell lines possessing amplified EGF-R genes with that of clonal NIH/3T3 cell lines containing the EGF-R coding sequence and exhibiting an EGF-dependent transformed phenotype (18). Human tumor cell lines, A431 and MDA-MB468, have been shown to exhibit EGF-R gene amplification (10,23-26) accompanied by overexpression of the EGF-R protein (26,27). By immunological analysis, the levels of the 170-kd EGF-R protein in A431 and MDA-MB468 cells were markedly elevated over that in M413 human embryo lung fibroblasts, which contain the unamplified EGF receptor gene. The elevated levels of EGF-R protein detected in the tumor lines were similar to that observed in NIH-EGF-R Cl A and Cl B cell lines, as detected both by immunoprecipitation of the EGF-R with a specific antibody and by a saturation binding assay of ^{125}I-EGF. Thus, human tumor cell lines that overexpressed the EGF-R gene demonstrated levels of EGF-R similar to those capable of conferring the EGF-dependent transformed phenotype in a model system (18).

IMPLICATIONS

Overexpression of membrane receptor-like molecules of the erbB proto-oncogene family is observed in the presence or absence of gene amplification in human mammary tumors at high frequency (10,13). Overall, 19 % of the patients exhibited erbB-2 gene amplification and 26 % showed erbB-2 overexpression in the absence of gene amplification. Samples with the highest levels of membrane protein consistently harbored erbB-2 gene amplification. Similar alterations were detected for the EGF receptor in mammary tumors, although at lower frequency. Gene amplification of erbB-2 with high protein expression as well as overexpression in the absence of gene amplification was detected in patients with stage I mammary cancer. In addition, in 7 patients with stage II-IV breast cancer the presence of identical alterations of the EGF receptor or erbB-2 in primary tumor and lymph node metastasis from the same patient suggests that erbB proto-oncogene alterations have likely developed prior to metastasis and were maintained in tumor progression. Supportive evidence derives from the observations that not a single discordant finding of overexpression registered among paired primary and metastatic lesions. Therefore, erbB-2 or EGF receptor alterations in human mammary neoplasia appear to be associated with the initiation of tumor growth or to act as growth-promoting factors at a relatively early tumor stage prior to metastasis. In none of the patients analyzed was expression of erbB-2 and EGF receptor altered simultaneously. Furthermore, no evidence for structural abnormalities of either protein product was obtained, indicating that a structurally normal coding sequence was overexpressed in mammary tumors (13).

The finding, that erbB-2 or EGF receptor levels are frequently elevated in human mammary tumors is paralleled by the in vitro observation, that the simple overexpression of an otherwise unaltered molecule, involved in the control of the normal cell proliferation, can lead to the acquisition of the malignant phenotype (14,18). We showed, in fact, that the human erbB-2 gene can be activated as an oncogene by its overexpression in NIH/3T3 cells (14). Thereby, the level of the erbB-2 product was shown to be critical in determining its transforming ability. An SV40-driven erbB-2 cDNA construct lacked detectable focus-forming ability despite the fact that NIH/3T3 cells containing this construct exhibited readily detectable levels of the erbB-2 protein. When the same erbB-2 cDNA was placed under LTR control, a further five-to ten-fold increase in expression of the erbB-2 product was associated with the acquisition of transforming properties by the gene. Similarly, introduction of an EGF-R expression vector, induced the appearance of a ligand-dependent transformed phenotype in NIH/3T3 cells (18).

Interesting differences emerged from the analysis of the transformed phenotypes induced by the EGF-R and the erbB-2 protein. In the former case, the overexpression of EGF-R was capable of inducing malignant transformation of NIH/3T3 cells only when the cells were grown in the presence of the physiological ligand (EGF) for the receptor (18). In the latter case, transformation seemed to be ligand-independent (14). In fact, transfected NIH/3T3 cells overexpressing the erbB-2 product were still capable of altered growth in chemically defined medium supplemented with EGF, FGF, and insulin, all of which have been excluded as exogenous ligands for this receptor-like protein. This raises intriguing questions about the mechanisms of transformation by these two related receptors.

We demonstrated increased ligand sensitivity for NIH/3T3 cells expressing high levels of EGF-R (18). Control NIH/3T3 cells showed a 4- to 5-fold increase in DNA synthesis upon EGF addition. However, NIH/3T3 clones that overexpressed

EGF receptors at levels 500- to 1000-fold over that of control cells demonstrated a markedly amplified response to EGF, exhibiting 80- to 100-fold increases in DNA synthesis. They also demonstrated responsiveness to the ligand at EGF concentrations which failed to stimulate control NIH/3T3 cells. Thus, our findings support the concept that EGF receptor overexpression amplifies normal EGF signal transduction. Since the ligand for the erbB-2 protein has yet to be identified, it is not possible to exclude that erbB-2 transformed cells, themselves, might produce the ligand for this receptor protein. Alternatively, an increased number of receptors may cause transformation either by raising the level of constitutive tyrosine kinase activity to a threshold required for growth stimulation or by facilitating receptor-receptor interactions that may be a prerequisite for their activation. We also demonstrated that EGF receptor gene overexpression was much less effective than overexpression of normal erbB-2 coding sequence in inducing the transformed phenotype. These findings support the hypothesis that the erbB-2 gene product is coupled to a distinct and more potent growth signaling pathway than the erbB/EGF receptor in NIH/3T3 cells. Investigation of recombinants between the EGF-receptor and erbB-2 coding sequences should make it possible to identify those regions that confer more potent transforming activity to the erbB-2 protein.

Accumulating evidence from in vivo observations and in vitro studies suggests that overexpression of growth factor receptor molecules of the erbB proto-oncogene family is linked to the pathway of certain human malignancies, including a high percentage of mammary tumors. In these tumors erbB-2 or EGF receptor overexpression is present relatively early in tumor development, while such alterations apparently are maintained during tumor progression (13). Other investigators have reported an inverse correlation of erbB-2 gene amplification and disease-free survival in breast cancer patients, suggesting a predictive nature of erbB-2 gene amplification for an aggressive disease course in human mammary neoplasia (28). Our laboratory has shown that erbB-2 or EGF receptor coding sequences, when overexpressed in NIH3T3 cells at protein levels comparable to those detected in mammary tumors with receptor gene amplification, are capable of conferring the transformed phenotype (10,13,14,18). Taken together, these observations implicate growth factor receptor gene amplification and overexpression in the development of human malignancies.

REFERENCES

1. J.M. Bishop, *Ann. Rev. Biochem.* **52**, 301 (1983).
2. R.A. Weiss, N. Teich, H. Varmus, J. Coffin, *Molecular biology of tumor viruses* (Cold Spring Harbor Laboratory, Cold Spring Harbor, New York, 1984).
3. J. Downward, Y. Yarden, E. Mayes, et al., *Nature* **307**, 521 (1984).
4. C.J. Sherr, C.W. Rettenmier, R. Sacca, M.F. Roussel, A.T. Look, E.R. Stanley, *Cell* **41**, 665 (1985).
5. C.R. King, M.H. Kraus, S.A. Aaronson, *Science* **229**, 974 (1985).
6. A.L. Schechter, M.C. Hung, L. Vaidyanathan, et al., *Science* **229**, 976 (1985).
7. K. Semba, N. Kamata, K. Toyoshima, T. Yamamoto, *Proc. Natl. Acad. Sci. USA.* **82**, 6497 (1985).
8. L. Coussens, T.L. Yang-Feng, Y.C. Liao, et al., *Science* **230**, 1132 (1985).
9. T. Yamamoto, S. Ikawa, T. Akiyama, et al., *Nature* **319**, 230 (1986).
10. M.H. Kraus, N.C. Popescu, S.C. Amsbaugh, C.R. King, *EMBO. J.* **6**, 605 (1987).
11. C.I. Bargmann, M.C. Hung, R.A. Weinberg, *Cell* **45**, 649 (1986).
12. M.H. Kraus, Y. Yuasa, S.A. Aaronson, *Proc. Natl. Acad. Sci. USA.* **81**, 5384 (1984).
13. H. Lacroix, J.D. Iglehart, M.A. Skinner, M.H. Kraus, *Oncogene* in press.
14. P.P. Di Fiore, J.H. Pierce, M.H. Kraus, O. Segatto, C.R. King, S.A. Aaronson, *Science* **237**, 178 (1987).

15. I. Macpherson, L. Montagnier, *J. Virol.* **23**, 291 (1964).
16. T. Akiyama, C. Sudo, H. Ogawara, K. Toyoshima, T. Yamamoto, *Science* **232**, 1644 (1986).
17. D.F. Stern, P.A. Heffernan, R.A. Weinberg, *Mol. Cell Biol.* **6**, 1729 (1986).
18. P.P. Di Fiore, J.H. Pierce, T.P. Fleming, et al., *Cell* **51**, 1063 (1987).
19. A. Gazit, J.H. Pierce, M.H. Kraus, P.P. Di Fiore, C.Y. Pennington, S.A. Aaronson, *J. Virol.* **60**, 19 (1986).
20. Y.H. Xu, N. Richert, S. Ito, G.T. Merlino, I. Pastan, *Proc. Natl. Acad. Sci. USA.* **81**, 7308 (1984).
21. T.A. Libermann, H.R. Nusbaum, N. Razon, et al., *Nature* **313**, 144 (1985).
22. C.R. King, M.H. Kraus, L.T. Williams, G.T. Merlino, I.H. Pastan, S.A. Aaronson, *Nucleic. Acids. Res.* **13**, 8477 (1985).
23. A. Ullrich, L. Coussens, J.S. Hayflick, et al., *Nature* **309**, 418 (1984).
24. G.T. Merlino, Y.H. Xu, S. Ishii, et al., *Science* **224**, 417 (1984).
25. C.R. Lin, W.S. Chen, W. Kruiger, et al., *Science* **224**, 843 (1984).
26. J. Filmus, M.N. Pollak, R. Cailleau, R.N. Buick, *Biochem. Biophys. Res. Commun.* **128**, 898 (1985).
27. M.M. Wrann, C.F. Fox, *J. Biol. Chem.* **254**, 8083 (1979).
28. D.J. Slamon, G.M. Clark, S.G. Wong, W.J. Levin, A. Ullrich, W.L. McGuire, *Science* **235**, 177 (1987).

SESSION III

ESTROGEN AND PROGESTERONE RECEPTOR ANALYSIS AND ACTION IN BREAST CANCER

Geoffrey L. Greene*, Paul Gilna* and Peter Kushner#

*The Ben May Institute, The University of Chicago, Chicago, Illinois 60637, and #Metabolic Research Unit, University of California San Francisco, California 94143

INTRODUCTION

The elucidation of the molecular mechanisms responsible for the hormonal regulation of cell proliferation in breast cancer has been the object of intense research. Because most breast cancers are initially dependent upon estrogens for continued growth, much of this research has focused on the role of estrogen receptor (ER) in the control of gene expression and mitosis[1], and on its use as marker for hormone responsiveness and prognosis.[2] In addition, progesterone receptor (PR), as both a mediator of hormonal responses and as a product of estrogen action on breast cancer cells, has been studied extensively as a tumor marker[3] and in terms of its regulation by estrogen agonists and antagonists[4]. Although its function in breast cancer is unknown, the presence as well as the induction of PR has been coupled to estrogen-induced proliferative responses in breast cancer cells. An improved understanding of the function and regulation of expression of these transcription factors is emerging from studies of the structure, composition and dynamics of the receptor proteins and the genes that encode them. The recent cloning and molecular analysis of all of the known steroid receptors has led to the definition of common functional domains and a proposed mechanism by which they interact with responsive genes, via cis-acting DNA enhancer elements, in normal and neoplastic tissues[5]. For ER and PR, these studies have been aided by the availability of a number of monoclonal antibody probes directed against specific regions of each receptor[6,7]. In addition, the same antibodies have been used to develop validated quantitative and histochemical immunoassays for ER and PR in a variety of hormone-responsive tissues and related cancers[8,9,10]. These assays have proved particularly useful in the evaluation of ER and PR in breast tumor extracts, in frozen and paraffin-embedded tumor sections, and in needle biopsies. The focus of this paper is on the current knowledge of ER and PR structure, composition and dynamics in breast cancer cells as a function of agonist and antagonist binding.

THE STEROID RECEPTOR FAMILY

The estrogen and progesterone receptors, like all of the steroid receptors, are members of a large family of trans-activating transcription factors that are activated by a ligand and bind with high affinity and specificity to short DNA enhancer elements called hormone response elements (HREs). Interaction of steroid-receptor complexes with responsive genes in vivo can result in either up or down regulation of transcription, depending upon the target gene and the tissue[5]. The molecular mechanisms by which either pathway occurs are still obscure, although it is generally believed that receptor-DNA complexes recruit, or allow the recruitment of, other transcription factors that comprise a functional transcription complex. This process might involve protein-protein interactions between receptor and other factors, resulting in the formation of DNA loops[11] to accommodate long stretches of DNA between promoters and HREs, or possibly by altering the local chromatin organization to permit access of other transcription factors; obviously, both events could occur. Although it is widely believed that an allosteric alteration of receptor structure occurs following hormone binding, exposing the DNA-binding domain, the nature of this change is not understood. The participation of other proteins, such as the heat shock protein hsp90, may be important in stabilizing the inactive form of receptor, as has been suggested for glucocorticoid receptor.[12] However, to date, despite extensive *in vitro* data that demonstrates the association of several members of this family with hsp90 in cell free systems, there is no *in vivo* evidence to link the hormone-binding receptor protein with hsp90 or any other protein prior to ligand-induced activation. It has also been suggested that nonhistone protein acceptor sites [13] (part of nuclear matrix?) play a key role in receptor action, possibly by directing receptor to a target gene. Although such sites have been described, they have not yet been linked in an obligatory manner to a functional transcription complex. Another unresolved issue is the role of phosphorylation in receptor function or dynamics. At least two levels of phosphorylation have been described. For estrogen receptor, and possibly for glucocorticoid receptor, it appears that phosphorylation on tyrosine[14] may be required to activate hormone binding. However, this observation remains controversial. A second level of phosphorylation would be the hormone-induced phosphorylation on multiple serine residues[15] that has been described for rabbit, chicken and human PR and for vitamin D receptor and glucocorticoid receptor. At this point, no functional role for this phosphorylation has been defined. However, it does not appear to influence receptor activation or binding to DNA or, for PR, processing of receptor, although an effect on GR recycling has been proposed. It is more likely that phosphorylation may be affecting interaction of these receptors with the transcriptional machinery. Finally, the nature of agonist- *vs* antagonist-receptor interaction is poorly understood at present. It seems likely that an altered conformation of receptor occurs in the presence of an antagonist, which could affect DNA binding, interaction with other transcription factors, phosphorylation, or interaction with hsp90. At least for PR, the pattern of phosphorylation appears to be the same in T47D human breast cancer cells when cells are exposed to either a progestin or antagonist[16], although the level of phosphorylation is higher in the presence of antagonist, suggesting that phosphorylation may be sensitive to agonist/antagonist differences. Obviously, there are still a number of key dynamic and molecular aspects of receptor activity that are not resolved at this time.

STRUCTURE AND PROPERTIES OF HUMAN ER

The isolation, sequencing and expression of a 2.1 kb cDNA containing all of the translated sequence for ER mRNA from MCF-7 human breast cancer cells has provided a wealth of information about the composition and functional domains of ER[17]. An open reading frame of 1785 nucleotides encodes a protein of 595 amino acids with Mr 66,200. This ORF is contained in a 6.6 kb mRNA that includes 4.3 kb of 3' untranslated sequence and approximately 230 nucleotides of 5' untranslated sequence. The long untranslated 3' sequence is characteristic of all of the steroid receptors and its function is unknown, although HREs have been found in this region of the rat glucocorticoid receptor mRNA[18]. A schematic representation of the human ER protein is shown in Fig. 1. The positions of all proline, cysteine, and basic (lys/arg) residues are indicated. It is noteworthy that a significant proportion of the prolines are in the amino terminal portion of the protein, as is also the case for PR. The consequences of this clustering of prolines are not yet known. However, the secondary structure of this portion of the receptor must be considerably altered from an *a*-helix in this region. This is also the region of greatest immunogenicity for PR and GR, but not ER, which may be due in part to its structural organization, as well as to a generally lower sequence homology in this region among receptors from different species. A comparison of

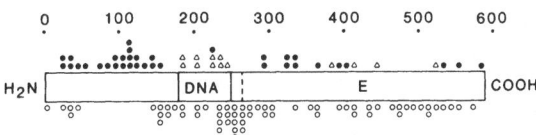

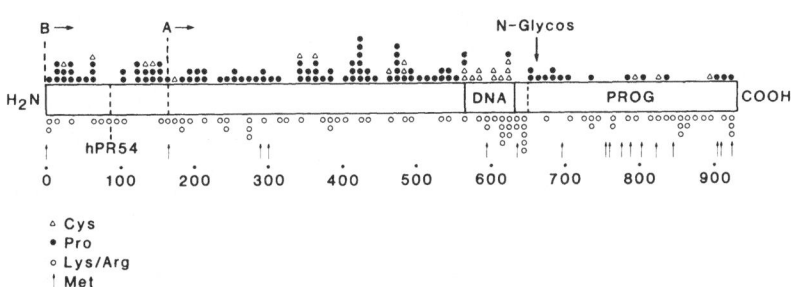

△ Cys
● Pro
○ Lys/Arg
↕ Met

Fig. 1. Schematic amino acid comparison between MCF-7 human estrogen receptor (upper) and T47D human progesterone receptor (lower). The two representations are aligned to make the 66-amino acid DNA-binding domains coincide. Details are given in the text.

amino acid sequences among all members of the steroid receptor family, coupled with functional analyses of *in vitro* generated mutants, has identified regions essential for the three major functions of steroid receptors, namely ligand binding, DNA binding, and transcriptional activation. The most highly conserved region is now known to be the DNA-binding domain and it is this region that has been used to define the members of a superfamily of regulatory proteins that includes the steroid receptors. For ER, 9 of the 13 cysteines are clustered in a 66 amino acid region which is now known to represent that portion of the DNA binding domain that is responsible for receptor-specific binding to HREs on target genes. These 9 cysteines are completely conserved among all of the steroid receptors, as are another 11 residues in this domain. Also characteristic of this region is the heavy concentration of basic amino acids (lys/arg) that may participate in DNA binding. This region can be further divided into two subregions analagous to the zinc coordinated 'fingers' found in the *Xenopus* transcription factor IIIA. The hydrophobic region in the carboxy terminal portion of the ER molecule contains not only the ligand binding domain, but also a ligand-dependent transcription activating region, as well as at least one possible translocation signal. In addition, it is probably this general region, by analogy to GR, that interacts with the hsp90 heat shock protein *in vitro,* although this has not been demonstrated for ER. The amino terminal portion of ER may also be required for maximal ER transcriptional activity and may contain a promoter-specific transcription activating region[19].

INTERACTION OF ER WITH DNA

As described above, the DNA binding domain of each steroid receptor appears to contain all of the information needed for target-specific interaction with an appropriate HRE, although the nature of this interaction remains to be better defined. It has recently been suggested that the first finger motif is responsible for sequence specificity and that the second finger may stabilize protein-DNA interaction through nonspecific DNA binding[20]. For estrogen receptor, the known response elements (EREs), such as those found in the *Xenopus* vitellogenin A1 and A2 genes and the chicken vitellogenin A2 gene, are palindromic sequences with 5 bp stems separated by a 3 bp spacer[21]. Similar sequences are found in the regulatory regions of the chicken ovalbumin gene and the rat prolactin gene. A consensus sequence for these EREs is shown in Fig. 2. Single copies of these elements are able to confer significant estrogen inducibility to reporter genes containing heterologous promoters, such as the chloramphenicol acetyltransferase (CAT) gene fused to the thymidine kinase promoter, when transfected into ER-containing cells. That these EREs are extremely specific for ER is evident from the inability of the closely related EREs of the vitellogenin B1 and B2 genes, each of which contains one or two nucleotide substitutions, to regulate transcription in the presence of ER. In recent gel shift experiments, the specific, high affinity interaction of purified MCF-7 ER (>90% pure) with the perfect palindromic vitellogenin A2 ERE contained in a 27-mer synthetic oligonucleotide was demonstrated[22]. A single A to G conversion within one stem of the palindromic ERE reduced the binding affinity 5- to 10-fold, indicating that ER-ERE binding is highly sequence-specific. The precise DNA contact sites involved in ER binding to the vitellogenin A2 ERE were determined by a methylation interference footprinting technique. In this case the probe was a 128-bp fragment obtained from a restriction digest of an ERE-tk-CAT plasmid containing a 21-mer vitellogenin A2 ERE in both orientations. A comparison of free probe and probe complexed with purified MCF-7 ER showed that methylation of all G residues of both strands within the conserved stems of the ERE strongly

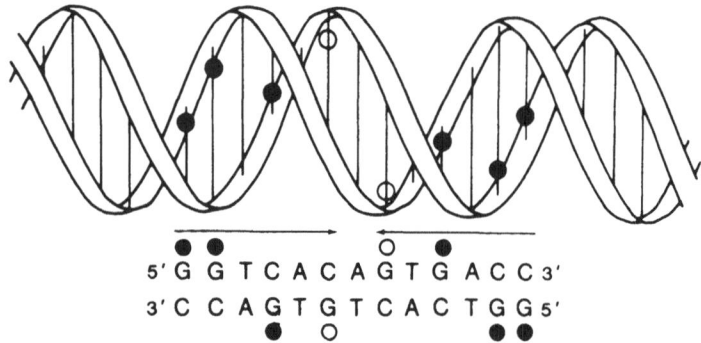

Fig. 2. Schematic representation of putative purine contact sites for the binding of ER to the double helical estrogen response element (ERE) of the vitellogenin A2 gene. Filled and open circles show strong and weak methylation interference sites, respectively. Reproduced from Klein-Hitpass *et al.*[22]

interferred with ER binding; methylated Gs within the 3-bp spacer only weakly interferred with receptor binding and methylated A residues had no effect. When projected onto DNA helices, a symmetrical distribution of G residues is observed, coincident with the dyad symmetry of the ERE, as shown in Fig. 2. Thus, the contact sites are located within one and one half successive turns of the major groove and are accessible from one face of the helix. Thus, both halves of the ERE palindrome appear to be in contact with the receptor complex, which suggests the formation of a complex containing a head to head dimer of ER bound to the ERE, with each monomer recognizing one half of the palindrome. These results are consistent with extensive *in vitro* data that indicates the formation of a 5 S homodimer of ER when receptor is activated[23]. Purified ER has also been characterized as an activated dimer. Finally, the 5-10-fold loss in affinity of ER for the ERE that occurs when only one half of the palindrome is modified suggests that the assembly of receptor dimers on a single ERE is a cooperative process.

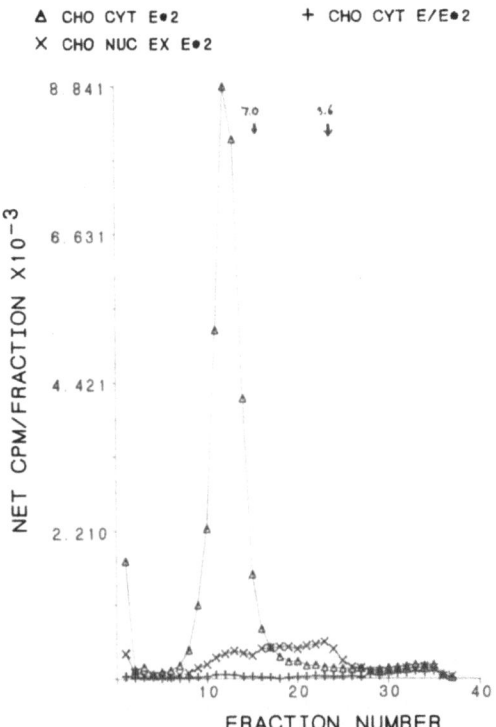

△ CHO CYT E•2   + CHO CYT E/E•2
X CHO NUC EX E•2

Fig. 3. Sedimentation analysis of human estrogen receptor expressed by MCF-7 ER cDNA in CHO-K1 cells. Sedimentation profiles in low-salt gradients (10 mM KCL) of cytosol (△—△) or nuclear extract (X—X) labeled with 10 nM [3H]estradiol, or cytosol (+—+) labeled with 10 nM [3H]estradiol plus 1 uM unlabeled estradiol for 60 min at 4oC. Unbound estradiol was removed by treatment with dextran-coated charcoal and aliquots (200 μl) were layered onto linear 10 to 30% sucrose gradients (3.5 ml), and centrifuged at 2oC for 15 hr at 253,000g. Successive 100-μl fractions were collected and counted in scintillation mixture. [14C]Ovalbumin (3.6 S) and [14C]IgG (7.0 S) were used as sedimentation markers in parallel gradients. For more details, see ref. 17, Fig. 2.

EXPRESSION OF HUMAN ER IN HETEROLOGOUS CELLS

To determine whether the 2.1 kb MCF-7 ER cDNA (OR8) would code for the synthesis of functional human ER in a heterologous system, the OR8 cDNA was inserted into a pBR vector containing a metallothionein promoter and SV40 enhancer sequence. This plasmid was then used to transform Chinese hamster ovary cells (CHO-K1), and cell homogenates from cloned, stable transfectants were analyzed for the expression of human ER in a form capable of binding estradiol17. Sedimentation analysis of a low-salt extract labeled with [3H]estradiol revealed the presence of a receptor-[3H]estradiol complex which sedimented at 8-9S in 10 mM KCl (Fig. 3) and at 4S in 0.4 M KCl (not shown). This complex reacted with three different monoclonal ER antibodies to form 8S immune complexes. One of these antibodies is specific for primate ER (D75P3γ). Specific steroid binding was abolished by the addition of excess radioinert estradiol or diethylstilbestrol. A high salt extract (0.4 M KCl) contained low levels of ER (Fig. 3) unless cells were first exposed to estradiol. Extracts of untransformed CHO-K1 cells did not contain any significant amount of endogenous ER. The formation of 8-10S salt-sensitive receptor-hormone complexes in hypotonic extracts of responsive cells is a hallmark of steroid receptors, although the biologic significance of these multimeric complexes has not been established. It is interesting that, although CHO-K1 cells appear to express little or no endogenous ER, the human ER expressed by OR8 cDNA in these

123

cells forms an 8-9S complex when occupied by [3H]estradiol under hypotonic conditions. This suggests either that this complex is a multimer of steroid-binding subunits or that associated nonsteroid-binding components are present in nontarget cells. Because it is now known that steroid receptors isolated from natural target cells associate with hsp90 heat shock protein *in vitro*[24], and that the hsp90 protein is both ubiquitous and abundant, it is likely that the expressed human ER is associating with hamster hsp90 in extracts from transfected cells. It is noteworthy that the cells used for the experiment depicted in Fig. 3 contained approximately 1.5-2.0 x 10[6] molecules of ER per cell, as judged by a whole cell binding assay, which is approximately 30 to 50-fold higher than the ER levels found in MCF-7 cells. However, all of the labelled receptor is present as an 8-9S complex, demonstrating the relative abundance of hsp90, or possibly another protein, in these cells. A schematic representation of the possible composition of the different forms of ER observed *in vitro* is shown in Fig. 4. Regardless of whether the unoccupied receptor is present in the cytoplasm or nucleus of a target cell, it is proposed to exist as a complex consisting of one steroid-binding protein, a dimer of hsp90, and possibly one or more small RNA molecules, as has been reported for unactivated rat glucocorticoid receptor[25]. Also shown in this model is the presence of phosphorylation sites on both the hsp90 and receptor proteins. As mentioned earlier, tyrosine phosphorylation of ER has been reported, and we have observed estrogen-induced phosphorylation of ER expressed in CHO cells. The formation of a 5S homodimer of ER upon steroid-, heat- or purification-induced activation was discussed above. In regard to the subcellular location of ER in the absence of hormone, a wealth of data now supports the idea that this receptor, and probably all other characterized members of this family except glucocorticoid receptor, is a nuclear protein[8]. As shown in Fig. 5, overexpressing CHO cells transfected with human ER cDNA show a nuclear localization of ER when stained with the H222 antibody by an indirect immunoperoxidase technique in cells that were grown in phenol red-free medium containing charcoal-stripped serum. Little or no specific ER staining is observed in the cytoplasm of these cells, unless the cell is undergoing mitosis. Thus, the translocation signal(s) encoded within the ER molecule does not appear to require hormone to be active, unlike the glucocorticoid receptor[26].

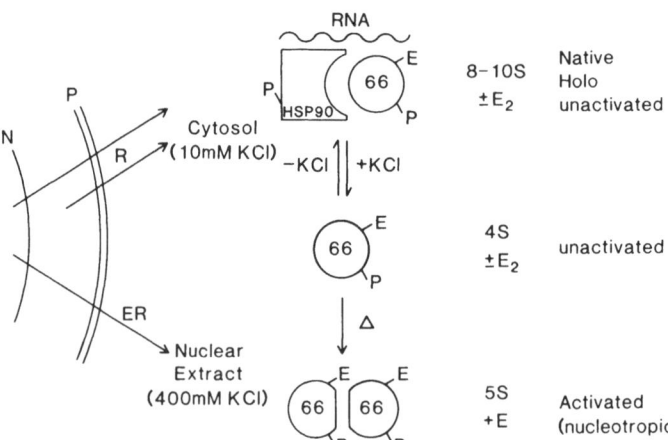

Fig. 4. Model of various *in vitro* forms of estrogen receptor isolated from a hormone-responsive cell. E = estrogen; E2 = estradiol; P = phosphorylation site(s); Δ = heat. See text for details.

Finally, evidence for the presence of a functional human ER in these CHO cells is provided by

The purification of human PR by steroid affinity chromatography and/or immunoadsorption, and the characterization of 14 rat and mouse monoclonal antibodies has been recently described[27]. PR from T47D human breast cancer cells consists of two steroid-binding forms (A: 88-93 kDa; B: 109-119 kDa) that appear to derive from a single mRNA open reading frame[27]. These forms can be identified by covalent labelling with [3H]R5020, by western blot analysis, or by silver staining of purified PR, as shown in Fig. 6 (silver stain not shown). Highly purified PR migrates as 93 kDa and 119 kDa progestin-binding proteins in SDS gels. In all, 13 monoclonal antibodies have been obtained that recognize epitopes shared by both forms of PR. One mouse immunoglobulin (KC146) is completely specific for the larger B form. Interestingly, the epitope for this antibody is present on all PRs tested, including the B form from chicken oviduct, whereas nine other antibodies recognize only human or nonhuman primate PR and the remaining four cross react with rabbit PR (Table 1). Interestingly, two antibodies (KD67 and KD68) do not recognize PR in monkey oviduct and thus appear to be specific for human PR. This discrimination between a human and nonhuman primate steroid receptor has not been observed previously for any of the characterized receptor antibodies. A T47D cDNA clone (hPR54)[28] containing about 90% of the open reading frame for the full length B form of PR, and a human genomic clone containing the remainder of the open reading frame and approximately 1.9 kb of 5' untranslated sequence have been isolated, sequenced, and partially characterized. A schematic representation of the predicted 933-amino acid B form (Mr 99,000) of PR[29] is shown in Fig. 1. When aligned with human ER *via* the DNA-binding domains, all of the additional PR sequence appears as an extension of the amino terminal portion of the molecule. Like ER, the PR protein contains a high proportion of prolines in the amino terminal half of the receptor, as well as a cluster of 10 cysteines in the DNA-binding domain, 9 of which are conserved with respect to ER, and a cluster of basic residues in and around the DNA-binding domain. The amino acid sequence homology between human ER and PR is about 56% in the 66-amino acid DNA binding domain and about 28% in the hormone-binding region. There is little homology between ER and PR 5' to the DNA binding domain. The sequence start site for hPR 54 is identified in Fig. 1 by a dashed line.

An issue that still remains unresolved is the relationship and derivation of the two reported hormone-binding forms of mammalian and avian PR. Among the members of the steroid receptor transcription factor family, only PR and possibly androgen receptor are reported to exist in two ligand-binding forms. Estimates of PR molecular weights vary from 78-95 kDa for the smaller A form and from 108-120 kDa for the larger B form. Recent gene cloning data for chicken, rabbit, and human PR indicate the existence of only one gene for these PRs, although multiple forms of PR mRNA have been observed. However, all available data suggests that only one transcript is translated to produce the two PR forms. The two most likely explanations for the appearance of A in cell-free extracts are: 1) that A is a proteolytic fragment of B, with cleavage occurring at a point approximately 20-25 kDa in from the amino terminus, as suggested for rabbit and human PR[27], or 2) that A is derived by translation of PR mRNA from an internal methionine, as suggested for chicken PR[30,31]. The equivalent putative translation start sites for the B and A forms of T47D PR are identified in Fig. 1. Although rabbit and human PR have been reported to occur exclusively as 110-kDa species in extracts or translation mixtures containing protease inhibitors, T47D and chicken oviduct PR have been reported to exist in both forms under all tested conditions. In fact, we have never observed the conversion of T47D B to A in any cell-free system. An alternative explanation is that the cleavage of B to A occurs *in vivo*. Mutagenic analysis of the methionines involved may help resolve this issue.

---

the results of experiments in which CHO cells were transfected with both an ER expression plasmid and a reporter ERE-tk-CAT plasmid. CAT activity was significantly induced when co-transfected cells were treated with estradiol.

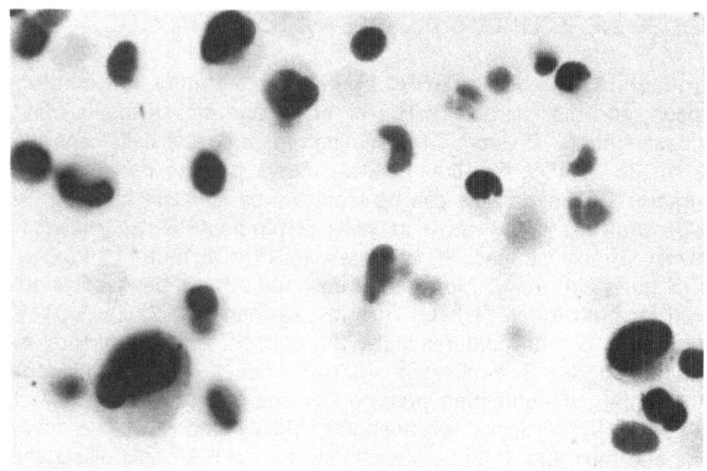

Fig. 5. Immunocytochemical staining of expressed ER in CHO cells transfected with MCF-7 ER cDNA[17]. Cells were grown in monolayer culture in DMEM/F12 medium, released with 1mM EDTA and centrifuged in a chambered glass slide previously coated with poly-L-lysine, to form an adherent monolayer. Attached cells were fixed with picric acid-paraformaldehyde and stained by the indirect immunoperoxidase technique[8] with H222 IgG[6]. There is no counterstain.

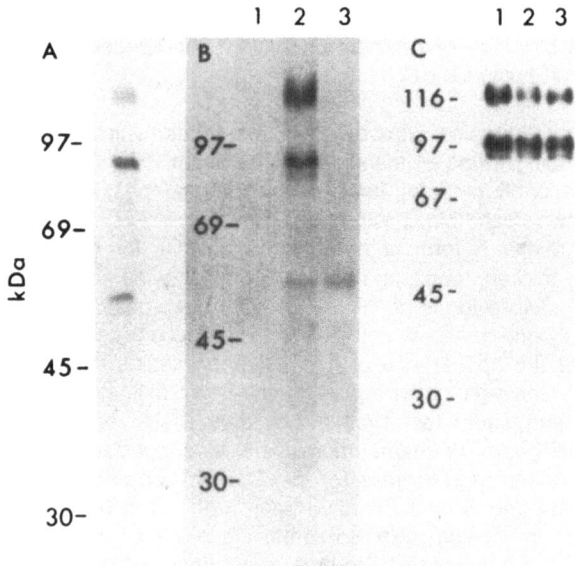

Fig. 6. Identification of human PR steroid-binding forms in partially purified PR complex (A) and in T47D cytosol (B) by covalent labeling with [3H]R5020, and by immunoblot analysis (C) with monoclonal antibody KD68. PR was photoaffinity labeled with [3H]R5020 in the presence (lane 3) or absence (lane2) of a 200-fold excess of radioinert ORG 2058. Proteins were separated by SDS-PAGE and analyzed by radioautography (A and B) or by immunoblotting (C) with KD68 IgG after transfer to nitrocellulose. Lane 1 (B and C) contains labeled, but unphotolyzed, PR. Reproduced from ref. 7.

In regard to PR phosphorylation, we are still attempting to define what factors alter the level of receptor phosphorylation, what amino acids are involved, and what role phosphorylation plays in receptor action and dynamics. In a collaborative study carried out with Kanury Rao and Fred Fox[32], we first established that at least the B form of T47D PR incorporates ^{32}P under steady state conditions; serine was the only amino acid labeled. EGF, TPA or dibutyryl cAMP had no significant effect on the level of phosphorylation. However, 10 nM progesterone resulted in a 2-fold increase in incorporation of [32]P. We still wish to know whether any tyrosine phosphorylation occurs, as proposed for ER, and what regions of the receptor protein are being phosphorylated, as well as how phosphorylation is affected by steroid antagonists, if at all.

REGULATION OF PR EXPRESSION

The regulation of progesterone receptor expression by estrogens, progestins and their antagonists is a useful model for studying hormonal regulation of gene expression in general. In collaboration with Benita Katzenellenbogen[4], we have studied the effects of some of these ligands on PR protein and mRNA levels in several breast cancer cell lines. By Northern blot analysis with human PR cDNA probes, PR mRNA appears as five species of 11.4, 5.8, 5.3, 3.5, and 2.8 kb; these species are absent in the PR-negative MB-231 and LY2 cell lines. In T47D cells, both the receptor and its mRNA levels are reduced by 90% within 48 hr of treatment with the synthetic progestins R5020 or ORG2058. In contrast, treatment with RU38,486, a progestin antagonist, reduces receptor and mRNA only transiently. In MCF-7 cells, PR mRNA and protein are virtually absent in the absence of estrogens. Treatment with estradiol induces both, in parallel, about 10 to 40-fold within three days. Antiestrogens (eg. LY117018) block this effect completely. Interestingly, progestins and progestin antagonists both reduce receptor and mRNA levels, although only by 40-60%. Clearly, the regulation of PR expression is different in the two cell lines. However, there is a close correlation between protein and mRNA levels and the changes appear to be directly mediated by the ligands, presumably via their cognate receptors. We will try to establish the molecular nature of this regulation with cloned PR gene sequences and purified or expressed ER.

As part of our effort to understand the structural and molecular aspects of PR gene regulation by several receptor-ligand complexes, we are currently isolating and characterizing genomic DNA for human PR. At present, we have a 6 kb fragment, obtained by hybridization screening of a human chromosome 11 library, that appears to contain the first two exons of PR translated sequence and 2-3 kb of 5' flanking sequence. This genomic DNA clone is being mapped and sequenced. Comparisons will then be made with other known hormone response elements to locate any consensus sequences in the PR gene. In addition, portions of the flanking region will be linked to a reporter gene (CAT) with a tk promoter so that we can begin to study the interaction of ER and PR with putative response elements.

ACKNOWLEDGEMENTS

These studies were supported by Abbott Laboratories, the American Cancer Society (BC-86) and the NCI (CA-02897).

REFERENCES

1. R.B. Dickson, M.E. MacManaway and M.E. Lippman, Estrogen-Induced Factors of Breast Cancer Cells Partially Replace Estrogen to Promote Tumor Growth, Science 232:1540 (1986).

2. E.R. DeSombre, P.P. Carbonne, E.V. Jensen, W.L. McGuire, S.A. Wells, J.L. Wittliff and

M.B. Lipsett, Special Report: Steroid Receptors in Breast Cancer, N. Engl. J. Med. 301: 1011 (1979).

3. G.M. Clark, W.L McGuire, C.A. Hubay, O.H. Pearson and J.S. Marshall, Progesterone Receptor as a Prognostic Factor in Stage II Breast Cancer, N. Engl. J. Med. 309: 1343 (1983).

4. L.D. Read, C.E. Snider, J.S. Miller, G.L. Greene and B.S. Katzenellenbogen, Ligand-Modulated regulation of Progesterone Receptor Messenger Ribonucleic Acid and Protein in Human Breast Cancer Cell Lines, Mol. Endocrinol. 2: 263 (1988).

5. R.M. Evans, The Steroid and Thyroid Hormone Receptor Superfamily, Science 240: 889 (1988).

6. G.L. Greene, N.B. Sobel, W.J. King and E.V. Jensen, Immunochemical Studies of Estrogen Receptors, J. Steroid Biochem. 20: 51 (1984).

7. G.L. Greene, K. Harris, R. Bova, R. Kinders, B. Moore and C. Nolan, Purification of T47D Human Progesterone Receptor and Immunochemical Characterization with Monoclonal Antibodies, Mol. Endocrinol. 2: 714 (1988).

8. G.L. Greene and M.F. Press, Immunochemical Evaluation of Estrogen Receptor and Progesterone Receptor in Breast Cancer, in: "Immunological Approaches to the Diagnosis and Therapy of Breast Cancer", R. L. Ceriani, ed., Plenum, New York (1987).

9. M.F. Press and G.L. Greene, Localization of Progesterone Receptor with Monoclonal Antibodies to the Human Progesterone Receptor, Endocrinology 122: 1165 (1988).

10. L.B. Kinsel, J.L. Flowers, J. Konrath, G.S. Leight, G.L. Greene, and K. S. McCarty, Heterogeneity vs Asynchrony of Receptor Expression in Breast Cancer as Determined by Monoclonal Antibodies, in: "Immunological Approaches to the Diagnosis and Therapy of Breast Cancer, R.L. Ceriani, ed., Plenum, New York (1987).

11. B. Theveny, A. Bailly, C. Rach, M. Rach, E. Delain, and E. Milgrom, Association of DNA-Bound Progesterone Receptors, Nature 329: 79 (1987).

12. D.B. Mendel, J.E. Bodwell, B. Gametchu, R.B. Harrison and A. Munk, Molybate-Stabilized Nonactivated Glucocorticoid-Receptor Complexes Contain a 90-kDa Non-Steroid-Binding Phosphoprotein that is Lost on Activation, J. Biol. Chem. 261: 3758 (1986).

13. A. Goldberger, B.A. Littlefield, J. Katzman and T.C. Spelsberg, Monoclonal Antibodies recognize the Nuclear Binding Sits of the Avian Oviduct Progesterone Receptor, Endocrinology 118: 2235 (1986).

14. F. Auricchio, A. Migliaccio, M. Di Domenico and E. Nola, Oestradiol Stimulates Tyrosine Phosphorylation and Hormone-0Binding Activity of its Own Receptor in a Cell-free System, EMBO J. 6: 2923 (1987).

15. H. Loosefelt, F. Logeat, M.T. Vu Hai and E. Milgrom, The Rabbit Progesterone Receptor: Evidence for a Single Steroid-Binding Subunit and Characterization of Receptor mRNA, J. Biol. Chem. 259: 14196 (1984).

16. G.L. Greene, Estrogen and Progesterone Receptor Composition, Expression and Analysis in Breast Cancer, 60th Annual Meeting of the Endocrine Society, Indianapolis, Abstr. p. 12.

17. G.L. Greene, P. Gilna, M. Waterfield, A. Baker, Y. Hort and J. Shine, Sequence and Expression of Human Estrogen receptor Complementary DNA, Science 231: 1150 (1986).

18. S. Okret, L. Poellinger, Y. Dong, and JA Gustafsson, Down-regulation of Glucocorticoid Receptor mRNA by Glucocorticoid Hormones and Recognition by the Receptor of a Specific Binding Sequence Within a Receptor cDNA clone, Proc. Natl. Acad. Sci. USA 83: 5899 (1986).

19. V. Kumar, S. Green, G. Stack, M. Berry, J.R. Jin and P. Chambon, Functional Domains of the Human Estrogen Receptor, Cell 51: 941 (1987).

20. S. Green, V. Kumar, I. Theulaz, W. Wahli and P. Chambon, The N-Terminal DNA-Binding 'Zinc Finger' of the Oestrogen and Glucocorticoid Receptors Determines Target Gene Specificity, EMBO J. 7: 3037 (1988).

21. L. Klein-Hitpass, G.U. Ryffel, E. Heitlinger and A.C.B. Cato, A 13 bp Palindrome is a Functional Estrogen Responsive Element and Interacts Specifically with Estrogen Receptor, Nuc. Acids. Res. 16: 647 (1988).

22. L. Klein-Hitpass, S.Y. Tsai, G.L. Greene, J.H. Clark, M.J. Tsai and B. O'Malley, Specific Binding of Estrogen Receptor to the Estrogen receptor Element, submitted, Mol. Cell. Biol. in press (1988).

23. M.A. Miller, A. Mullick, G.L. Greene and B. Katzenellenbogen, Characterization of the Subunit Nature of Nuclear Estrogen Receptors by Chemical Cross-linking and Dense Amino Acid Labeling, Endocrinology 117: 515 (1985).

24. S. Schuh, W. Yonemoto, J. Brugge, V.J. Baur, R.M. Riehl, W.P. Sullivan and D.O. Toft, A 90,000-Dalton Binding Protein common to both Steroid Receptors and the Rous Sarcoma Virus Transforming Protein pp60 vsrc, J. Biol. Chem. 260:14292 (1985).

25. A.L. Unger, R. Uppaluri, S. Ahern, J.L. Colby and J.L. Tymoczko, Isolation of Ribonucleic Acid from the Unactivated Rat Liver Glucocorticoid Receptor, Mol. Endocrinol. 2:952 (1988).

26. D. Picard and K.R. Yamamoto, Two Signals Mediate Hormone-Dependent Nuclear Localization of The Glucocorticoid Receptor, EMBO J. 6:3333 (1987).

27. M. Misrahi, H. Loosefelt, M. Atger, C. Meriel, V. Zerah, P. Dessen and E. Milgrom, Organization of the Entire Rabbit Progesterone Receptor mRNA and of the Promoter and 5' Flanking Region of the Gene, Nuc. Acids Res. 16: 5459 (1988).

28. P. Gilna, T. Zaruchi-Schulz and G.L. Greene, Cloning and Characterization of Human Progesterone Receptor, 69th Annual Meeting of the Endocrine Society, Indianapolis, Abstr. 1.

29. M. Misrahi, M. Atger, L. d'Auriol, H. Loosefelt, C. Meriel, F. Fridlansky, A. Guiochon-Mantel, F. Galibert and E. Milgrom, Complete Amino Acid Sequence of the Human Progesterone Receptor Deduced from Cloned cDNA, Biochem. Biophys. Res. Comm. 143: 740 (1987).

30. M.A. Carson, M.J. Tsai, O.M. Conneely, B.L. Maxwell, J.H. Clark, A.D. W. Dobson, A. Elbrecht, D.O. Toft, W.T. Schrader and B.W. O'Malley, Structure Function Properties of the Chicken Progesterone Receptor A Syntheisized from Complementary Deoxyribonucleic Acid. Mol. Endocrinol. 1: 791 (1987).

31. H. Gronemeyer, B. Turcotte, C. Quirin-Stricker, M.T. Bocquel, M.E. Meyer, Z. Krozowski, J.M. Jeltsch, T. Lerouge, J.M. Garnier and P. Chambon, The Chicken Progesterone Receptor: Sequence, Expression and Functional Analysis. EMBO J. 6: 3985 (1987).

32.K. Rao, W. Piralta, G.L. Greene and C. F. Fox, Cellular Progesterone Receptor Phosphorylation in Response to Ligands Activating Protein Kinases, Biochem. Biophys. Res. Comm.146:1357 (1987).

MONOCLONAL ANTIBODIES AGAINST STEROID RECEPTORS AND STEROID-INDUCED

PROTEINS

Martine Perrot-Applanat, Jean-François Prud'homme, Mai-Thu Vu Hai, André Jolivet, Frédéric Lorenzo, and Edwin Milgrom

INSERM U. 135 "Hormones et Reproduction"
Faculté de Médecine Paris Sud
94275 Le Kremlin-Bicêtre Cedex, France

Introduction

Estrogens play an important role in the genesis of experimental and human breast cancers [1,2]. Once established, the tumors are frequently hormone-dependent, i.e. they regress or stop growing if deprived of estrogen[3]. In humans, about one-third of advanced breast cancers are thus susceptible to remission with endocrine therapy[4]. Criteria for the selection of patients that will respond to hormonal treatment have been the subject of intense study during the last 2 decades[5]. On the molecular level this had led to the development of analytical tools for the study of steroid receptors and steroid-induced proteins.

Initial studies correlated the presence of ER and PR with: a) a high probability of response to endocrine therapy; 75-80% of the patients respond to hormone treatment when both receptors are present, and b) a more favorable prognosis, i.e. a greater disease-free interval between PR positive and negative patients. Determination of ER and PR content has thus become widely used in the prognosis and treatment of this disease. In 1984-1986, the development of monoclonal antibodies to estrogen[6] and progesterone[7] receptors has allowed immunocytochemical studies of these receptors[8-11]. This method displays several advantages over the steroid-binding method: it does not depend on the association of radiolabeled steroid hormone with the receptor. ER and PR can be detected, even at low concentration, in tumors taken from patients in which endogenous hormone levels are elevated. The immunohistochemical technique also offers a tool for the study of tumor heterogeneity.

We have developed a panel of well characterized monoclonal antibodies against human and rabbit PR[7,12,13], useful for immunocytochemistry of PR in breast cancer[11] and in endometrium[14]. Results of the immunocytochemical staining for PR in breast cancers were compared with the results of determining PR content by steroid-binding assay.

In addition, the study of other estrogen-regulated messengers or proteins could be useful in the prediction of clinical response to hormone therapy. In this respect, the study of estrogen-induced proteins in MCF-7 breast cancer cells was investigated, in particular that of BCEI (also called pS2) whose messenger RNA is relatively abundant

(0.8%)[15,16]. The DNA complementary (cDNA) to this mRNA was cloned and sequenced; it codes for a protein of 84 amino acids[16,17]; it was coexpressed in E. coli with β-galactosidase cDNA, thus allowing the preparation of polyclonal and monoclonal antibodies against it.

During these studies we have also developed a method allowing a rapid mapping of epitopes for monoclonal antibodies.

MONOCLONAL ANTIBODIES TO PROGESTERONE RECEPTORS

Over 80 mouse monoclonal antibodies (mAb) have been raised against the purified rabbit and human progesterone receptors[7,12,13]. These antibodies have been extensively characterized and shown to be highly specific by various methods, including precipitation of [3H] progestin-PR complexes with a second antibody, displacement of complexes after centrifugation on density gradients, and Western blot analysis on target and non-target tissues[11,12,13]. They have also been used to clone the receptor cDNA[18].

As previously shown[19,20], the PR consists mainly of a 110,000 daltons (110 kDa) species together with a 79,000 daltons (79 kDa) and 65,000 daltons (65 kDa) forms which we believe arise from proteolytic degradation of the 110 kDa form. Immunoblot experiments or ELISA tests with purified 110 kDa ("B form"), 79 kDa ("A form") and 65 kDa forms of PR allowed the antibodies to be classified into 3 categories: those recognizing the 3 forms, those recognizing A and B forms and those recognizing only the B form. No antibody recognized only the A form or only the 65 kDa fragment.

Epitope mapping. The precise mapping of epitopes recognized by monoclonal PR antibodies has been performed using a new method of epitope mapping[12]. This technique involves the introduction of the cDNA encoding the complete PR into the expression vector pGEM4, transcription with Sp6 polymerase and translation by a reticulocyte lysate in the presence of either [35S]-methionine or [3H]-leucine. Acellular transcription-translation of the cloned cDNA is performed in conditions where spontaneous or artificial premature termination of translation occurs, giving rise to C-terminally truncated receptor protein. The last step involves immunoprecipitation of the C-terminally truncated proteins with the antibody studied. Immunoprecipitation was observed by electrophoresis and fluorography for the largest polypeptides. When the antigenic site is deleted immunoprecipitation no longer occurs. Obviously, this method can only be applied to continuous epitopes.

This method has been initially used for the study of mAb raised against the rabbit PR[12]. All monoclonals fell into 4 groups recognizing 4 different immunogenic domains, localized as follows: between amino acids 1-60, between amino acids 101-110; between amino acids 295 and 325, after amino acid 370. The antibodies which react only with the intact rabbit receptor ("B form") belong to the two groups recognizing epitopes localized at the N-terminus of the protein (upstream from amino acid 110). The antibodies which recognize the 110 kDa and 79 kDa receptor forms, but not the 65 kDa form correspond to the epitope localized between amino acids 295 and 325. These results suggest that the N-terminus of the 79 kDa form is localized between amino acids 110 and 295, and the N-terminus of the 65 kDa form between amino acids 325 and 370. All these domains contain a major hydrophilic region and were in the N-terminal half of the protein. No antibodies were directed against the cysteine-rich basic region known to be involved in DNA binding, nor against the C-terminal end of the receptor which is responsible for its steroid binding properties. This is probably due to the very high conservation of these regions of the protein in different species. Competition experiments using [125I] receptor and antibodies interacting with two different immunogenic domains confirmed the map of the epitopes[12].

Identical experiments have been performed with the human PR[13] and the results are similar to those observed with rabbit PR.

Table 1 shows the class, the immunoblot reactivity and the location of epitopes of 8 selected monoclonals against rabbit and human PR. Most antibodies against PR were also analyzed by immunocytochemistry on human and rabbit tissues[9,11]. Our results show a good correlation between Western blot and immunocytochemical analysis (Table 1). This observation suggests that the affinity of these antibodies is very high, making it possible to label this rare antigen, when it is present in situ.

IMMUNOSTAINING OF PROGESTERONE RECEPTORS (AND ESTROGEN RECEPTORS) IN BREAST CANCERS

Materials and Methods

Tumors. The tumors were obtained from 52 patients with primary breast carcinomas, treated at the Centre René Huguenin (Saint Cloud, France). In each case, one fragment of the tumor was used for routine histological examination. It was graded according to the classification of Bloom and Richardson[21]. Two other fragments were trimmed of adhering fat and necrotic tissue, quickly frozen in liquid nitrogen, and stored until analyzed. Both biochemical analysis of ER and PR content by steroid-binding assay[22] and immunocytochemical staining for PR were performed on these tumor samples. In 22 cases, a tumor specimen had been also routinely fixed and embedded in paraffin.

Among 50 biopsy samples examined, 42 were diagnosed as being predominantly infiltrating ductal carcinomas (with or without intraductal carcinoma), 6 were infiltrating lobular carcinomas, 1 was medullary carcinoma, and 1 mucinous carcinoma. Two other biopsies were from male patients.

Immunostaining. In the first phase of this work, using mAB anti-PR we have developed an immunocytochemical method suitable for detecting PR on frozen sections from human tissues[11], especially in breast cancer biopsies. Staining was done with the peroxidase antiperoxidase technique, which involves incubation of the sections with mouse receptor antibodies (12 µg/ml) followed by goat antibodies to mouse IgG which serves as a bridge between bound mouse antibodies and mouse PAP complex added subsequently. All of the formaldehyde-containing fixatives (picric acid-formaldehyde, formalin, periodate-lysine-paraformaldehyde and to a lesser extent glutaraldehyde) were found to yield suitable immunostaining for PR. The maximal staining intensity for PR varied according to which monoclonal PR antibody was used. Strong staining was obtained with the mouse IgG mAbs Let (64, 126,456,548) and Li (417, 523, 533 and 386).

Tumors were classified as PR-immunocytochemically positive if they contained malignant cells showing nuclear staining regardless of the staining intensity and the proportion of positive epithelial cells. The average intensity of specific staining was graded as absent (-), weak but definitely detectable (+), moderate (++), and strong (+++).

Results and Discussion

Immunostaining of progesterone receptor. The immunocytochemical detection of PR was performed in 52 human breast tumors using mAb Let

Table 1. Characteristics of some monoclonal antibodies raised against the progesterone receptor (PR). The table shows a selection of 8 antibodies among the 80 monoclonal antibodies which were obtained.

Antibody	Class	Epitope n° of a-a	Western blotting of immunopurified receptor	Immunocytochemical staining	
				breast tumor	rabbit uterus
Mi 60-10	IgG$_{2a}$	370-396	+{3}	-	+
Let 126	IgG$_1$	22-60	+{1}	+	+
Let 456	IgG$_1$	22-60	+{1}	+	+
Let 548	IgG$_1$	295-325	+{2}	+	+
Li 169	IgG$_1$	1-121	+{1}	+	+
Li 386	IgG$_1$	208-296	+{3}	+	+
Li 417	IgG$_1$	208-296	+{2}	+	+
Li 216	IgG$_1$	371-455	+{3}	+	-

Series Mi and Let were obtained by immunization with rabbit PR (rPR). Serie Li was obtained by immunization with human PR (hPR). Western blot analysis was performed either with rPR (series Mi and Let) or hPR (serie Li). The number between square brackets indicates the number of receptor bands detected by immunoblot : {1}, one band (110 kDa); {2}, two bands (110 kDa and 79 kDa); {3}, three bands (110 kDa, 79 kDa and 65 kDa).

126*. Localization has shown an exclusively nuclear distribution in carcinoma breast cells (Fig. 1) and benign ductal or lobular epithelial cells (Figure 2.). No specific staining is seen in the surrounding connective tissue.

Specific PR immunostaining was found to be very heterogeneous: PR-positive tumors showed variations in intensity and distribution of staining among cells as well as in different areas of the same sections or in different samples from the same primary lesion. Those variations were also noted among non-malignant cells of breast ducts and in T47D breast cancer cells (Fig. 3). As already discussed in a previous study on rabbit and guinea pig progesterone target organs[9], this heterogeneity may be attributed either to receptor content variations which are cell cycle dependant or to variations due to the presence of both progesterone-responsive and non-responsive cells. Similar variations have been reported for ER by other investigators using immunohistochemical techniques[8]. The study of PR heterogeneity may provide additional information about the clinical unresponsiveness seen in about 20% of patients with PR-positive breast cancer.

In our series of 50 female breast tumors the presence or absence of nuclear staining did not seem to correlate with pathological classification (among the 42 invasive ductal carcinomas, 28 were positive and 14 were negative; 3 invasive lobular carcinomas were negative and 3 were positive). Among 24 positively stained tumors, 2 were classified as grade I (9%), 18 as grade II (75%), and 3 as grade III (12%). Among the 17 negative tumors, one was classified as grade I, 10 as grade II (60%) and 6 grade III (37%).

Correlation of immunoperoxidase staining with PR content. As shown in Table 2, 88% of all tumors with positive PR values had positive staining ; the percentage of positively stained cases rose to 96% among the tumors with PR content above 30 fmol per mg cytosol protein. The number of positive cells was also proportionally larger in tumors with high PR content. On the other hand, among 14 cases with PR-negative tumors by steroid-binding assay only one showed immunoreactivity (few labeled cells). Therefore, the PR immunocytochemical staining in frozen sections from breast carcinoma correlated well (92%) with the PR presence determined by the steroid-binding assay, except for 4 tumors: one of these tumors had a high concentration of PR; in this case we have no satisfactory explanation for the lack of immunostaining. It is possible that PR concentration was different in the fragment taken for the steroid-binding assay from that present in the three fragments taken for the immunocytochemical detection. Another reason for this discrepancy might reside in a loss of PR antigenicity due to fixation or due to an unexplained in vivo "modification" of receptor. Such hypotheses were also suggested by others for ER. In the other 3 cases where a discrepancy was observed, PR concentration was low (< 30 fmol/mg protein) and specific nuclear staining was absent. A likely explanation may reside in the fact that tumors containing low amounts of receptor often contain few cells that are receptor positive: such cells present in the large tumor fragment used for the steroid-binding assay would account for the measurement of the PR content, whereas they might not be detected by immunohistological examination. This explanation is supported by the examination of tumors containing similar concentrations of PR (<30 fmol/mg protein) and where only a small number of cells were immunostained.

In addition, two male breast cancers (with PR content of 13 and 68 fmol PR/mg protein) were analyzed by the immunoperoxidase method and

---

*now sold by Transbio (France) under INSERM licence.

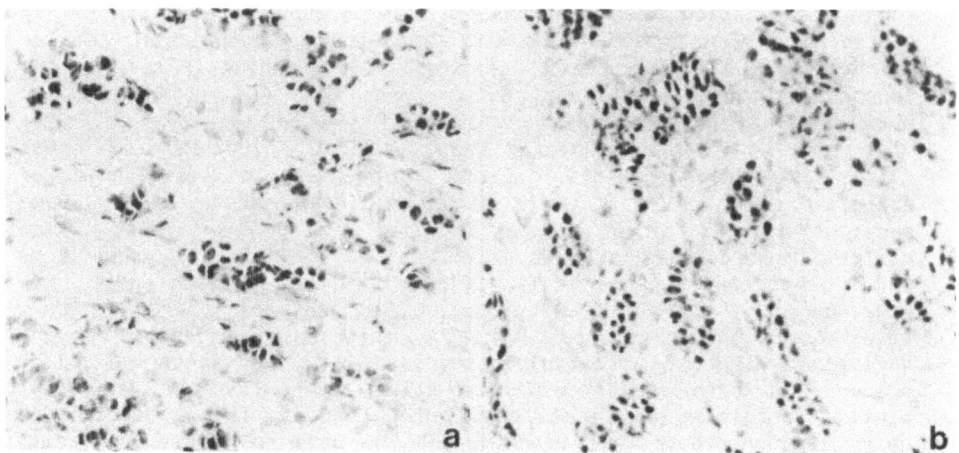

Fig. 1. Immunostaining with anti-progesterone receptor monoclonal antibody is limited to the nuclei of carcinoma cells. Frozen section from infiltrating ductal carcinoma of the breast.

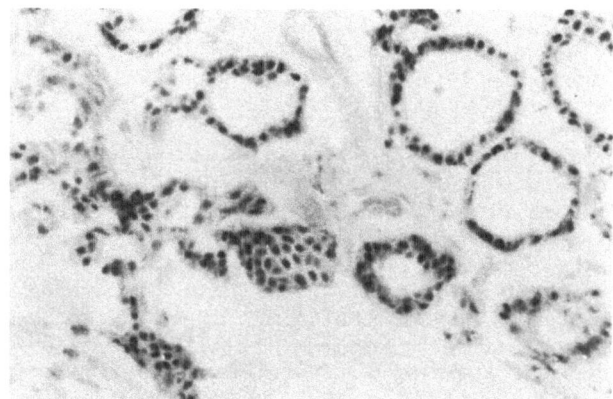

Fig. 2. Presence of nuclear immunostaining for PR in the non carcinoma ductal cells, at the periphery of a carcinoma.

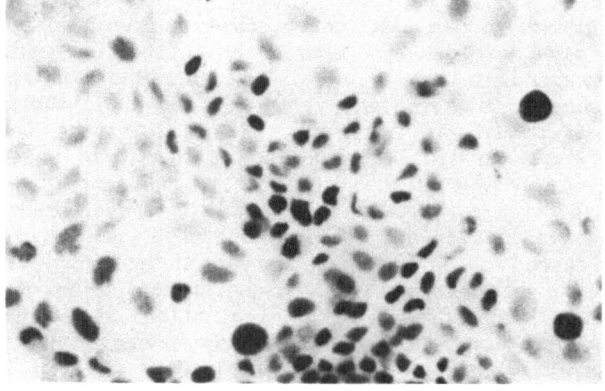

Fig. 3. Immunocytochemical staining for PR in human breast cancer cell line T47D.

Table 2. Immunoperoxidase staining of PR in frozen sections and PR content in 50 human breast cancers

PR immunostaining PR concentration fmol/mg protein	N° of tumors	n° of cases	
		positive	negative
< 10 (Negative)	14	1	13
10-30 (borderline)	8	5	3
> 30 (positive)	28	27	1
Total	50	33	17

found to be PR positive; this finding could be correlated with the fact that a high percentage (83%) of primary breast cancers in males seem to have estrogen receptors[23].

Immunoperoxidase detection of PR (and ER) in paraffin sections. The immunocytochemical detection of PR was also performed on paraffin-embedded sections from human breast cancers, with similar distribution of PR (nuclear and heterogeneous) in carcinoma cells (Perrot-Applanat et al., submitted for publication).

These immunocytochemical methods allow the detection of both PR and ER on adjacent frozen or paraffin sections from the same tissues (11 , Perrot-Applanat et.al., submitted for publication). ER was detected in paraffin-embedded tissues by the use of monoclonal anti-ER antibodies (ERICA kit) and the DNAse pretreatment method described by Shintaku and Said[24]. Various combinations of ER and PR content that were determined by steroid-binding assay were also detected by the double immunocytochemical assay. Only one tumor biochemically classified as ER negative/PR positive was studied. It was found to be immunocytochemically ER positive. The biopsy was taken from a woman who had received tamoxifen. This observation shows that immunocytochemistry may detect false negative results. In conclusion, this immunocytochemical method on paraffin sections now allows the observation of tumors embedded in paraffin years ago, thus providing opportunities for retrospective studies.

ESTROGEN-INDUCED PROTEIN IN BREAST CANCER

The study of BCEI or pS2, an estrogen-induced protein in MCF-7 breast cancer cells[15,16] was investigated. The cDNA clones prepared from mRNA induced by estrogen were identified by differential hybridization of RNAs from estrogen-treated and non treated[16], or tamoxifen treated MCF-7 cells[15]. One of the cDNAs corresponds to a relatively abundant mRNA[16], specific for BCEI and coding for a 84 amino acids polypeptide[16].

Polyclonal and monoclonal antibodies against this protein were prepared as follows: the cDNA of this estrogen-induced protein was expressed in E. coli in pUR290-292 β-galactosidase vector system25. A fusion protein was electrophoretically purified and injected into rabbits. A second fusion protein of β-galactosidase and pS2/BCEI deleted for the putative signal peptide and dG tail was purified by a

DEAE-cellulose column. Immunization of mice with this 30% pure chimeric-protein has permitted to prepare 7 monoclonal antibodies against the pS2/BCEI protein. Two were purified and characterized. The hybridoma screening assay was realized by ELISA tests using the electrophoretically purified β-galactosidase, fusion protein and a serum free culture medium from estradiol-treated MCF-7 cells as coated antigens.

The specificity of the monoclonal antibodies was determined by direct Western blotting or indirectly after immunoprecipitation.

Using these monoclonal antibodies, various biochemical and immunocytochemical studies are now being performed to clarify the possible function and distribution of this protein. The BCEI gene encodes an 84 amino acid protein that is secreted after signal peptide cleavage[27]. Since the pS2 gene is specifically expressed under estrogen transcriptional control in some breast cancer cells[16, 26-28], these antibodies may also be useful in investigating whether the pS2 protein can serve as a specific marker for the diagnosis and prognosis of estrogen-dependant breast cancers. Striking similarities with growth factors, notably EGF[29] were observed and should be clarified.

References

1. T.L. Dao, 1964, Carcinogenesis of mammary gland in rat. Prog. Exp. Tumor Res., 5:157.
2. B.E. Henderson, R.K. Ross, M.C. Pike, and J.T. Casagrande, 1982, Endogenous hormones as a major factor in human cancer. Cancer Res., 42:3239.
3. G.T. Beatson, 1896, On the treatment of inoperable cases of carcinoma of the mamma: Suggestions for a new method of treatment with illustrative cases. Lancet, ii:104.
4. E.V. Jensen, and E.R. DeSombre, 1977, The diagnostic implications of steroid binding in malignant tissues. Adv. Clin. Chem., 19:57.
5. J.C. Henderson, and G.P. Canellos, 1980, Cancer of the breast. The past decade. N. Engl. J. Med., 302:17.
6. G.L. Greene, C. Nolan, J.P. Engler, E.V. Jensen, 1980, Monoclonal antibodies to human estrogen receptor. Proc. Natl. Acad. Sci. USA, 77:5115.
7. F. Logeat, M.T. Vu Hai, A. Fournier, P. Legrain, G. Buttin, and E. Milgrom, 1983, Monoclonal antibodies to rabbit progesterone receptor: crossreaction with other mammalian progesterone receptors. Proc. Natl. Acad. Sci. USA, 80:6456.
8. W.J. King, and G.L. Greene, 1984, Monoclonal antibodies localize oestrogen receptor in the nuclei of target cells. Nature, 307:745.
9. M. Perrot-Applanat, F. Logeat, M.T. Groyer-Picard, and E. Milgrom, 1985, Immunocytochemical study of mammalian progesterone receptor using monoclonal antibodies. Endocrinology, 116:1473.
10. W.J. King, E.R. DeSombre, E.V. Jensen, and G.L. Greene, 1985, Comparison of immunocytochemical and steroid-binding assays for estrogen receptor in human breast tumors. Cancer Res., 45:293.
11. M. Perrot-Applanat, M.T. Groyer-Picard, F. Lorenzo, A. Jolivet, M.T. Vu Hai, C. Pallud, F. Spyratos, and E. Milgrom, 1987, Immunocytochemical study with monoclonal antibodies to progesterone receptor in human breast tumors. Cancer Res., 47:2652.
12. F. Lorenzo, A. Jolivet, H. Loosfelt, M.T. Vu Hai, S. Brailly, M. Perrot-Applanat, and E. Milgrom, 1988, A rapid method of epitope mapping. Application to the study of immunogenic domains and to the characterization of various "forms" of rabbit progesterone receptor. Eur. J. Biochem., 176:53.

13. M.T. Vu Hai, A. Jolivet, V. Ravet, F. Lorenzo, M. Perrot-Applanat, M. Citerne, and E. Milgrom, 1988, Novel monoclonal antibodies against human uterine progesterone receptor. Mapping of receptor immunogenic domains. Submitted for publication.

14. E. Garcia, P. Bouchard, J. De Brux, J. Berdah, R. Frydman, G. Schaison, E. Milgrom, and M. Perrot-Applanat, 1988, Use of immunocytochemistry of progesterone and estrogen receptors for endometrial dating. J. Clin. Endocrinol. Metab., 67:80.

15. P. Masiakowski, R. Breathnach, J. Bloch, F. Gannon, A. Krust, and P. Chambon, 1982, Cloning of cDNA sequences of hormone-regulated genes from the MCF-7 human breast cancer cell line. Nucleic Acids Res., 24:7895.

16. J.F. Prud'homme, F. Fridlansky, M. Le Cunff, M. Atger, C. Mercier-Bodard, M.F. Pichon, and E. Milgrom, 1985, Cloning of a gene expressed in human breast cancer and regulated by estrogen in MCF-7 cells. DNA, 4:11.

17. S.B. Jakowlev, R. Breathnach, R. Jeltsch, J.M. Masiakowski, and P. Chambon, 1984, Sequence of the pS2 mRNA induced by estrogen in the human breast cancer cell line MCF-7. Nucleic Acids Res., 12:2861.

18. H. Loosfelt, M. Atger, M. Misrahi, A. Guiochon-Mantel, C. Mériel, F. Logeat, R. Bénarous, and E. Milgrom, 1986, Cloning and sequence analysis of rabbit progesterone-receptor complementary DNA. Proc. Natl. Acad. Sci. USA, 83:9045.

19. H. Loosfelt, F. Logeat, M.T. Vu Hai, and E. Milgrom, 1984, The rabbit progesterone receptor. Evidence for a single steroid-binding subunit and characterization of receptor mRNA. J. Biol. Chem., 259:14196.

20. F. Logeat, R. Pamphile, H. Loosfelt, A. Jolivet, A. Fournier, and E. Milgrom, 1985, One-step immunoaffinity purification of active progesterone receptor. Further evidence in favor of the existence of a single steroid binding subunit. Biochemistry, 24:1029.

21. H.J.G. Bloom, and W.W. Richardson, 1957, Histological grading and prognosis in breast cancer. Br. J. Cancer, 11:359.

22. EORTC Breast Cancer Cooperative Group. 1980, Revision of the standards for the assessement of hormone receptors in human breast cancer. Eur. J. Cancer, 16:1513.

23. T.K. Mayer, and R.A. Mooney, 1988, Laboratory analyses for steroid hormone receptors, and their applications to clinical medicine. Clinica Chimica Acta, 172:1.

24. I.P. Shintaku, and J.W. Said, 1987, Detection of estrogen receptors with monoclonal antibodies in routinely processed formalin-fixed paraffin sections of breast carcinoma. Am. J. Clin. Pathol. 87:161.

25. U. Ruther, and B. Muller-Hill, 1983, Easy identification of cDNA clones. EMBO J., 2:1791.

26. F.E.B. May, and B.R. Westley, 1986, Cloning of estrogen-regulated messenger RNA sequences from human breast cancer cells. Cancer Res., 46:6034.

27. A.M. Nunez, S. Jakowlev, J.P. Briand, D. Gaire, A. Krust, M.C. Rio, and P. Chambon, 1987, Characterization of the estrogen-induced pS2 protein secreted by the human breast cancer cell line MCF-7. Endocrinology, 121:1759.

28. A.M.C. Brown, J.M. Jeltsch, M. Roberts, and P. Chambon, 1984, Activation of pS2 gene transcription is a primary response to estrogen in the human breast cancer cell line MCF-7. Proc. Natl. Acad. Sci. USA, 81:6344.

29. M.E. Baker, 1988, Estrogen-induced pS2 protein is similar to pancreatic spasmolytic polypeptide and the kringle domain. Biochem. J., 253:307.

TEN YEAR SURVIVAL PATTERNS IN PRIMARY BREAST CANCERS COMPARED TO HORMONE RECEPTOR ANTIGEN DETECTION BY MONOCLONAL ANTIBODIES

***Petra Kiene, *Laura Kinsel, **John Konrath, **Geoffrey Greene, *George Leight, *Edwin Cox, *Kenneth S. McCarty, Sr. and *Kenneth McCarty, Jr.

*Duke University, Durham, N. C.; **Univ. of Chicago, Abbott Laboratories, Chicago, IL. and ***Univ. of Hamburg

ABSTRACT

The prognostic significance of immunocytochemical methods for estrogen (ER) and progesterone (PgR) receptor analyses was studied in 257 patients with primary breast cancer followed up to ten years. H222 antibody was used for ER and JZB39 used for PgR. ER positive (>10 fmol/mg prot) tumors using ligand assays showed disease free interval (DFI) advantage for 3 years but none after three years. H222 positive tumors were associated with survival advantage throughout the ten year period (p=0.004). PgR (by ligand analysis) advantage was only seen in the first 3.5 years. JZB39 positive tumors showed significant survival advantage through the ten year period (p=0.04). Both ER and PgR correlated with nuclear grade and histologic grade. Within histologic grades ER positive DFI advantage was observed only among HG II lesions (p=0.04). While separation within lymph node groups was observed in the initial period in each category, only the 1-3 node positive subgroup had distinct advantage throughout the period of follow-up. The data indicate that semi-quantitative immunocytochemical ER and PgR analyses contributes to the separation of prognostic groups among specific subgroups of primary breast cancer.

INTRODUCTION

Since steroid receptor assays have been available, they have been used in breast cancer patients to predict the probability of response to hormonal therapy (7), and have been suggested to be indicators of prognosis for survival and disease-free interval (DFI). Several studies have shown estrogen receptor (ER), determined by ligand binding assays, (ER-BIO) to indicate a better prognosis for patients with ER positive tumors (2,3,4,) observing the patients over a short follow-up up to 36 months. Other studies (5,6) with longer follow-up reported ER not to be a predictor of the disease course. The relationship between PgR and prognosis has been less well investigated, but also showing controversial results (7,8). The development of highly specific monoclonal antibodies against ER and PgR protein made the immunocytochemical detection of ER and PgR in frozen sections of tissue possible. Good correlations between the biochemical and the immunocytochemical assay have been demonstrated by several investigators (9,10). This is of special interest in view of the heterogeneity of breast tumors and their differences in receptor expression. Immunocytochemical assay of ER (ER-ICA) has been correlated to DFI and survival, showing predictive value in short and long term follow-up observation (11,12). Previous investigations have shown histologic and nuclear grade as a predictor for DFI and survival (13,14). The present report presents 257 patients with primary breast cancer followed up to ten years. Estrogen and progesterone receptors have been measured by multiconcentration titration analysis (biochemical) and by immunocytochemical assay, being correlated to DFI and survival. The patients' group was separated, using nuclear grade, histologic grade and axillary lymph node status as categories to determine whether receptor status adds information within specific prognostic subgroups.

MATERIALS AND METHODS

Patient Population

The cohort consists of 257 patients with primary breast cancer treated at Duke University Medical Center and Cabarrus Memorial Hospital from February 1976 to December 1980. ERBIO and ER-ICA were performed on all tumors, biochemical progesterone receptor (PgR-BIO) in 190 tumors and progesterone receptor immunocytochemical assay (PgR-ICA) in 211 tumors. One hundred and sixty-six patients were treated with modified radical mastectomy, 51 radical mastectomy, 16 simple mastectomy, while 24 patients underwent a diagnostic biopsy due to the presence of advanced disease, (beyond the regional nodes).

After surgery, 178 patients received no further therapy, 24 were treated with CMF chemotherapy, 7 with alkeran chemotherapy, 13 with radiation therapy, 16 with Tamoxifen, and 11 received other chemotherapy, while 1 was not definable. Seven patients were treated with combination therapy, consisting of Tamoxifen and radiation (2), CMF and radiation (2), or other chemotherapy and radiation (3). The patients were staged according to following categories:

    Stage 1: Negative lymph nodes
    Stage 2: 1-3 positive nodes
    Stage 3: > 4 positive nodes, and/or muscle or skin
              involvement
    Stage 4: distant metastases.

Other recorded parameters were: age, menopausal status, race, site and date of first recurrence, date of last follow-up examination or date of death.

Steroid Receptor Analyses

Tissue Preparation: Tissues were quick frozen after being washed in 0.005M HEPES, 0.010M TRIS, 0.0015 EDTA, 0.01 thioglycerol, and 0.02% sodium azide at a pH of 7.4; maintained at -80 degrees Celsius in airtight liquid N_2 capsules from the time of the excision until sectioned for immunocytochemical analysis.

Dextran-coated charcoal and/or sucrose density gradient methods were performed at the time the tissue was first received. Results equal or greater than 10 fmol/mg protein were considered to be positive.

Immunocytochemical analysis: Cryostat sections of fresh frozen tissue were fixed in 3.7% formaldehyde-phosphate-buffered saline, followed by immersion in 100% methanol at -10 degrees Celsius for four minutes. This was followed by one minute at -10 degrees Celsius in acetone. The primary antibodies H222 and JZB39 were used at concentrations of 5 ug/ml and 4 ug/ml. The blocking reagent was normal goat serum, the bridging antibody was goat anti-rat immunoglobin, and the peroxidase-anti-peroxidase complex was of rat origin. Control slides consisted of serial sections of breast cancer in which the monoclonal antibody was replaced by normal rat immunoglobulin. The antigen-antibody complex was developed using diaminobenzidine-H_2O_2. The slides were treated with poly-L-lysine to improve adhesion of the frozen section. The sections were counterstained with methyl green.

Scoring of Assays

Biochemical assays were summarized as femtomoles of estrogen or progesterone binding per milligram of cytosol protein. The immunocytochemical analysis was scored in a semi-quantitative fashion incorporating both the intensity and distribution of specific staining. The evaluations were recorded as percentages of positively stained target cells in each of four intensity categories, which were denoted as 0 (no staining), 1+= (weak, but detectable above control), 2+ (distinct), and 3+ (strong, with minimal light transmission through stained nuclei). For each tissue, a value designated the HSCORE was derived by summing percentages of cells stained at each intensity multiplied by the weighted intensity of staining:

$$HSCORE = \sum Pi \ (i+1)$$

when i=1,2,3, and Pi varies from 0 to 100%. An HSCORE of 75 or greater was considered positive.

The evaluation of the histologic grade was done with modification, according to the method of Fisher et al.(15), using a scale of 0-3. The category 0 indicates intraductal elements only, I is well differentiated, II is moderately differentiated and III for poor differentiation. Nuclear grades consisted of 1 (poorly differentiated), 2 (moderately differentiated), and 3 (well differentiated), category 2 was further separated into 2A and 2 B, with 2A representing a better differentiation than 2B. Pearson regression analysis, Cox-Mantel test, Kaplan-Meir Survival estimate and multivariant regression analysis were used for the statistical analyses.

RESULTS

The immunocytochemical evaluation, using monoclonal antibodies to estrogen (H222) and progesterone (JZB39) protein, showed specific staining localized to nuclei of the target cells. ER showed an intraobserver reliability of 0.94, PgR of 0.90, the interobserver reliability was 0.92 for ER and 0.83 for PgR. Correlating the biochemical assay and the immunocytochemical analysis, a relationship appeared between the log values of the biochemical assay and the HSCORE (ER-BIO/ER-ICA r=0.64; PgR-BIO/PgR-ICA r=0.57).

Results of all assays were correlated to survival and DFI. Determination of the ER content by immunocytochemical method (H222) showed significant separation (p=0.004), with advantage for the positive group in survival over ten years. ER-BIO showed small separation over the first five years, but converged after five years. PgR-BIO divided the

143

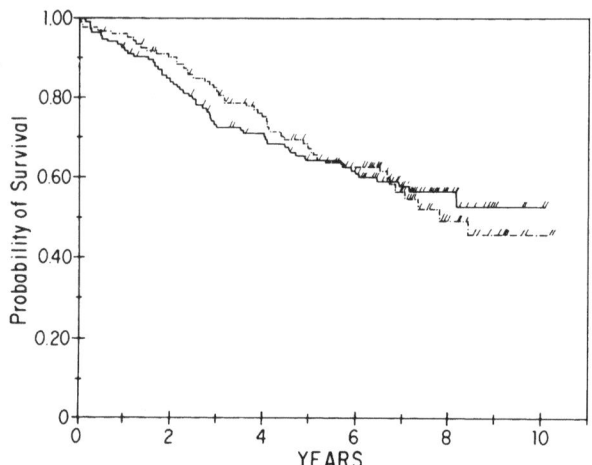

FIGURE 1. COMPARISON OF SURVIVAL IN PATIENTS WITH ER-BIO
POSITIVE (–•–•) VERSUS ER-BIO NEGATIVE (—) TUMORS.
P= NON-SIGNIFICANT. BIOCHEMICAL ASSAY IS POSITIVE IF
$\geq$ 10 FMOL/MG PROTEIN.

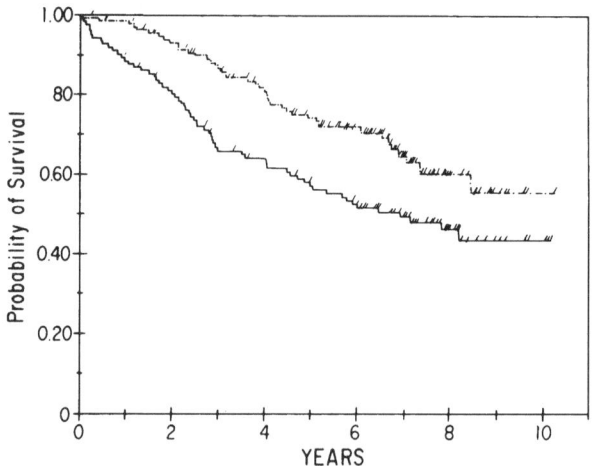

FIGURE 2. COMPARISON OF SURVIVAL IN PATIENTS WITH ER-ICA
POSITIVE (–•–•) VERSUS ER-ICA NEGATIVE (—) TUMORS;
P=0.004. IMMUNOCYTOCHEMICAL ASSAY IS POSITIVE IF HSCORE
$\geq$ 75.

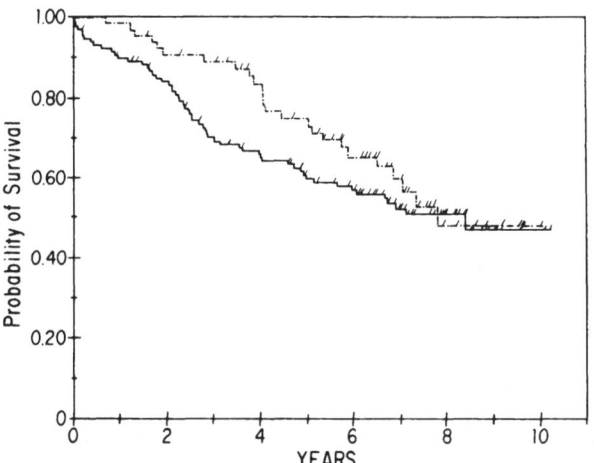

FIGURE 3: COMPARISON OF SURVIVAL IN PATIENTS WITH PGR-BIO
POSITIVE (—•—•) VERSUS PGR-BIO NEGATIVE (—) TUMORS.
P= NON SIGNIFICANT. BIOCHEMICAL ASSAY IS POSITIVE IF
$\geq$ 10 FMOL/MG PROTEIN.

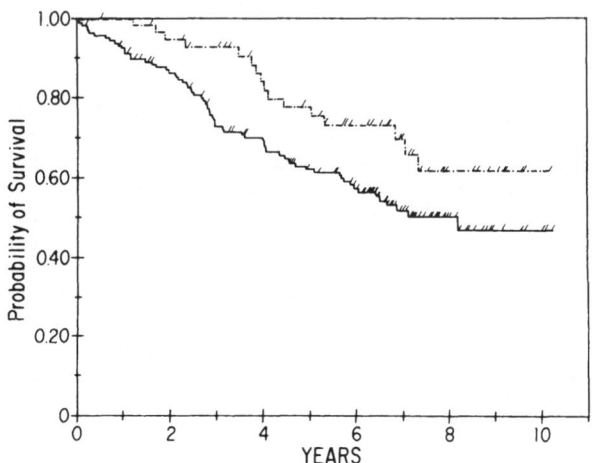

FIGURE 4: COMPARISON OF SURVIVAL IN PATIENTS WITH PGR-ICA
POSITIVE (—•—•) VERSUS PGR-ICA NEGATIVE (—) TUMORS.
P=0.04. IMMUNOCYTOCHEMICAL ASSAY IS POSITIVE IF HSCORE
$\geq$ 75.

groups through only 7 years, PgR-ICA was a significant indicator of survival (p=0.04). The DFI presented with similar trends. Immunocytochemical analysis of ER and PgR separated the cohort consistently over ten years, with advantage for the positive patients. ER-BIO positive tumors showed advantage to three years, PgR-BIO positive over 3.5 years, this advantage was reversed after these periods. Positive tumors showed no advantage for survival or DFI correlated to negative tumors, but two specific subgroups turned out to have predictive value for more favorable prognosis. In DFI, ER-BIO negative, ER-ICA positive tumors were seen with best prognosis, while ER-BIO positive, ER-ICA negative tumors did less well. The survival pattern gave similar results. No specific subgroup was seen using this evaluation for progesterone analysis. Combining ER-BIO and PgR-BIO to separate the cohort for survival, no significant advantage for any group appeared, while separation with immunocytochemical analysis ER-ICA and PgR-ICA positive tumors showed prognostic advantage. Poor prognosis was seen in ER-ICA negative, PgR-ICA positive tumors. While separation within axillary lymph node groups, using categories of negative nodes, one to three nodes positive, four and more involved or skin or muscle infiltration, significant advantage in survival appeared only using H222 in 1-3 nodes positive patients (p=0.03) and in DFI, using PgR-BIO in node negative patients (p=0.04). Separation by lymph node status shows significant differentiation for each group in DFI. Survival gave a similar distribution, but without significant relationship between 1-3 nodes positive versus more than 4 nodes involved.

Dividing the cohort using histologic grade, ER-BIO shows a significant relationship in moderately differentiated tumors (p=0.03), considering DFI. Among poorly differentiated tumors, ER-BIO separates this group in DFI for 3.5 years, in survival for 5 years, with advantage for receptor positive patients, while ER-ICA separates the groups through the ten years of followup, both for DFI and survival (without statistical significance). PgR analyses shows separation using PgR-BIO in DFI for 4 years, and in survival for 7 years.

DISCUSSION

Several studies have suggested sex steroid receptor analyses to have predictive value for DFI and survival in human breast cancer (2,3,4), while others (5,6) have failed to demonstrate a correlation between disease course and steroid receptor content. This study compares the outcome of patients with steroid receptor positive tumors versus those with negative tumors, measured by biochemical and immunocytochemical analyses. Correlations between these methods have been reported by several groups (9,10), but the biochemical ligand assays and the immunocytochemical assays are not identical. The threshold used to assign a tumor as receptor positive is critical both in ICA and for the ligand assay. Using the thresholds of $\geq$ 10 fmol/mg prot for the ligand assays and $\geq$ 75 HSCORE for the ICA's prognostic separation was noted for the ERICA through the 10 years of follow-up with only limited prognostic advantage for PgRICA and for ER and PgR by ligand assays (at these thresholds).

REFERENCES

1)   E.V. Jensen, G.E. Block, S. Smith, K. Kyser, E.R. DeSombre. Estrogen receptors and breast cancer response to adrenalectomy. Natl. Cancer Inst. Monog. 34:55-69, 1971.
2)   W.A. Knight, R.B. Livingston, E.J. Gregory, W.L. McGuire. Estrogen receptor as an independent prognostic factor for early recurrence in breast cancer. Cancer Res. 37: 4669-4671, 1977.

3) T. Cooke, R. Shields, D. George, P. Maynard, K. Griffiths. Oestrogen receptors and prognosis in early breast cancer. Lancet 1: 995-997, 1979.

4) J.C. Allegra, M.E. Lippman, R. Simon, E.B. Thompson, A. Barlock, L. Green, K.K. Huff, H.M.T. Do, S.C. Aitken, and R. Warren. Association between steroid hormone receptor status and disease-free interval in breast cancer. Cancer Treat. Reports 63:1271-1277, 1979.

5) R. Hilf, M.L. Feldstein, S.L. Gibson, and E.D. Savlov. The relative importance of estrogen receptor analysis as a prognostic factor for recurrence or response to chemotherapy in women with breast cancer. Cancer 45:1993-2000, 1980.

6) J.M.M. Raemaekers, L.V.A.M. Beex, A.J.M. Koenders, G.F.F.M. Pieters, A.G.H. Smals, T.J. Benraad, P.W.C. Kloppenborg and The Breast Cancer Group. Disease-free interval and estrogen receptor activity in tumor tissue of patients with primary breast cancer: analysis after long-term follow-up. Breast Cancer Res. Treat. 6:123-130, 1985.

7) R. Sutton, M. Campbell, T. Cooke, R. Nicolson, K. Griffiths and I. Taylor. Predictive power of progesterone receptor status in early breast carcinoma. Br. J. Surg. 74:223-226, 1987.

8) G.A. Gelbfish, A.L. Davidson, S. Kopel, B. Schreibman, J.S. Gelbfish, G.A. Degenshein, B.L. Herz and J.N. Cunningham. Relationship of estrogen and progesterone receptors to prognosis in breast cancer. Ann. Surg. 207:75-78, 1988.

9) K.S. McCarty, Jr., L.S. Miller, E.B. Cox, J. Konrath, K.S. McCarty, Sr. Estrogen receptor analysis. Correlation of biochemical and immunohistochemical methods using monoclonal antireceptor antibodies. Arch. Path. and Lab. Med. 109:716-721, 1985.

10) W.J. King, E.R. DeSombre, E.G. Jensen, G.L. Green. Comparison of immunocytochemical and steroid-binding assays for estrogen receptor in human breast tumors. Cancer Research 45:293-304, 1985.

11) S.M. Thorpe, C. Rose, B.B. Rasmussen, W.J. King, E.R. DeSombre, R.M. Blough, H.F. Mouridsen, N. Rossing and K.W. Andersen. Steroid hormone receptors as prognostic indicators in primary breast cancer. Breast Cancer Res. Treat 7:91-98, 1986.

12) E.R. DeSombre, S.M. Thorpe, C. Rose, R.R. Blough, K.W. Andersen, B.B. Rasmussen, and W.F. King. Prognostic usefulness of estrogen receptor immunocytochemical assays for human breast cancer. Cancer Res. 46:4256s-4264s, 1986.

13) B. Fisher, E.R. Fisher, C. Redmond, A. Brown, and Contributing NSABP Investigators. Tumor nuclear grade, estrogen receptor and progesterone receptor: their value alone or in combination as indicators of outcome following adjuvant therapy for breast cancer. Breast Cancer Res. Treat 7: 147-160, 1986.

14) H.J.G. Bloom, W.W. Richardson. Histological grading and prognosis in breast cancer. Br. J. Cancer 3: 359-377, 1957.

15) E.R. Fisher, R.M. Gregonis, B.R. Fisher. The pathology of invasive breast cancer. A syllabus derived from finding of the National Surgical Adjuvant Breast Project (Protocol No 4), Cancer 36:1-84, 1976.

SIGNIFICANCE OF STEROID RECEPTOR IMMUNOASSAY IN BREAST CANCER

Edward J. Keenan and Debra Corbin

Departments of Pharmacology, Surgery, and Medicine
School of Medicine
The Oregon Health Sciences University
Portland, Oregon

INTRODUCTION

Human breast cancers that contain estrogen (ER) and progesterone (PR) receptors are more likely to respond to antihormone therapy than are carcinomas that lack steroid receptors (1-10). This difference provides the basis for the present use of ER and PR assays in determining the endocrine dependence of breast cancers (8-11). The absence of steroid receptors in breast carcinoma tissue is also of prognostic significance in that receptor-negative tumors generally recur more quickly (12-14).

The commonly employed methods for measuring steroid receptors in cells depend upon the binding of radiolabeled hormone to unoccupied receptors found in the cytosolic fraction of tissue homogenates prepared in hypotonic buffers. The concentration of receptors determined by steroid binding assay (SBA) is therefore an approximation based upon the proportion of occupied and unoccupied receptors in a cytosol. In addition, the measured concentration is an estimate based upon the accuracy of the mathematical extrapolation of the radioligand binding data as frequently achieved by Scatchard plot analysis.

A further problem encountered in determining total steroid receptor concentration in tissues arises from the difficulty in extracting all steroid receptor forms from the nucleus into the cytosolic fraction when using homogenization buffers of low-ionic strength. Extraction of nuclear steroid receptors which are occupied by endogenous hormone requires treatment of nuclei with hypertonic buffer. Quantitation of these occupied receptors subsequently requires assay conditions which permit ligand exchange usually accomplished by elevating the incubation temperature (15). Such conditions may also promote degradation of these temperature-labile proteins and lead to underestimation of nuclear steroid receptor content.

The development of monoclonal antibodies to estrogen and progesterone receptors has provided the opportunity to study these proteins directly and to develop new methodologies to quantitate steroid receptors in the cytosolic and nuclear fractions of breast and other cancers (16-19). These new approaches include a semi-quantitative immunocytochemical procedure (20-23) as well as a quantitative enzyme-linked immunoassay (24-32).

In the present study the conventional steroid binding assay and recently developed immunoassay of estrogen and progesterone receptors were correlated in human breast cancers. In addition, the subcellular distribution of ER in breast tumors was established by immunoassay. Likewise, the effects of estrogen replacement therapy and antiestrogen treatment on concentrations of immunoreactive ER were studied in primary and recurrent breast cancers.

MATERIALS AND METHODS

Tumor specimens were obtained from patients with histologically verified primary or recurrent carcinoma of the breast undergoing biopsy or mastectomy. Fresh tissue specimens were placed on ice, frozen and subsequently maintained at -68 C until processing. Clinical information was sought to establish if patients were receiving exogenous hormones or hormone antagonists at the time of surgery. Some patients were receiving postmenopausal estrogen replacement therapy at diagnosis, which consisted of conjugated estrogen in doses ranging from 0.625-1.25 mg/day. Breast cancer patients who developed recurrent disease while being treated with tamoxifen, an antiestrogenic drug, were receiving 20-40 mg of the drug daily.

Frozen tissues weighing 0.5-2.5 g were minced with a scissors and homogenized (1:10,wt:vol) in TEDG-Mo buffer (0.05 M Tris-HCl, 1.5 mM sodium EDTA, 0.5 mM dithiothreitol, 10% glycerol and 10 mM sodium molybdate, pH = 7.5). Homogenization was accomplished using two bursts (10 seconds) of a precooled Polytron (Brinkman Instruments) at a setting of 5 with a 10-second cooling interval. Tissue homogenates and all reagents were maintained at 0-4 C during processing and assay.

Homogenates were centrifuged at 800 g for 10 minutes to provide a crude nuclear pellet. To prepare the cytosol fraction the supernatant was removed and centrifuged at 40,000 g for 20 minutes. The cytosol fractions for steroid receptor binding assay were then diluted with TEDG-Mo buffer to yield a protein concentration of 2-3 mg/ml as measured by the method of Lowry et al. (33). An aliquot of each cytosol was further diluted to a protein concentration of 0.5-1.0 mg/ml for quantitation of steroid receptors by immunoassay.

The crude nuclear pellets were washed once with TEDG-Mo buffer (5 ml) and a nuclear extract was obtained by resuspending the pellets in a hypertonic buffer, 0.6 M KCl-TEDG-Mo buffer (3 ml), and incubating for 60 minutes. Prior to recentrifugation (40,000 g, 20 min), the nuclear extracts were diluted 1:1 with TEDG-Mo buffer. The protein concentration of the nuclear extracts ranged from 0.5-1.0 mg/ml.

In order to quantitate estrogen receptor levels by steroid binding assay aliquots of cytosol (200 ul) were incubated with 17B-^{3}H-estradiol (spec. act. = 90-110 Ci/mmol, Amersham) ranging from 0.2-4.0 nM final concentration. This binding of radiolabeled estradiol represented total binding capacity. Nonspecific binding of 17B-^{3}H-estradiol was estimated by incubating parallel tubes containing excess, unlabeled diethylstilbestrol (400 nM). Equilibrium binding conditions were established by incubating cytosols for 16-20 hours at 0-4 C. Free and bound radiolabeled estradiol were separated by addition of dextran-coated charcoal. A 200 ul aliquot of charcoal slurry (0.05% dextran - 0.5% charcoal) was added and each tube was vortexed. After a 5-minute incubation, tubes were centrifuged at 1500 g for 10 minutes. Radioactivity in aliquots (200 ul) was quantitated by scintillation counting. The difference between radiolabeled estradiol binding in the absence and presence of unlabeled DES was considered specific 17B-^{3}H-estradiol binding. Specific binding ranged from 40-80% of total tritiated estradiol binding and was considered characteristic of binding to estrogen receptor if the equilibrium dissociation constant (K_D) ranged from 0.01-0.5 nM. The concentration of estrogen binding sites and the affinity of binding were established by Scatchard plot analysis (34).

A similar approach was utilized to quantitate progesterone receptors (PR) in cytosolic fractions. PR was labeled with a range of concentrations (0.5-10.0 nM) of tritiated promegestone (R-5020, spec. act. = 80-100 Ci/mmol, New England Nuclear). Nonspecific binding of radiolabeled R-5020 was estimated by incubating parallel tubes containing excess, unlabeled promegestone (1000 nM). Equilibrium binding conditions were established by incubating for 16-20 hours at 0-4 C. Bound tritiated R-5020 was separated from free radiolabel by adding dextran-coated charcoal and was quantitated as described above. Specific binding of ^{3}H-R5020 represented the difference between total and non-specifically bound radioligand. This binding was considered characteristic of association with progesterone receptor if the K_D for the binding ranged between 0.1 and 4.0 nM. The affinity and concentration of progesterone receptors was determined by Scatchard plot analysis.

ER and PR immunoassay kits were obtained from Abbott Laboratories (North Chicago, Illinois) and the assays were conducted according to the manufacturer's specifications. Breast tumor cytosols or nuclear extracts were incubated with plastic beads coated with either anti-ER or anti-PR monoclonal antibodies for 18 hours at 2-8 C. Immobilized steroid receptors were separated from unbound substances by washing and aspiration. A second specific ER or PR antibody conjugated to horseradish peroxidase was added and a complex of layered antibodies and receptor was formed. After a one hour incubation at 37 C for ER or at 2-8 C for PR, the beads were washed and enzyme substrate (hydrogen peroxide and o-phenylenediamine - 2 HCl) was added producing a colorimetric reaction which proceeded for 30 minutes (25 C) and was terminated by the addition of sulfuric acid (1N). The color intensity was proportional to the concentration of steroid receptor and was quantitated spectrophotometrically at 492 3

nM. Receptor concentration was determined from a standard
curve of human ER or PR run simultaneously.

RESULTS

Linear regression analysis of cytosolic ER levels
determined by steroid binding assay (SBA) and enzyme-linked
immunoassay (EIA) in 110 ER-positive (ER > 10 fmol/mg
protein) and ER-negative primary breast cancers revealed a
strong correlation (r = 0.99) and the slope of the
regression line equaled 0.99. A comparison of the cytosolic
ER concentrations in the ER-positive tissues as quantitated
by SBA and EIA is presented in Table 1. Both assays revealed
approximately 4-fold higher concentrations of cytosolic ER in
primary tumors obtained from older patients (>50 years) as
compared to younger patients. The concentration of
cytosolic ER measured in older and younger patients was
similar by either SBA or EIA. Menopausal estrogen
replacement therapy was not associated with a significant
difference in the concentrations of cytosolic ER in primary
breast cancers when compared to ER levels in the untreated
older patient population. EIA and SBA of ER detected similar
levels of cytosolic ER in tumors which were diagnosed in
patients receiving menopausal estrogen replacement. In
contrast, evaluation of recurrent disease sites from patients
receiving tamoxifen, an antiestrogenic drug, revealed a
discrepancy between SBA and EIA in the quantitation of
cytosolic ER. SBA failed to detect ER (> 10 fmol/mg protein)
in these tissues. However, significant concentrations (174 $\pm$
43 fmol/mg protein) of immunoreactive ER were revealed in
each of the specimens.

TABLE 1

Cytosolic Estrogen Receptor Concentrations in Human
Breast Cancer as Quantitated by Steroid Binding
Assay (SBA) and Immunoassay (EIA)

Age/Treatment	N	Cytosolic Estrogen Receptor (fmol/mg protein)	
		SBA	EIA
< 50 years	22	41 $\pm$ 6	51 $\pm$ 7
> 50 years	53	181 $\pm$ 25	185 $\pm$ 21
Estrogen	21	118 $\pm$ 19	137 $\pm$ 21
Tamoxifen	6	< 10	174 $\pm$ 43

Data expressed as $\bar{X}$ + SEM

The subcellular distribution and total concentration of
ER in primary and recurrent breast cancers as determined by

EIA are presented in Table 2. In contrast to cytosolic ER
levels no distinct age-related differences in nuclear ER
concentration were observed in primary breast cancer.
However, a proportionately lower fraction of the total ER was
found in the nuclear extracts of tumors from older patients.
Only 20% of the total ER was associated with the nuclear
fraction in tumors obtained from patients older than 50 years
of age. Furthermore, estrogen replacement therapy was not
associated with increased levels of salt-extractable nuclear
ER. In addition to significant levels of immunoreactive
cytosolic ER detected in metastatic tumor sites obtained from
patients receiving tamoxifen at the time of cancer
progression, EIA also revealed substantial levels of nuclear
ER in these specimens (2.5 ± 0.8 pmol/g).

TABLE 2

Subcellular Distribution of Estrogen Receptors
in Human Breast Cancer Determined by Immunoassay

Age/Treatment	N	Estrogen Receptor (pmol/g)		
		Cytosol	Nucleus	Total
< 50 years	5	0.3 ± 0.06	0.6 ± 0.2	0.9 ± 0.2
> 50 years	7	2.5 ± 0.5	0.6 ± 0.1	3.1 ± 0.5
Estrogen	32	2.1 ± 0.3	0.5 ± 0.1	2.5 ± 0.3
Tamoxifen	6	4.4 ± 1.8	2.5 ± 0.8	6.9 ± 2.4

Data expressed as $\bar{X}$ + SEM

Analysis of total ER levels, i.e. cytosolic and nuclear,
demonstrated that the concentrations of immunoreactive ER in
primary tumors from older patients were approximately 3-fold
higher than observed in tumors from younger patients (Table
2). Estrogen replacement therapy did not influence total ER
levels. The total concentration of ER in recurrent disease
sites obtained from patients receiving antiestrogen therapy
was higher than observed in primary cancers obtained from
young as well as older patients (Table 2).

In contrast to the effects upon tumor ER content, estrogen
replacement therapy was associated with approximately 3-fold
higher levels of cytosolic PR as determined by SBA (Table 3).
Concentrations of cytosolic PR in metastatic sites obtained
from patients receiving tamoxifen were also elevated and were
similar to PR levels observed in patients receiving estrogen
replacement at the time of diagnosis.

Linear regression analysis of cytosolic PR determined in
44 specimens by SBA and EIA revealed a strong correlation
($r = 0.97$) with a slope of regression equal to 1.10. A
comparison of cytosolic PR concentrations in PR-positive
(PR > 10 fmol/mg protein) specimens as determined by SBA and
EIA is shown in Table 4. Similar concentrations of cytosolic

PR were detected by both assays. Furthermore, cytosolic PR levels in primary tumors were not influenced by patient age.

TABLE 3

Effect of Estrogen Replacement Therapy or Tamoxifen on Cytosolic Progesterone Receptor Concentrations in Human Breast Cancer.

Treatment	N	Cytosolic Progesterone Receptor (pmol/g)
None	11	2.8 ± 1.1
Estrogen	31	12.4 ± 4.7
Tamoxifen	4	15.8 ± 9.7

Data expressed as $\bar{X}$ + SEM

TABLE 4

Cytosolic Progesterone Receptor Concentrations in Human Breast Cancer as Quantitated by Steroid Binding Assay (SBA) and Immunoassay (EIA)

Age	N	Cytosolic Progesterone Receptor (fmol/mg protein)	
		SBA	EIA
< 50 years	8	152 ± 44	189 ± 58
> 50 years	20	101 ± 28	95 ± 27

Data expressed as $\bar{X}$ + SEM

DISCUSSION

The immunoassay of steroid receptors is a rapid, reproducible, sensitive and specific approach to the quantitation of these proteins in normal and neoplastic tissues. Since the immunological evaluation of steroid receptors is independent of the state of receptor occupancy, immunoassay is also useful in assessing the influences of hormones and hormone antagonists on the apparent subcellular distribution of steroid receptors as well as in regulating steroid receptor concentration.

It is clearly evident from the present study that the enzyme-linked immunoassay (EIA) of cytosolic estrogen and progesterone receptors in human breast cancers is quantitatively equivalent to estimates derived from conventional steroid binding assay (SBA). While patient age influences both the SBA and EIA of cytosolic ER, PR values in

the soluble fraction are not affected by patient age.
Cytosolic ER levels in breast tumors from younger patients
(< 50 years) are approximately one-third the concentration of
ER detected in primary breast cancers from postmenopausal
patients.

Employing immunoassay to quantitate nuclear ER extracted
with hypertonic buffer reveals similar levels of receptor in
both age groups. Consequently, the lower concentrations of
cytosolic ER seen in tumors from younger patients are
seemingly unrelated to the accumulation of nuclear ER that
might be mediated by the plasma estrogens present in the
premenopausal state. Instead the age-related differences in
ER content in breast cancer must be attributed to an as yet
unrecognized cellular regulatory process. This likelihood is
further supported by results of the present studies in which
postmenopausal estrogen replacement therapy did not
significantly influence total ER content as evaluated by
immunoassay. Nor did estrogen treatment increase the immunoreactive nuclear ER concentration compared to untreated
postmenopausal patients.

The role of estrogen in these carcinomas is suggested
by the 3-fold higher levels of cytosolic PR, an estrogen-
dependent protein, which are present in tumors obtained from
patients receiving estrogen replacement therapy at the time
of diagnosis. The inability to detect increased levels of
immunoreactive ER in nuclear salt extracts despite the
apparent induction of PR by estrogen replacement therapy may
be related to the retention of a salt resistant form of ER
perhaps in association with the nuclear matrix (35). The
fact that the SBA and EIA measure similar concentrations of
cytosolic and salt-extractable nuclear ER in tumors from
estrogen-treated patients suggests that conjugated estrogens
(principally estrone) do not produce prolonged occupancy of
ER. Estrone does exhibit a significantly lower affinity for
ER as compared to 17B-estradiol which would contribute to an
increased tendency for estrone to dissociate from the
estrogen receptor (15).

In distinct contrast only the ER immunoassay detected
significant levels of cytosolic ER in tumor tissue obtained
from patients whose tumors progressed while being treated
with tamoxifen, an antiestrogenic drug. The ER binding assay
failed to detect cytosolic ER in these specimens. One
explanation for this observation is the occupancy of ER by
tamoxifen or a metabolite in a manner which is not readily
reversible. Consequently, the cytosolic ER is identified
immunologically but binding of radiolabeled estradiol is
precluded. If the immunoreactive ER present in these
tissues is a complex of the antiestrogen and receptor then
its primary localization in the cytosolic fraction suggests
that the complex is loosely associated with nuclei prior to
cell disruption. Current evidence supports the view that ER
is principally if not exclusively localized to nuclei but
exists in either a low or high affinity form within the
nucleus (36). Presumably the low affinity, nuclear
antiestrogen-ER complex is extracted into the cytosolic
fraction during in vitro studies utilizing hypotonic assay
buffers. In studies using rat uterine ER tamoxifen
administration has previously been shown to induce an altered

155

form of cytosolic ER which is also only revealed by immunoassay (38). However, it has been recently suggested that tamoxifen and its active metabolite, 4-hydroxytamoxifen, enhance the immunoreactivity of ER to one of the monoclonal antibodies (H222) used in the ER immunoassay (37).

Significant levels of ER are also present as a salt-extracted form in the nuclear fraction derived from tumors in patients progressing while receiving tamoxifen. Therefore, the total ER content of these sites is approximately 2-fold higher than observed in primary breast carcinomas arising in untreated patients of comparable age (> 50 years). It is not presently clear if tumor relapse in patients receiving tamoxifen is related to an increase in cellular ER induced in response to antiestrogen treatment. Such a phenomenon could conceivably lead to increased sensitivity of the tumor cells to estrogen or to an incomplete antiestrogen-mediated blockade of receptor function. It is interesting that recent evidence indicates that tamoxifen treatment increases plasma levels of estrogen in some breast cancer patients (39). Consequently, a combination of increased tumor cell ER and circulating estrogens could contribute to override antiestrogenic drug action and result in estrogen-mediated tumor relapse.

Consistent with the concept that initial breast tumor relapse occurring during tamoxifen therapy might be driven by estrogen is the observation in the present studies that cytosolic PR levels are elevated in these tumors. In fact the levels of PR in the cytosol are comparable to those concentrations observed in tumors obtained from patients receiving estrogen replacement. It should be emphasized that, at present, caution should be exercised in making comparisons of the ER and PR content between primary and recurrent breast cancers since differences in the degree of tumor cellularity in primary and metastatic tissue could contribute to differences in steroid receptor concentrations when normalized for tissue weight.

Immunoassay of ER and PR facilitates quantitation of total cellular receptor since the immunological assay is independent of endogenous hormone or exogenously administered drugs. This methodology represents a suitable and practical approach to the study of ER and PR and to the clinical utilization of ER and PR in establishing the endocrine dependence of neoplastic diseases. Importantly, this technology provides a valuable means of defining the factors which regulate ER and PR in normal and malignant tissues and may provide the basis for understanding the failure of anti-estrogen therapy in some breast cancer patients.

REFERENCES

1. E.V. Jensen, G.E. Block, S. Smith, K. Kyser, and E.R. DeSombre, Estrogen receptors and breast cancer response to adrenalectomy, Natl Cancer Inst Monograph 34:55-70, (1971).

2. H. Maass, B. Engel, H. Hohmeister, F. Lehmann, and G. Trams, Estrogen receptors in human breast cancer tissue, Am J Obstet Gynecol 113:377-382, (1972).

3. E. Engelsman, J.P. Persijn, C.B. Korsten, and F.J. Cleton, Oestrogen receptors in human breast cancer tissue and response to endocrine therapy, Br Med J 2:750-752, (1973).

4. B.S. Leung, W.S. Fletcher, T.D. Lindel, D.C. Wood, and W.W. Krippaehne, Pedictability of response to endocrine ablation in advanced breast carcinoma, Arch Surg 106:515-519, (1973).

5. E.D. Savlov, J.L. Wittliff, R. Hilf, and T.C. Hall, Correlations between certain biochemical properties of breast cancer and response to therapy: A preliminary report, Cancer 33:303-309, (1974).

6. W.L. McGuire, P.P. Carbone, and E.P. Vollmer (eds.), "Estrogen Receptors in Human Breast Cancer", Raven Press, New York (1975).

7. C.K. Osborne, M.G. Yochmowitz, W.A. Knight III, W.L. McGuire, The value of estrogen and progesterone receptors in the treatment of breast cancer, Cancer 46:2884-2888, (1980).

8. K. Seibert, M. Lippman, Hormone receptors in breast cancer, Clinics in Oncology 1:735-794, (1982).

9. J.L. Wittliff, Steroid hormone receptors in breast cancer, Cancer 53:630-643, (1984).

10. E.R. DeSombre, P.P. Carbone, E.V. Jensen, W.L. McGuire, S.A. Wells Jr., J.L. Wittliff, and M.B. Lipsett, Steroid receptors in breast cancer, N Engl J Med 301:1011-1012, (1979).

11. W.L. McGuire and G.M. Clark, Role of progesterone receptors in breast cancer, Seminars in Oncology 12:12-16, (1985).

12. W.A. Knight, R.B. Livingston, E.J. Gregory, and W.L. McGuire, Estrogen receptor as an independent prognostic factor for early recurrence in breast cancer, Cancer Res 37:4669-4671, (1977).

13. P.V. Maynard, R.W. Blamey, C.W. Elston, J.L. Haybittle, and K. Griffiths, Estrogen receptor assay in primary breast cancer and early recurrence of the disease, Cancer Res 38:4292-4295, (1978).

14. R. Hahnel, T. Woodings, and A.B. Vivian, Prognostic value of estrogen receptors in primary breast cancer, Cancer 44:671-675, (1979).

15. J.H. Clark and E.J. Peck, "Female Sex Steroids: Receptors and Function", Springer-Verlag, New York (1979).

16. G.L. Greene, C. Nolan, J.P. Engler, and E.V. Jensen, Monoclonal antibodies as probes for estrogen receptor detection and characterization, J Steroid Biochem 16:353-359, (1982).

17. G.L. Greene, C. Nolan, J.P. Engler, and E.V. Jensen, Monoclonal antibodies to human estrogen receptor, Proc Natl Acad Sci, U.S.A., 77:5115-5119, (1980).

18. G.L. Greene, F.W. Fitch, and E.V. Jensen, Monoclonal antibodies to estrophilin: Probes for the study of estrogen receptors, Proc Natl Acad Sci, U.S.A., 77:157-161, (1980).

19. G.L. Greene, N.B. Sobel, W.J. King, and E.V. Jensen, Immunochemical studies of estrogen receptors, J Steroid Biochem 20:51-56, (1984).

20. W.J. King, E.R. DeSombre, E.V. Jensen, and G.L. Greene, A comparison of immunocytochemical and steroid-binding assays for estrogen receptor in human breast tumors, Cancer Res 45:293-304, (1985).

21. L.P. Pertshuk, K.B. Eisenberg, A.C. Carter, and J.G. Feldman, Immunohistologic localization of estrogen receptors in breast cancer with monoclonal antibodies, Cancer 55:1513-1518, (1985).

22. K.S. McCarty Jr., L.S. Miller, E.B. Cox, J. Konrath, and K.S. McCarty Sr., Estrogen receptor analysis. Correlation of biochemical and immunohistochemical methods using monoclonal antireceptor antibodies. Arch Pathol Lab Med 109:716-721, (1985).

23. E.R. DeSombre, S.M. Thorpe, C. Rose, R.R. Blough, K.W. Andersen, B.B. Rasmussen, and W.J. King, Prognostic usefullness of estrogen receptor immunocytochemical assays for human breast cancer, Cancer Res 46:4256s-4264s, (1986).

24. C. Nolan, L.W. Przywara, L.S. Miller, V. Suduikis, and J.T. Tomita, A sensitive solid-phase enzyme immunoassay for human estrogen receptor, in: "Current Controversies in Breast Cancer," F.C. Ames, G.R. Blumenschein and E.D. Montague, eds., University of Texas Press, Austin (1984).

25. V.C. Jordon, H.I. Jacobson, and E.J. Keenan, Determination of estrogen receptor in breast cancer using monoclonal antibody technology: Results of a multicenter study in the United States, Cancer Res 46:4237s-4240s, (1986).

26. M.J. Duffy, L. O'Slorain, B. Waldron, and C.Smith, Estradiol receptors in human breast carcinomas assayed by use of monoclonal antibodies, Clin Chem 32:1972-1974, (1986).

27. J.A. Holt and J. Bolanos, Enzyme-linked immunochemical measurement of estrogen receptor in gynecologic tumors, and an overview of steroid receptors in ovarian carcinoma, Clin Chem 32:1836-1843, (1986).

28. S.M. Thorpe, Monoclonal antibody technique for detection of estrogen receptors in human breast cancer: Greater sensitivity and more accurate classification of receptor status than the dextran-coated charcoal method, Cancer Res 47:6572-6575, (1987).

29. C.M. Smyth, D.E. Benn, and T.S. Reeve, An enzyme immunoassay compared with a ligand-binding assay for measuring progesterone receptors in cytosols from breast cancers, Clin Chem 34:1116-1118, (1988).

30. J.T. Wu and L.W. Wilson, Progesterone receptor: Stability studies and correlation between steroid binding assay and enzyme immunoassay, Clin Chem 34:1987-1991, (1988).

31. S.M. Thorpe, Immunological quantitation of nuclear receptors in human breast cancer: Relation to cytosolic estrogen and progesterone receptors, Cancer Res 47:1830-1835, (1987).

32. B.G. Mobbs and I.E. Johnson, Use of an enzymeimmunoassay (EIA) for quantitation of cytosolic and nuclear estrogen receptor, and correlation with progesterone receptor in human breast cancer, J Steroid Biochem 28:653-662, (1987).

33. O.H. Lowry, N.J. Rosebrough, A.L. Farr, and R.J. Randall, Protein measurement with the Folin phenol reagent, J Biol Chem 193:265-275, (1951).

34. G. Scatchard, The attractions of proteins for small molecules and ions, Ann NY Acad Sci 51:660-672, (1949).

35. E.R. Barrack and D.S. Coffey, Biological properties of the nuclear matrix: Steroid hormone binding, Recent Prog Horm Res 38:133-195, (1982).

36. M.R. Walters, Steroid hormone receptors and the nucleus, Endocrine Rev 6:512-543, (1985).

37. M.Nakao, B. Sato, M. Koga, K. Noma, S. Kishimoto, and K. Matsumoto, Identification of immunoassayable estrogen receptor lacking hormone binding ability in tamoxifen-treated rat uterus, Biochem and Biophys Res Comm 132:336-342, (1985).

38. P.M. Martin, Y. Berthois, and E.V. Jensen, Binding of antiestrogens exposes an occult antigenic determinant in the human estrogen receptor, Proc Natl Acad Sci, U.S.A., 85:2533-2537, (1988).

39. R.F. Pommier, E.A. Woltering, E.J. Keenan, and W.S. Fletcher, The mechanism of hormone-sensitive breast cancer progression on antiestrogen therapy, Arch Surg 122:1311-1316, (1987).

H23 MONOCLONAL ANTIBODY RECOGNIZES A BREAST TUMOR ASSOCIATED

ANTIGEN: CLINICAL AND MOLECULAR STUDIES

I. Tsarfaty*, S. Chaitchik**, M. Hareuveni*,
J. Horev*. A. Hizi[+], D.H. Wreschner* and I. Keydar*

*Department of Microbiology, the George S. Wise
Faculty of Life Sciences, Tel Aviv University, Tel
Aviv, Israel, [+]Department of Histology and Cell
Biology, Sackler School of Medicine, Tel Aviv
University, **Department of Oncology, Tel Aviv Medical
Center Sackler School of Medicine, Tel Aviv University

ABSTRACT

A monoclonal antibody (MoAb) H23 was generated in our laboratory
against particles released by the T47D cell line. H23 MoAb
recognized specific antigens in 90% of 590 breast tumor biopsies
tested by the indirect immunoperoxidase test. Furthermore, the H23
MoAb detects antigens in sera and body fluids of patients with
breast carcinoma. The level of serum antigen in 546 individuals
tested correlates with the clinical status of the disease and with
poor survival. The cDNA coding for the epitope recognized by H23
MoAb was isolated from a cDNA expression library and its sequence
and orientation established. The nucleotide sequence showed that
the cDNA insert was composed of 60 bp tandem repeats. We have
analyzed the RNA isolated from primary human tumors, and it was
demonstrated that breast carcinomas expressed the highest levels of
mRNA species hybridizing with this cDNA. The gene coding for the
cDNA was isolated from a genomic library and encompasses 7.5 kb. A
2.3 kb segment of this gene was found to be an array of tandem 60 bp
repeat units whilst the remaining parts of the gene do not contain
these repeats. The fact that these non-repeat sequences hybridize
to identical mRNA species, has led to ongoing studies aimed at their
further characterization.

INTRODUCTION

Tumor specific markers are invaluable for diagnostic,
prognostic, as well as for therapeutic purposes. Breast cancer
being one of the leading causes of death, influenced many
researchers in looking for a specific marker for this neoplasia.
Over the past years, several MoAbs directed against tumor associated
antigens have been established with different degrees of specificity
for breast tumor cells (1,2). Several immunogens have been used to
generate MoAbs reactive with human tumors such as milk fat globule
membranes and human mammary tumor cell lines. (3-6). Human-mouse
hybridomas were prepared also using either lymph nodes from
mastectomized patients (7), or lymphocytes from donors containing

high titers of antibodies to MMTV or HuMTV (8,9). The T47D cell
line established in our laboratory after induction with steroid
hormones, produce particles (HuMTV) with some retroviral
properties: buoyant density, presence of single stranded RNA and
reverse transcriptase activity. Since the T47D cells as well as the
particles are recognized by the MoAb against MMTV gp52 (10), we
decided to purify this fraction on a sucrose gradient and to use it
as an immunogen to generate MoAbs.

In this paper we describe one of the resulting hybridomas,
designated H23, producing γ1 mouse IgG, its clinical application
and its use in molecular studies.

MATERIALS AND METHODS

Generation of the H23 monoclonal antibodies

The H23 MoAbs were raised against particles secreted by the T47D
cell line into culture medium and purified on sucrose gradient
(10). Splenocytes from the immunized mice were fused with mouse
myeloma X63-Ag8.653 cells according to the procedure described by
Kohler and Milstein (11). The hybridomas obtained were screened for
their ability to produce mouse immunoglobulins recognizing the HuMTV
antigens (I.K. et al. in press).

The indirect immunoperoxidase technique (IPT)

Immunohistochemical staining was performed on paraffin embedded
5μ thick tissue sections (12). The tissue blocks were received
from the pathology departments of 2 different hospitals: The
Ichilov Medical Center and the Sheba Medical Center. The human
tissues included either biopsies or surgically removed tumors. The
H23 MoAb IgG was used at a concentration of 10 ug/ml in PBS and the
secondary antibody - peroxidase conjugated anti-mouse IgG (Sigma) at
50 ug/ml in PBS. Cells were scored positive only if the staining
was cytoplasmic.

Enzyme linked immunosorbent assay (ELISA)

Nunc immunoplate wells were coated with 200 ul of MoAb H23 at a
concentration of 10 ug/ml in 0.05 M sodium bicarbonate buffer pH 9.6
and incubated for two hours at 37°C followed by extensive washing in
PBS containing 0.1% Brij-35 at 4°C. Patient sera or body fluids
(200 ul) were added at dilutions of 1:2, 1:4, 1:8, 1:16 and 1:32 in
PBS and the plates were incubated at 4°C over night. After
extensive washing as above, alkaline phosphatase conjugated H23 MoAb
was added and incubated 2 h at 37°C. After thorough washing 200 ul
of substrate (0.6 mg/ml p-nitrophenyl phosphate) was added to each
well. The product of the enzymatic reaction was determined from the
absorbance at 405 nm. HuMTV was used as reaction was determined
from the absorbance at 405 nm. HuMTV was used as the positive
control. The results were automatically recorded from the Dynatech
spectrophotometer on to an IBM PC computer. The antigen level at
each dilution was expressed as the ratio between the A405 of the
sample tested and that of the HuMTV antigen control. The antigen
level in the undiluted sample was calculated as the geometrical mean
of these ratios obtained at the five dilutions.

Statistical evaluation of the data obtained from the ELISA test
was based on the Student t-test. The survival analysis was
performed by the life table method according to computer program SAS

"lifereg" using the IBM 370 computer of the TAU Computer Center. Sera from healthy women was obtained from 3 kibbutzim, and the patients' sera from the Department of Oncology at the Ichilov Medical Center.

RNA analysis

RNA was extracted from tumor frozen tissues surgically removed using the guanidine thiocyanate/cesium chloride method. Poly-A RNA was purfied by oligo (dT) cellulose chromotography. For dot blot analysis 15 ug of each sample of total RNA was applied with gentle vacuum in 200 ul of 2X SSC (1X SSC is 0.15M NaCl and 0.015M sodium citrate) to a Gelman nylon membrane using the BRL dot blot apparatus. The RNA samples were covalently bound to the nylon membrane by UV irradiation followed by baking at 80°C under vacuum. The blots were prehybridized and probed at 42°C for 16 hours in 40% formamide, 5X SSC, 0.1% polyvinylpyrillidone, 0.1% Ficoll, 0.2% SDS and 100 ug/ml denatured salmon sperm DNA with cDNA inserts labelled by nick translation to a specific activity of $2-5 \times 10^8$ cpm/ug. A final concentration of $1-2 \times 10^6$ cpm (Cerenkov counts/ml) was used. Following hybridization, the blots were washed at 65° for 2-4 hours with several changes of 2X SSC, 0.2% SDS followed by stringent washing at 65°C (2x30 min) with 0.2X SSC, 0.5% SDS. Quantification of the hybridization intensity was performed with LKB 222-020 Ultrascan XL II laser densitometer. Bound probes were removed by washing of blots in hybridization buffer at 70°C for 60 min and the membranes were then rehybridized with a different probe under similar conditions.

RESULTS AND DISCUSSION

Detection of antigen in breast tumor cells by H23 MoAb

The H23 MoAb was first characterized by its ability to recognize the T47D cells and the released particles. H23 MoAb reacted with antigens localized on the live cell membranes as demonstrated by the FACS assay. Furthermore, the antigen seems very stable since it can be demonstrated in the cell cytoplasm of T47D cells embedded in paraffin (I.K. et al., in press). Given the stability of this antigen during fixation and paraffin embedding a large survey of 812 patients' paraffin block sections was performed using the indirect immunoperoxidase technique (IPT).

Given the high percentage of breast tumor detection by the immunoperoxidase technique, it was obvious to enquire about the location of this antigen on the live tumor cells. Tumor cells were collected from pleural effusions of patients with metastatic breast cancer and from the effusion of patients with carcinoma of the lung. The live cells were assayed with FITC labelled H23 MoAb. The breast tumor cells showed fluorescence on the cell membrane. No fluorescence was detected on the lung tumor cells. Furthermore, the fluorescent staining was abolished when H23 MoAb was preabsorbed with the HuMTV antigens (data not shown).

Does H23 MoAb recognize antigens in body fluids?

It is likely that an antigen found on the cell membrane might be shed off into the surrounding fluid. To determine if H23 MoAb can detect antigens in body fluids, an ELISA assay was performed with patient sera and healthy female sera. Fig. 2 represents the results obtained.

163

Table 1. Indirect Immunoperoxidase Staining of Human Malignant and Normal Tissues with the H23 MoAb

Total cases tested: 812

	Positive
Normal breast tissue	0/45
Normal tissues (other than breast)	0/22
Benign breast tissue	1/56
Breast adenocarcinomas	532/590
Breast metastases to: lymph node	19/19
ovary	5/5
lung	4/4
bone	1/1
Carcinomas of other organs:	
colon	0/26
kidney	0/4
ovary	0/3
skin	0/3
thyroid	0/3
lung	0/2
prostate	0/1
liver	0/1
uterus	0/9
stomach	0/9
bladder	0/9

Table 1 demonstrates that we were able to detect the antigen in 532 cases out of 590 cases studied (90.2%). Most of the cases under study were infiltrating ductal carcinomas. The other histological types were intraductal, infiltrating lobular, medullary and tubular carcinomas. As for the 58 breast carcinomas in which we did not detect antigen, we could not find any correlation to a given histological type or to the clinical stage of the disease. The amount of cells stained and the intensity of staining varied and does not seem to correlate with histological type. In all 29 metastatic cases the cytoplasmic antigen was detected in the tumor cells. None of the other cases listed in Table 1 showed detectable cytoplasmic antigen, although in several cases, we could observe some apical dark lining that we did not score as positive. One benign tumor, an epitheliosis, showed clear cytoplasmic staining. The other benign breast tumors of the following histological types (fibrocystic, fibroadenomas, papillomatosis and sclerosis adenosis) did not contain detectable cytoplasmic antigen. Neither did we detect cytoplasmic antigen in normal tissues or in the 70 malignancies other than breast tested. Fig. 1 shows an example of the immunoperoxidase staining of an infiltrating ductal carcinoma section.

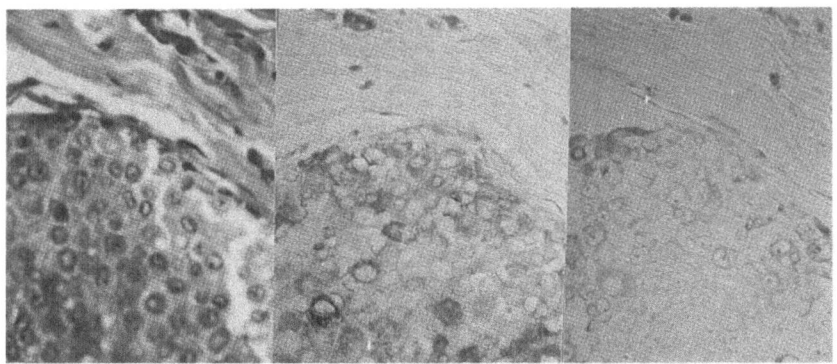

Fig 1. Indirect immunoperoxidase test on infiltrating ductal carcinoma sections with the H23 MoAb. A. H α E staining; B. IPT staining - note the cytoplasmic staining; C. H23 MoAb preabsorbed with HuMTV antigen - note abolishment of staining. (x250)

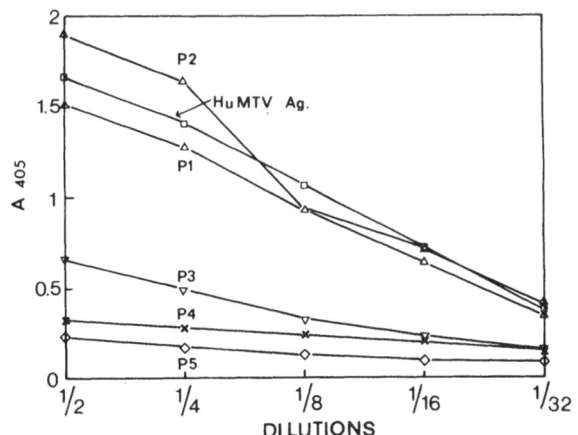

Fig 2. ELISA of H23 MoAb with human sera. The sera was diluted and analyzed by ELISA with H23 MoAb (see methods). HuMTV antigen − positive control. P1, P2-breast cancer patients with metastases.

P3-breast cancer patient without known metastases. P4-healthy
woman. P5-a patient with lung carcinoma.

Sera of patients with breast cancer contained higher levels of
antigen as compared to the healthy counterparts. The results
obtained in the preliminary ELISA assays encouraged us to undertake
a large study of plasma, sera and other body fluids (pleural
effusions or ascitic fluids) from patients with carcinoma of the
breast without known metastases (M0), breast cancer patients with
known metastases (M1), and age matched healthy woman (H0). The
levels of antigen recognized by H23 MoAb (in the 3 different groups)
were compared, and correlated with the clinical status and survival
of the breast cancer patients.

Table 2 represents the p values for the pairwise comparison of
antigen levels between the different groups

Groups	Number of individuals	P values for pairwise comparison
Healthy women (HO)	401	HO vs. MO <0.02
Breast Ca. patients without known metastases (MO)	360	HO vs. M1 <0.0001
Breast Ca. patients with metastases (M1)	127	MO vs. M1 <0.0001

The most striking finding was that the antigen levels in the M1
(breast cancer with metastases) population was elevated as compared
to the antigen levels detected in the M0 (breast cancer patient with
no evidence of metastases) with a p<0.0001.

Fig. 3 represents the survival curves of breast carcinoma patients according to highest grade obtained during the follow-up of the patients (70 months).

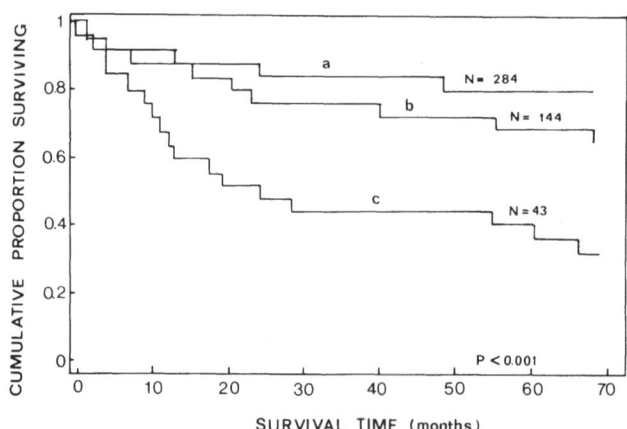

Fig 3. Survival rate of breast cancer patients according to the
antigen levels detected by H23 MoAb in their sera. The survival
analysis was performed on a group of 471 patients according to the
period of time they lived following the maximum antigen level
detected in their sera (70 months follow-up).

The population was divided into 3 groups according to the antigen levels detected. Group a (284) patients had antigen levels that were not different from those seen in the healthy population, whilst groups b (144 patients) and c (43 patients) represents patients with moderately and highly elevated antigen levels, respectively. It can be seen that there is a high correlation between the antigen level detected and survival rate, thus demonstrating that the level of antigen may be a prognostic indicator for survival of breast cancer patients. Breast tumor associated antigens found in the circulation of patients with this neoplasia were reported by several groups (13, 14, 15). It has to be defined whether these antigens are all coded for by one gene or possibly a family of similar genes.

Isolation of the cDNA and gene coding for the H23 Recognized Antigen

In addition to the detection of antigens in the body fluids of breast carcinoma patients and in their tumor cells, the H23 MoAb was used for isolating a cDNA fragment coding for the antigenic epitope. This cDNA was then used for isolating a genomic fragment that codes for this antigen.

The cDNA was identified by screening with H23 MoAb. A λ gt11 cDNA expression library prepared with mRNA isolated from T47D human breast carcinoma cells was kindly supplied by Prof. Chambon. This procedure resulted in H23 immunoreactive clones. Preliminary investigations had indicated that mRNA species hybridizing with one of the cDNA inserts thus obtained (designated 3b) were overexpressed in breast carcinoma tissue. A more extensive analysis involving samples from 8 malignant breast tumors, 5 benign breast tissues and 15 non-breast tumors and adjacent "normal" tissue of epithelial origin (including stomach, colon, bladder, lung and kidney) demonstrated that, on the average, cDNA insert hybridizing mRNA species were expressed 7 to 8 fold in the breast carcinomas compared to the other samples. (Fig. 4) Some individual breast tumor RNA samples demonstrated a hybridization signal that was 20 - 25 fold higher to that seen in adjacent "normal" breast tissue (M.H. et al., submitted).

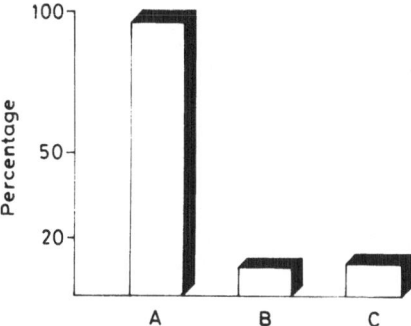

Fig 4. Analysis of dot blot hybridization with 3b cDNA of RNA samples isolated from benign and malignant breast tissue and other
(Continued)

Nucleotide sequencing of the cDNA inserts revealed that they were completely composed of 60 bp tandem repeating units. This unit was GC rich with strand preference for the C or G nucleotides. A similar although not identical sequence has been recently published (16). We do not know whether the differences arise because we are dealing with a different epitope or whether the two cDNAs code for similar but distinct proteins.

A cDNA, pMUC 10, that also codes for a breast tumor associated antigen and contains a 60 bp tandem repeat unit has been also reported (17), but as no sequence data was presented, we cannot make a direct comparison. We determined which cDNA strand codes for the antigen epitope by probing a Northern blot containing tumor RNA with synthetic oligo-nucleotides complementary to either strand of the repeat unit. This analysis showed that only one synthetic strand hybridized to mRNA species and gave an identical hybridization pattern to that observed with the complete cDNA insert (D.H.W. et al., submitted).

In order to isolate and thus characterize the gene coding for the tumor antigen, genomic libraries prepared from T47D and MCF7 human breast carcinoma cell lines were screened with the cDNA inserts described above (I.T. in preparation). A 7.5 kb gene was thus isolated and characterized by restriction enzyme mapping and partial nucleotide sequencing. A 2.3 kb fragment of this gene was also completely composed of a 60 bp tandem repeating unit. Obviously this fragment gave an identical Northern blot hybridization to that seen following probing with the cDNA insert (I.T. et al., in preparation). However, other non-repeat genomic fragments also hybridized to the same mRNA species, and we are thus presently characterizing the non-repeat elements both of the gene and cDNA (D.H.W. et al., in preparation).

CONCLUSIONS

H23 MoAb was generated against particulate antigens released by T47D human breast carcinoma cells. This antibody specifically recognized 90.2% of all malignant breast tumors examined. This antibody also detects antigen in the sera of breast cancer patients. The antigen levels correlate with the clinical status of the disease and with survival. Using this MoAb we were able to isolate cDNA and the gene coding for the antigen. Although the H23 MoAb was generated against particulate antigens, we do not have any evidence that the antigen is virally coded.

---

epithelial non-breast tissues. Total RNA from different human tissues was dot blotted and probed with the 3b cDNA insert or, for standardization, a cDNA insert coding for part of human 18S ribosomal RNA (DHW, unpublished). Total RNA extraction dot blotting, hybridization and washing conditions were as described in Materials and Methods. The blots were exposed to Agfa Curix x-ray films at -70°C. The autoradiographs were scanned by laser densitometry using a LKB laser densitometer and the absorbance values obtained with the 3b cDNA probe were divided by the levels observed following 18S cDNA probing. This procedure resulted in a normalized arbitrary unit for each sample. The values obtained for the breast carcinoma samples were summed and the mean value set at 100 (column A). The mean values obtained with RNA from benign breast tissues (column B) or from epithelial non-breast tissues tumor (column C) were expressed as a percentage relative to the breast carcinoma samples.

Acknowledgements

This work was supported by: Teva Industries, Simko Chair for Breast Cancer Research, Frederico Fund for Tel Aviv University and Mr. Toby Green, London. I.T. and M.H. were the recipients of an EMBO short term Fellowship and D.H.W. is the recipient of a Koret Foundation Fellowship, California. We thank Amir Prat and Yael Villa for help in the statistical analyses.

REFERENCES

1. J. Schlom, D. Colcher, P.A. Hold, F. Greiner, M. Weeks, P.B. Fisher, P. Noguchi, S. Peskta, and D. Kufe, 1985, Adv. in Cancer Res., 43:143.
2. F. Greiner, P. Horan-Hand, D. Colcher, M. Weeks, A. Thor, P. Noguchi, S. Peskta, and J. Schlom, 1987, J. Lab. Clinical Med., 109:244.
3. J. Taylor-Papadimit,iou, J. Peterson, J., Arklie, R.L. Burchell, R.L., Ceriani, and W.F. Bodmer, 1981, Int. J. Cancer, 28:17.
4. R.L. Ceriani, J. Peterson, J.Y. Lee, R. Moncada, and E.W. Blank, 1983, Somatic Cell Genet., 9:415.
5. D. Kufe, G. Inghiami, M. Abe, D. Hayes, H. Gusti-Wheeler, and J. Schlom, 1984, Hybridoma, 3:223.
6. J. Hilkens, J. Hilgers, F. Buijs, P.H. Hageman, D. Schol, G. Van Doornewaard, and J. Van den Tweel, 1984, In: Protides of the Biological Fluids. 31, H. Peeters ed. Pergamon Press.
7. J. Schlom, D. Wunderlich, and Y.A. Teramoto, 1984, Proc. Nat. Acad. Sci., (USA) 77:6841.
8. I. Keydar, I. Tsarfaty, N.I. Smorodinsky, E. Sahar, Y. Shoenfeld, and S. Chaitchik, 1987, In: New Experimental Modalities in the Control of Neoplasia, ed. P. Chandra, Plenum Press, Ch 9.
9. Y. Shoenfeld, A. Hizi, R. Tal, N.I. Smorodinsky, G. Lavy, C. Mor, S. Schteren, I. Mammon, J. Pinhas, and I. Keydar, 1987, Cancer, 59:43.
10. I. Keydar, T. Ohno, R. Nayak, R. Sweet, F. Simoni, F. Weiss, S. Karby, R. Mesa-Tejada, and S. Spiegelman, 1984, Proc. Nat. Acad. Sci., (USA) 81:4188.
11. J. Kolher, and C. Milstein, 1975, Nature, 256:495.
12. I. Keydar, G. Selzer, S. Chaitchik, M. Hareuveni, S. Karby, and A. Hizi, 1982, Eur. J. Cancer & Clin. Oncol., 18:1321.
13. D.F. Hayes, T. Ohno, M. Abe, H. Sekine, and D.W. Kufe, 1985, Clin. Invest., 75:1671.
14. L.D. Papsidero, G.A. Chrogan, M.J. O'Connell, L.A. Valenzuela, T. Nemoto, and T.M. Chu, 1983, Cancer Res., 43:1741.
15. L.D. Papsidero, T. Nemoto, G.A. Chroghan, and T.M. Chu, 1984, Cancer Res., 44:4653.
16. J. Siddiqui, M. Abe, D. Hayes, E. Shani, E. Yunis, and D. Kufe, 1988, Proc. Natl. Acad. Sci., USA 85:2320.
17. D.M. Swallow, S. Gendler, B. Griffiths, G. Corney, J. Taylor-Papadimitriou, and M. Bramwell, 1987, Nature London, 328:82.

COMPLEMENTATION OF MONOCLONAL ANTIBODIES DF3 AND B72.3

IN REACTIVITY TO BREAST CANCER

Noriaki Ohuchi[1], Minoru Akimoto[1], Shozo Mori[1], Donald W. Kufe[2] and
Jeffrey Schlom[3]

[1]Second Department of Surgery, Tohoku University School of Medicine
Sendai 980, Japan. [2]Dana-Farber Cancer Institute, Boston, MA 02115
Laboratory of Tumor Immunology and Biology, NCI, NIH, MD 20892

INTRODUCTION

Monoclonal antibodies (MAbs) developed thus far against human
carcinomas have led to a more systemic study of human breast tumors.
The reactive antigens include a wide variety of cellular products such
as receptors, oncogene products, and tumor-associated antigens (TAAs)
which can be utilized to "fingerprint" cell populations. The utilization of antibodies as immunologic probes to detect and phenotype cell
populations in tissue preparations have moved rapidly from the research
area to the clinical application. The MAbs are also increasingly being
utilized in serum assays to detect circulating TAAs in patients with
breast carcinoma.

MAb DF3 was generated by the immunization of mice with a membrane-
enriched fraction of human metastatic mammary carcinoma (1). This
MAb recognizes high molecular weight (330,000-450,000 d) glycoprotein
determinants (2,3,4). The antigen was found on the surface of live
mammary carcinoma cells, MCF-7 and BT-20 (1). The biochemical analysis
has demonstrated that the DF3 antigen is a glycoprotein with the MAb
DF3 binding site involving the glycosidic linkage between protein and
carbohydrate moieties (2). The MAb DF3 has previously shown a
differential reactivity to cytoplasmic antigen in carcinoma versus
antigen concentrated on luminal surface of benign lesions of the breast.
We have also described utilizing the immunohistochemical analysis that
in situ carcinomas and atypical hyperplasias express elevated levels of
the DF3 antigen as compared to benign breast disease without atypia (5).
Serum assays utilizing MAb DF3 have been developed to identify the high
molecular weight circulating antigen in the plasma of patients with
breast cancer (6,7,8). Among them CA15-3 immunoradiometric assay
(IRMA) is a two site IRMA utilizing MAbs 115D-8 (which recognizes MAM-6
antigen (9)) and DF3, and is a sensitive assay for monitoring the
clinical course of patients with breast cacner (10).

MAb B72.3, prepared against a membrane-enriched fraction of human
mammary carcinoma biopsy, has been shown to be reactive with a wide
range of human epithelial malignancies including breast, colorectal,
gastric, lung, ovarian, and endometrial carcinomas (11-17). The
antigen reactive with B72.3, TAG-72, has been purfied from the LS-174T

human colon cancer xenograft and can be characterized as a high molecular weight ($>10^6$d) glycoprotein with characteristics of a mucin (12,18). The TAG-72 antigen has been shown to be distinct immunologically and biochemically from CEA and the TAAs recognized by MAbs 19-9, DUPAN-2, and OC125 (19,20). A novel IRMA, CA72-4, has recently been developed utilizing two MAbs CC-49 (18) and B72.3 which recognize antigen determinants on the TAG-72. The elevated levels of serum TAG-72 was found in patients with gastrointestinal, ovarian, breast and other epithelial malignancies (21).

The potential applications of MAbs in the management of patients with breast cacner may include immunohistopathological analysis of tissue samples to detect tumor cells, serum assays to monitor tumor burden, and targeting of tumor lesions in vivo. Since the DF3 antigen and the TAG-72 antigen have been shown to be different the MAbs DF3 and B72,3 may capture the respective antigenic epitope(s) expressed in tissue specimen as well as serum of the patients with breast cancer. In the light of the degree of antigenic heterogeneity observed in most human carcinomas the use of mixtures of MAbs reactive with different antigen may be essential for the application of MAbs as immunological adjuncts to detect or treat breast cancer. This study was initiated to determine whether the two distinct antigens, DF3 and TAG-72, were expressed on the same breast carcinoma specimens, and to determine whether more carcinoma cells were able to be detected by the combination of the MAbs as compared to carcinoma cells reactive with each individual MAb. Serum levels of the TAG-72 and the antigen recognized by CA15-3 were also investigated to determine whether the two distinct antigens were complementarily expressed in patients with breast cancer.

MATERIALS AND METHODS

Serum Samples

Serum samples from 52 patients with breast carcinoma (34 with primary carcinoma and 18 with recurrent carcinoma) and 23 with benign breast disease were obtained at the Second Department of Surgery, Tohoku University School of Medicine and the Department of Surgery, Sendai City Hospital, Sendai, Japan. All of these samples were coded and stored at -70°C until use.

Tissues

Surgical specimens were obtained from the patients whose serum samples were investigated for radioimmunometric analyses. Formalin-fixed, paraffin-embedded breast tissues were collected from 24 out of the 34 patients with primary breast carinoma and 12 out of the 18 patients with recurrent carcinoma. All of the tissues were obtained at primary operations, and no tissues at metastatic sites were included in this study.

Monoclonal Antibodies

The MAb DF3 (IgG$_1$) was produced by the immunization of BALB/c mice with a partially purified membrane-enriched fraction of a human metastatic breast carcinoma (1). The MAb B72.3 (IgG$_1$) was also generated against a membrane-enriched fraction of human metastatic breast carcinoma (11), and is immunoreactive with a high molecular weight glycoprotein complex designated tumor-associated glycoprotein, TAG-72. The antigen was purified from a xenograft of human colon carcinoma cell line, LS-174T, using Sepharose CL-4B chromatography and

B72.3 antibody affinity columns. The purified TAG-72 was used as an immunogen to generate B72.3 second generation MAb CC-49 (18).

Radioimmunoassays

The CA15-3 assay kits (Centocor, Malvern, PA) were used to determine circulating CA15-3 antigen level. Twenty microliters of either a patient sample or positive control were added to 1000 μl of diluent. Two-hundred microliters of the diluted specimen, positive control and each CA15-3 standard were incubated with MAb 115D-8-coated polyethyrene beads for two hours at room temperature. The beads were washed and incubated with 200 μl of ^{125}I-MAb DF3 at 4°C for 16 hours. The beads were again washed, and counts/min/bead were determined by gamma counting. The CA15-3 antigen level was determined by comparison with a curve generated with standard solutions provided in the kit.

The CA72-4 (Centocor, Malvern, PA) is a novel quantitative immuno-radiometric assay system utilizing two monoclonal antibodies CC-49 (18) and B72.3 which recognize the TAG-72 antigen (21). The assay was performed as follows; 100 μl of phosphate buffer and 100 μl of serum or standard (normal human plasma containing TAG-72 antigen) was aliquoted into a reaction tray. Polyethylene beads coated with MAb CC-49 were added to the reaction tray and incubated for 4 hours at 37°C. The beads were washed with distilled water, then 200 μl of ^{125}I-labeled MAb B72.3 was added to each well containing a bead. The serum samples were incubated for 20 hours at 4°C, the beads were washed with distilled water, and the number of counts bound was determined in a gamma counter. Bound radio-activity was converted to CA72-4 units/ml by reference to a standard curve generated by linear regression. All standards, positive controls and serum samples were counted concurrently.

Immunohistochemical Assays

Formalin-fixed, paraffin-embedded breast tissues were investigated for expression of DF3 and TAG-72 antigens utilizing avidin-biotin complex immunohistochemical method. Three-micrometer sections were deparaffinized in xylene and rehydrated in graded alcohols, and the endogenous peroxidase activity was blocked with the use of methanol containing 0.3% H_2O_2. The sections were washed in phosphate buffered saline (PBS), and treated with 10% normal horse serum. This reagent and all subsequent reagents were diluted in PBS containing 0.1% bovine serum albumin at pH 7.4. Serial sections were independently treated with first MAb DF3 (at 0.1 μg/ml) or MAb B72.3 (at 40 μg/ml) for 16 hours at 4°C. The primary antibodies were removed, then the sections were rinsed in PBS, followed by incubation in biotinylated horse anti-mouse IgG (Vector Lab. Inc., Burlingame, CA). The slides were again rinsed in PBS, then incubated with avidin-DH and a biotinylated horse-radish H complex (ABC) for 30 minutes. After rinse in PBS, the sections were treated with 3-amino-9-ethylcarbazole (AEC: Sigma, St. Louis, MO). The sections were washed and briefly counterstained with hematoxylin.

Scoring Methods for Immunohistochemical Evaluation

Immunohistochemically stained tissues were scored in the following manner. The percentage reactivity was determined by approximating the number of reactive cells with each MAb, and dividing by the total number of cells x 100. A cell was considered reactive if the cytoplasm, cell membrane, or both displayed a distinct reddish-brown precipitate visualized under light microscopy indicative of reactive antigen. At least 5 microscopic fields or more than 200 epithelial cells for each specimen were evaluated.

Table 1. Average Values and Positve Rates of Serum CA15-3 and CA72-4
in Patients with Carcinoma and Benign Disease of the Breast

| | Number tested | Mean CA15-3 (U/ml) | Mean CA72-4 (U/ml) | Positive rates in | |
				CA15-3 (≥23 U/ml)	CA72-4 (≥4 U/ml)
Carcinomas	52	70.3	18.9	30.8%	36.5%
Primary	34	50.1	3.5	17.6%	29.4%
Stage I	12	8.6	2.3	0.0%	8.3%
Stage II	10	17.3	4.0	20.0%	30.0%
Stage III	9	42.2	3.9	22.2%	44.4%
Stage IV	3	348.7	5.1	66.7%	66.7%
Recurrent	18	108.4	48.0	55.6%	50.0%
Benign diseases	23	12.5	2.3	4.3%	4.3%

RESULTS

Serum Levels of CA15-3 and CA72-4 in Patients with Breast Carcinoma and Benign Breast Disease

The levels of circulating DF3 antigen in the serum of patients were determined by the use of CA15-3 radioimmunometric assay. The CA15-3 RIA system comprises of two MAbs, i.e., first MAb 115D-8 and second MAb DF3. Therefore, the antigen detected by CA15-3 RIA is the one specifically reactive with MAb DF3. The average values of serum CA15-3 in patients with breast cancer at various stage and those with benign breast disease are listed in Table 1. Elevated levels of serum CA15-3 were found in patients with breast carcinoma, especially those with advanced primary carcinoma (stages III and IV) and recurrent carcinoma, as compared to those with benign breast disease. The distribution of CA15-3 levels in sera from 430 healthy individuals (316 males and 114 females) has recently been investigated, and the mean + 2SD (standard deviation) of CA15-3 was found to be 22.9 units/ml (22). When less than 23 units/ml was taken as the cut-off level for the CA15-3 serum assay, the elevated CA15-3 was found in 30.8% of the patients with breast carcinoma (n=52); 17.6% with primary carcinoma (n=34) and 55.6% with recurrent carcinoma (n=18), whereas only one patient with cystsarcoma phyllodes among the patients with benign breast disease (n=23) examined demonstrated elevated level of CA15-3 (Table 1).

The serum TAG-72 antigen levels in patients with benign and malignant breast disease condition were measured by the use of CA72-4 RIA system. The mean CA72-4 concentration in serum samples from 514 healthy individuals was 1.9 units/ml, and the cut-off value for CA72-4 was determined as 4.0 units/ml according to the mean + 2SD, 3.9 units/ml

Table 2. Correlation Between Serum Levels of CA15-3 and CA72-4 in 52 Patients with Breast Carcinoma

		CA-15-3	
		<23 U/ml	≥23 U/ml
CA72-4	<4 U/ml	24/52 (46.1%)	9/52 (17.3%)
	≥4 U/ml	12/52 (23.1%)	7/52 (13.4%)

(21). As shown in Table 1, the average value of CA72-4 in patients with breast carcinoma was 18.9 units/ml, much higher than that (2.3 units/ml) in patients with benign breast disease. The elevated levels of TAG-72 antigen were found in 36.5% of patients with breast carcinoma; 29.4% with primary carcinoma and 50.0% with recurrent carcinoma, while only one patient with intraductal papilloma among the patients with benign disease showed elevated level of TAG-72. In patients with breast carcinoma at early stage, however, both levels of serum DF3 and TAG-72 were relatively low, suggesting that either CA15-3 or CA72-4 RIA system may not be useful for the screening purpose of circulating TAAs in patients with early breast cancer.

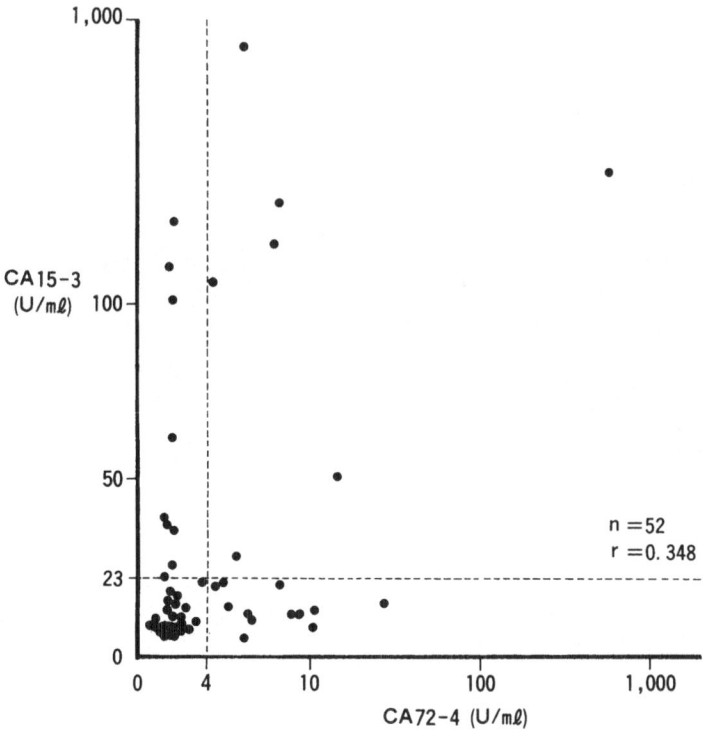

Figure 1. Serum levels of CA15-3 and CA72-4 in 52 patients with breast carcinoma. The correlation coefficient (r) between the levels of CA15-3 and those of CA72-4 was 0.348.

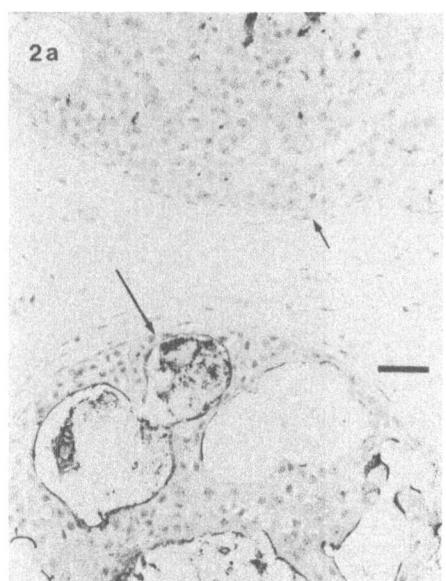 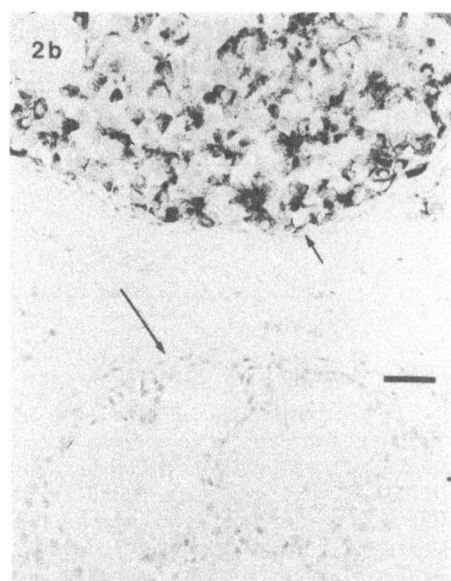

Figure 2. Immunohistochemical reactivities of MAbs DF3 (a) and B72.3 (b) with serial sections of an intraducal carcinoma of the breast. Counterstained with hematoxylin. Note the differential reactivity with MAb B72.3 from the reactivity with MAb DF3. The carcinoma cell population indicated by short arrow is strongly reactive with MAb B72.3, while the cell population indicated by long arrow is completely negative. In contract, the cell population indicated by long arrow is strongly reactive with MAb DF3 (Scale bar = 50 um).

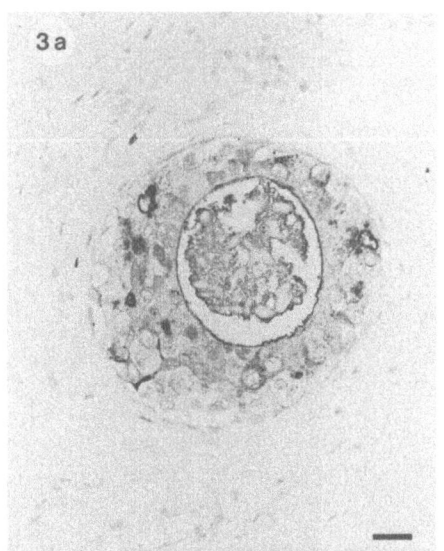 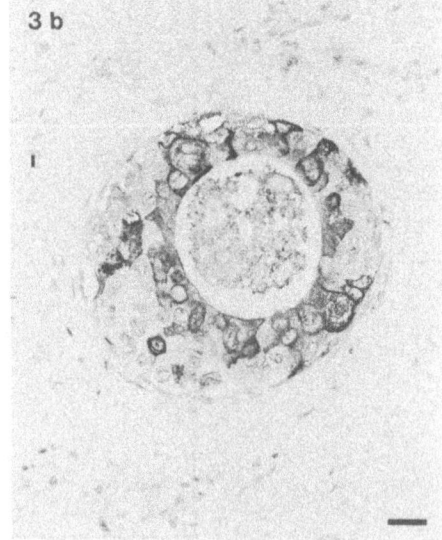

Figure 3. Immunohistochemical reactivities of MAbs DF3 (a) and B72.3 (b) with serial sections of an invasive ductal carcinoma with a predominant intraductal component. Note the strong, but heterogeneous reactivity of MAb B72.3 with the cytoplasms of carcinoma cells which are focally reactive with MAb DF3 (Scale bar = 20 um).

Correlation Between CA15-3 and CA72-4 Levels in Serum of Patients with Breast Carcinoma

The distribution of serum levels of CA15-3 and CA72-4 in the same patients with breast carcinoma were illustrated in Figure 1. The mutual relation between CA15-3 and CA72-4 values was analyzed, and the correlation coefficient (r) was found to be 0.348, indicating that there was no close relationship between the two parameters. Elevated serum levels of either CA15-3 or CA72-4 were found in 21 of 52 patients (40.3%) with breast carcinoma, whereas only 7 patients (13.5%) demonstrated elevated levels of both CA15-3 and CA72-4 (Table 2). Consequently, neither CA15-3 nor CA72-4 was elevated in 24 of 52 patients (46.1%) with breast carcinoma. It should be emphasized, however, that 15 of 18 (83.3%) patients with recurrent breast carcinoma demonstrated elevated levels of CA15-3 and/or CA72-4.

Immunohistochemical Reactivity of MAbs DF3 and B72.3 with Breast Carcinomas

Serial sections from surgically resected breast carcinoma specimens were reacted with MAb DF3 or B72.3 using ABC immunohistochemical method to determine whether breast carcinoma cells express DF3 or TAG-72 antigen at cellular level. Figures 2a and 3a illustrate the immunohistochemical reactivity of MAb DF3 with tissue sections of breast carcinoma, and Figures 2b and 3b show the reactivity of MAb B72.3 with the serial sections, respectively. MAb DF3 was generally reactive with cytoplasm and/or apical surface of breast carcinoma cells, the pattern in contrast to luminal reactivity observed in benign or normal mammary epithelial cells (5). The percentage cellular reactivity of MAb DF3 with breast carcinomas was shown in Figure 4. All of 36 breast carcinomas were immunoreactive with MAb DF3, with 27 of 36 (75.0%) demonstrated ≥20% of carcinoma cells reactive. There was no statistical difference between primary breast carcinomas without recurrence and those with recurrence in the reactivity with MAb DF3.

MAb B72.3 was reactive with apical surface and/or cytoplasm of breast carcinomas and was generally not reactive with benign or normal mammary epithelial cells (13). Thirty-two of 36 (88.9%) breast carcinomas were reactive with MAb B72.3, with 16 of 36 (44.4%) demonstrated ≥20% of carcinoma cells reactive. No difference between the carcinomas without recurrence and those with recurrence were observed in terms of immunohistochemical reactivity with MAb B72.3.

Correlation Between MAbs DF3 and B72.3 Immunohistochemical Reactivities with Breast Carcinomas

As illustrated in Figures 2 and 3, MAb DF3 was reactive with breast carcinoma cells in different fashion from MAb B72.3, i.e., MAb DF3 reacted with one carcinoma cell population, while MAb B72.3 reacted with other cell population. It is interesting to note that both MAbs generally demonstrate a heterogeneous reactivity with breast carcinoma cell populations. The percentage cellular reactivites of MAbs DF3 and B72.3 were obtained from the serial sections treated with individual MAb (Figure 4), and the mutual relationship between the two groups in reactivities of MAbs DF3 and B72.3 with the same tissues were analyzed. There was no correlation between the two MAb reactivities since the correlation coefficient (r) was found to be 0.405. This result indicates that the antigen reactive with MAb DF3 is distinct from the antigen reactive with MAb B72.3, and that the use of combination of MAbs is important for more comprehensive reactivity of carcinoma cells of the breast.

DISCUSSION

Breast carcinomas express a variety of tumor-associated antigens including carcinoembryonic antigen (CEA). MAbs which recognize DF3, TAG-72, MAM-6, epithelial membrane antigen (EMA), human mammary epithelial antigen (HME), human milk fat globule membrane antigen (HMFGM) and other antigens have been developed (23,24,25). Among them the MAb DF3 reacts with a high molecular weight glycoprotein involving the carbohydrate moiety linked to the protein with 0-glycosidic bonds (2) detectable in human breast carcinomas and human milk (1,5,26). Abe and Kufe (4) have recently described by immunoblotting and competitive

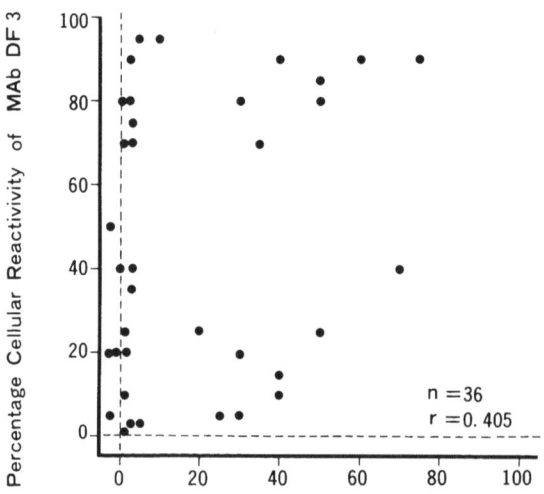

Figure 4. Percentage immunohistochemical reactivities of MAbs DF3 and B72.3 with breast carcinomas using formalin-fixed, paraffin-embedded serial sections. The correlation coefficient (r) between the percentage reactivity of MAb DF3 and that of MAb B72.3 was 0.405.

blocking assays that MAbs DF3, F36/22 (prepared against MCF-7 breast carcinoma cell line (27)), and 115D-8 react with related but not identical glycoproteins, thus these MAbs all recognizing a family of high molecular weight tumor-associated antigen. In contrast, the MAb B72.3 recognizes a novel high molecular weight glycoptein, TAG-72, in which oligosaccharides are linked through serine and threonine. The TAG-72 antigen has been shown to be distinct biochemically, immunologically, and in terms of expression from CEA and the antigens detected by other anti-TAA MAbs such as DU-PAN-2, 19-9, OC-125, the anti-HMFGM MAbs and DF3 (19,20,28). MAb DF3 has shown strong reactivity to the surface of MCF-7 and BT-20 mammary carcinoma cell lines, but has not shown reactivity to LS-174 T colon carcinoma cell line (1), whereas MAb B72.3

has shown strong reactivity to the LS-174 T cells which express TAG-72 antigen, but no binding to BT-20 cells in live cell RIAs (29).

We have utilized immunohistochemical method for the two distinct tumor associated antigens, DF3 and TAG-72, and have defined the non-coordinate expression of two antigens on the serial sections of breast carcinomas. By means of double-staining techniques using the combination of avidin-biotin peroxidase complex and avidin-biotin alkaline phosphatase complex immunohistochemical methods we have also defined the complemental expression of the two antigens on the same tissue sections (manuscript in preparation). These results thus indicate that the combination of MAbs (which recognize distinct tumor-associated antigens) may be important for more comprehensive reactivity of breast carcinoma, and may contribute to immunohistochemical detection of more carcinoma cells on tissue section.

The radioimmunometric assays utilizing MAbs DF3 or B72.3 were performed to detect the DF3 and TAG-72 antigens in serum of the patients with breast carcinoma. CA72-4 is a novel quantitative RIA system utilizing two MAbs B72.3 and CC-49, which both recognize the TAG-72. We have recently investigated the serum levels of TAG-72 antigen in patients with benign and malignant disease condition as well as healthy individuals, and defined the elevated levels of TAG-72 antigen in patients with gastrointestinal, ovarian, breast carcinomas and other epithelial malignancies as compared to those in patients with benign disease (21). The average value of CA72-4 in patients with carcinoma was 37.9 units/ml, much higher than that (2.6 units/ml) in patients without carcinoma. In this study we have described the levels of TAG-72 antigen in serum of patients with carcinoma and benign disease of the breast. The elevated TAG-72 was found in 29.4% of patients with primary breast carcinoma, 50.0% with recurrent breast carcinoma, and only 4.3% with benign breast disease, suggesting that the serum CA72-4 RIA may be useful as a novel tumor marker for monitoring serum TAG-72 antigen in patients with breast carcinoma. The positive rates in serodiagnosis of breast cancer patients using CA72-4 and CA15-3 increased to 53.9%, with 83.3% positive in patients with recurrent breast cancer. When combined with an RIA utilizing the anti-CEA antibody, 63.5% of breast cancer patients demonstrated elevated levels of at least one of the three antigens, TAG-72, DF3, and CEA (data not shown). These results thus clearly indicate that the MAbs DF3 and B72.3 have complementation in reactivity to breast carcinomas and the combination of MAbs which recognize different TAAs may be useful as immunological adjuncts for detection of breast carcinoma. It should be emphasized, however, like other tumor markers for epithelial malignancy which have been developed, that the CA72-4 and CA15-3 RIA systems are not sensitive enough to detect the respective serum antigens in patients with early stages of breast carcinoma.

In view of the degree of antigenic heterogeneity which has been observed in most human epithelial malignancies, the use of mixtures of MAbs reactive with different tumor-associated antigens, or reactive with distinct epitopes on the same antigen molecule, is essential for the application of MAbs in immunohistochemical and immunocytochmical analyses, serum assays, MAb-guided in situ immunoscintigraphy, and MAb-guided immunotherapy of breast carcinoma. Extensive investigations to determine if these anti-TAA MAbs can be used as in vivo tumor targeting for either diagnostic or therapeutic adjuncts will be required.

REFERENCES

1. D. W. Kufe, G. Inghirami, M. Abe, D. Hayes, H. Justi-Wheeler, and J. Schlom, Differential reactivity of a novel monoclonal antibody (DF3) with human malignant versus benign breast tumors. Hybridoma 3: 223 (1984).

2. H. Sekine, T. Ohno, and D. W. Kufe, Purification and characterization of a high molecular weight glycoprotein detectable in human milk and breast carcinomas. J. Immunol. 135;3610 (1985).

3. E. L. Friedman, D. F. Hayes, and D. W. Kufe, Reactivity of monoclonal antibody DF3 with a high molecular weight antigen expressed in human ovarian carcinomas. Cancer Res. 46:5189 (1986).

4. M. Abe, and D. W. Kufe, Identification of a family of high molecular weight tumor-associated glycoproteins. J. Immunol. 139:257 (1987).

5. N. Ohuchi, D. L. Page, M. J. Merino, M. J. Viglione, D. W. Kufe, and J. Schlom, Expression of tumor-associated antigen (DF3) in atypical hyperplasias and in situ carcinomas of the human breast. J. Natl. Cancer Inst. 79:109 (1987).

6. D. F. Hayes, H. Sekine, T. Ohno, M. Abe, K. Keefe, and D. W. Kufe, Use of a murine monoclonal antibody for detection of circulating plasma DF3 antigen levels in breast cancer patients. J. Clin. Invest. 75:1671 (1985).

7. R. Tobias, C. Rothwell, J. Wagner, A. Green, and Y. S. Liu, Development and evaluation of a radioimmunoassay for the detection of a monoclonal antibody defined breast tumor associated antigen 115D-8/DF3. J. Am. Assoc. Clin. Chem. 31:986 (1985).

8. A. van Dalen, J. M. G. Bonfrer, H. Dupree, K. H. Heering, D. L. van der Linde, and W. J. Nooijen, CA15-3 as a marker in the follow-up of patients with breast cancer, in: "Tumor marker" G. Wust, ed., Steinkopff Verlag, Darmstadt, Germany, pp.182 (1987).

9. J. Hilkens, F. Buijs, J. Higers, Ph. Hageman, J. Calafat, A. Sonnenberg, and M. van der Valk, Monoclonal antibodies against human milk-fat globule membranes detecting differentiation antigens of the mammary gland and its tumors. Int. J. Cancer 34: 197 (1984).

10. D. F. Hayes, V. R. Jr. Zurawski, and D. W. Kufe, Comparison of circulating CA15-3 and carcinoembryonic antigen levels in patients with breast cancer. J. Clin. Oncol. 4:1542 (1986).

11. D. Colcher, P. Horan Hand, M. Nuti, and J. Schlom, A spectrum of monoclonal antibodies rective with human mammary tumor cells. Proc. Natl. Acad. Sci. USA 78;3199 (1981).

12. V. G. Johnson, J. Schlom, A. J. Paterson, J. Bennet, J. L. Magnani, and D. Colcher, Analysis of a human tumor-associated glycoprotein (TAG-72) identified by a monoclonal antibody B72.3. Cancer Res. 46:850 (1986).

13. A. Thor, N. Ohuchi, C. A. Szpak, W. W. Johnston, and J. Schlom, Distribution of oncofetal antigen tumor-associated glycoprotein (TAG-72) identified by a monoclonal antibody B72.3. Cancer Res. 46:3118 (1986).

14. N. Ohuchi, A. Thor. M. Nose, M. Kyogoku, and J. Schlom, Tumor-associated glycoprotein (TAG-72) detected in adenocarcinomas and benign lesions of the stomach. Int. J. Cancer 38:643 (1986).

15. A. Thor, F. Gorstein, N. Ohuchi, C. A. Szpak, W. W. Johnson, and J. Schlom, Tumor-associated glycoprotein (TAG-72) in ovarian carcinomas defined by monoclonal antibody B72.3. J. Natl. Cancer Inst. 76:995 (1986).

16. W. W. Johnston, C. A. Szpak, A. Thor, and J. Schlom, Phenotypic characterization of lung cancers in fine needle aspiration biopsies using monoclonal antibody B72.3. Cancer Res. 46:6462 (1986).

17. A. Thor, M. J. Viglione, R. Muraro, N. Ohuchi, J. Schlom, and F. Gorstein, Monoclonal antibody B72.3 reactivity with human endometrium: a study of normal and malignant tissues. Int. J. Gynecol. Pathol. 6:235 (1987).

18. R. Muraro, M. Kuroki, D. Wunderlich, D. J. Poole, D. Colcher, A. Thor, J. W. Greiner, J. Simpson, A. Molinoto, P. Noguchi, and J. Scholom, Generation and characterization of B72.3 second generation monoclonal antibodies reactive with the tumor-associated glycoprotein 72 antigen. Cancer Res. 48:4588 (1988).

19. N. Ohuchi, J. F. Simpson, D. Colcher, and J. Schlom, Complementation of anti-CEA and anti-TAG-72 monoclonal antibodies in reactivity to human gastric adenocarcinomas. Int. J. Cancer 40:726 (1987).

20. M. S. Lan, R. C. Bast, M. I. Colnagi, R. C. Knapp, D. Colcher, J. Schlom, and R. S. Metzgar, Co-expression of human cancer-associated epitopes on mucin molecules. Int. J. Cancer 39:68 (1986).

21. N. Ohuchi, S. Mori, E. Gero, D. Colcher, F. Mochizuki, T. Nishihira, K. Hirayama, N. Matoba, P. M. Kaplan, and J. Schlom, Serum levels of tumor-associated glycoprotein (TAG-72) in patients with carcinoma detected by CA72-4 radioimmunometric assay. (submitted for publication).

22. N. Ohuchi, Y. Taira, K. Takahashi, S. Sato, H. Matoba, M. Akimoto, and S. Mori, Comparison of serum levels of CA15-3 and cytoplasmic reactivity of monoclonal antibody DF3 in patients with breast cancer. (submitted for publication).

23. J. P. Sloane, and M. G. Ormerod, Distribution of epithelial membrane antigen in normal and neoplastic tissues and its value in diagnostic tumor pathology. Cancer 17:1786 (1981).

24. J. Taylor-Papadimitriou, J. A. Peterson, J. Arklie, J. Burchell, R. L. Ceriani, and W. F. Bodmer, Monoclonal antibodies to epithelium specific components of the milk fat globule membrane: production and reaction with cells. Int. J. Cancer 28:17 (1981).

25. R. L. Ceriani, J. A. Peterson, J. Y. Lee, R. Moncada, and E. W. Blank, Characterization of cell surface antigens of human mammary epithelial cells with monoclonal antibodies prepared against human milk fat globule. Somatic Cell Genet. 9:415 (1983).

26. A. Thor, M. J. Viglione, N. Ohuchi, J. F. Simpson, R. Steis, J. Cousar, M. Lippman, D. W. Kufe, and J. Schlom, Comparison of monoclonal antibodies for the detection of occult breast carcinoma metastases in bone marrow. Breast Cancer Res. Treat. 11:133 (1988).

27. L. D. Papsidero, G. A. Croghan, M. J. O'Connell, L. A. Vallenzuella, T. Nemoto, and T. M. Chu, Monoclonal antibodies (F36/22 and M7/105) to human breast carcinoma. Cancer Res. 43:1741 (1983).

28. N. Ohuchi, D. Wunderlich, J. Fujita, D. Colcher, R. Muraro, M. Nose, and J. Schlom, Differential expression of carcinoembryonic antigen in early gastric adenocarcinomas versus benign gastric lesions defined by monoclonal antibodies reactive with restricted antigen epitopes. Cancer Res. 47:3565 (1987).

29. P. Horan Hand, D. Colcher, D. Salomon, J. Ridge, P. Noguchi, and J. Schlom, Influence of spatial configulation of carcinoma cell populations in the expression of a tumor-associated glycoprotein. Cancer Res. 45.833 (1985).

DIFFERENTIAL EXPRESSION OF DF3 ANTIGEN BETWEEN PAPILLARY CARCINOMAS

AND BENIGN PAPILLARY LESIONS OF THE BREAST

Noriaki Ohuchi,[*][§] Maria J. Merino,[†] Darryl Carter,[‡]
Jean F. Simpson,[*] Susan Kennedy,[†] Donald Kufe,[¶]
and Jeffrey Schlom[*]

[*]Laboratory of Tumor Immunology and Biology and [†]Laboratory of
Pathology, National Cancer Institute, National Institutes of
Health, Bethesda, MD 20892; [‡]Department of Pathology, Yale
University School of Medicine, New Haven, CT 06510; and [¶]Dana
Farber Cancer Institute, Boston, MA 02115

ABSTRACT

Murine monoclonal antibody (MAb) DF3, prepared against a membrane-
enriched fraction of breast carcinoma metastasis, has previously shown
differential reactivity to breast carcinoma cells and normal or benign
breast epithelial cells. Using the avidin-biotin peroxidase complex
immunohistochemical method, we have examined cytoplasmic DF3 antigen
expression in breast papillary lesions to define whether the MAb DF3
distinguishes papillary carcinomas from benign papillary lesions. MAb DF3
reacted with antigen in the cytoplasm in 17 of 19 papillary carcinomas, 12
(63%) of which demonstrated significant levels of cytoplasmic DF3 expression (≥20% of carcinoma cells reactive). In contrast, none of the benign
lesions examined demonstrated more than 10% of epithelial cells reactive in
the cytoplasm. Specimens containing a spectrum of lesions from benign
papilloma through atypical hyperplasia to carcinoma showed a corresponding
general increase in DF3 antigen expression in the cytoplasm with the
transition of papilloma to carcinoma. These results suggest that papillary
carcinomas express DF3 antigen in the cytoplasm, and this may help to
distinguish them from benign papillary lesions on the basis of cytoplasmic
reactivity.

INTRODUCTION

Surgical treatment for papillary lesions of the breast, including
papillary carcinoma, papilloma, or papillomatosis (epitheliosis), should be
performed on the basis of precise histopathological diagnosis and biological behavior of given lesions. The relationship of benign papillary
lesions to carcinoma has been described using follow-up studies[1,2] and a
three-dimensional reconstruction study.[3] The histopathological differentiation of papillary carcinoma from benign papillary lesions has been
described.[4-7] It is still difficult, however, to diagnose papillary

[§]Present address: Department of Surgery, Tohoku University School of
Medicine, Sendai, 980 Japan.

carcinoma when no foci of invasive carcinoma cells are detected or the given tumor cells lack the complete criteria for the diagnosis of carcinoma in situ.[8] In our study, we were able to help differentiate papillary carcinoma from benign papillary lesions based on the expression of breast carcinoma-associated antigen.

The identification of human breast carcinoma-associated antigens and the development of monoclonal antibodies (MAbs) directed against these antigens have been the subject of much investigation.[9-16] Among them, MAb DF3, generated by using a membrane-enriched fraction of a human metastatic breast carcinoma as immunogen, recognized high molecular weight determinants (330,000 to 450,000) found in secretory breast epithelial cells and breast carcinomas.[17,18] The antigen reactive with this MAb was found on the surface of live mammary carcinoma cell lines (MCF-7 and BT-20) but was not found on the surface of colon carcinoma cell lines by using solid-phase radioimmunoassays.[17] Elevated levels of DF3 antigen have been found in the circulation of patients with breast carcinomas.[19] Furthermore, using a radioimmunometric method, Gion et al.[20] have recently demonstrated higher levels of DF3 antigen (CA15/3) in the cytosol of breast carcinoma than in normal breast tissues.

MAb DF3 has shown a strong differential reactivity to cytoplasmic antigen in breast carcinomas versus reactivity to antigen concentrated on apical borders of benign lesions and normal mammary epithelial cells by using immunohistochemical assays.[17] We have recently demonstrated elevated levels of cytoplasmic DF3 antigen expression in atypical hyperplasia as well as carcinoma in situ of the breast, compared with hyperplasia without atypia and nonproliferative disease.[21] This study was initiated to define if a difference exists on the basis of level of expression of tumor-associated antigen between malignant and benign papillary lesions of the breast.

MATERIALS AND METHODS

Monoclonal Antibodies

Murine IgG1 MAb DF3 was generated by an immunization of BALB/c mice with a partially purified membrane-enriched fraction of a human breast carcinoma metastasis to the liver.[17] The characterization of MAb DF3 has been described in detail elsewhere.[17,18] An isotype identical control MAb MOPC-21 (murine IgG1, Litton Bionetics, Charleston, SC) was used as a negative control for all tissue samples.

Tissues

Formalin-fixed, paraffin-embedded tissue specimens were obtained from 19 patients with papillary carcinoma and 16 patients with benign papillary lesions of the breast from the Department of Pathology, Yale University School of Medicine, New Haven, CT. The serial sections of each specimen were cut 5 μm thick and mounted on gelatin-coated glass slides. One section from each specimen was stained with hematoxylin and eosin (H&E) for histopathological diagnosis.

Histopathological Diagnosis

The differential diagnosis of papillary lesions was basically made using the criteria proposed by Kraus and Neubecker[4] and Azzopardi.[5] The criteria, including cellular atypia as well as structural atypia to differentiate intraductal carcinoma from benign papillary lesions, were described in detail elsewhere.[22] Benign papillary lesions were classified into intraductal papilloma and epithelial hyperplasia in terminal duct-lobular unit. Intraductal papillomas include central and peripheral types of papillomas[3,23] that are comparable to ductal and terminal duct hyperplasias of Wellings et al.[24] Epithelial hyperplasias are hyperplastic lesions without fibrovascular cores and are similar to fenestrated epitheliosis of Azzopardi,[5] terminal duct hyperplasias of Wellings et al.,[24] and papillomatosis of Haagensen et al.[25]

Immunohistochemical Methods

Formalin-fixed, paraffin-embedded breast tissue specimens were examined for DF3 antigen expression by using avidin-biotin peroxidase complex (ABC) immunohistochemical methods. Five-micrometer sections mounted on gelatin-coated glass slides were deparaffinized in xylene and rehydrated in graded alcohols. Endogenous peroxidase activity of tissue sections was blocked by using methanol containing 0.3% H_2O_2. After washing in phosphate-buffered saline (PBS) at pH 7.4, the sections were pretreated with 10% normal horse serum for 15 min. This and all subsequent reagents were diluted with PBS containing 0.1% bovine serum albumin (BSA) at pH 7.4. After the pretreatment, the sections were incubated with primary MAb DF3 ascites at 1:10,000 dilution for 30 min at room temperature. Serial sections of each specimen were incubated with an isotype identical negative control MOPC-21 at 20 μg/ml. The first MAbs were removed, then the sections were rinsed in PBS, followed by incubation with a second antibody, biotinylated horse anti-mouse IgG (Vector Labs Inc., CA). The slides were washed in PBS and incubated with avidin-DH:horseradish H complex (ABC) for 30 min. After another rinse in PBS, the sections were treated with 0.06% diaminobenzidine (Sigma, St. Louis, MO) with 0.01% H_2O_2 for 5 min. After a final rinse in PBS, the sections were briefly counterstained with hematoxylin, dehydrated in graded alcohols, cleared in xylene, and mounted under a coverslip with Permount to be examined under a light microscope.

Counting Methods for Immunohistochemical Reactivity

The percentage of MAb DF3-reactive cells was given as an estimation of the number of epithelial cells reactive with MAb DF3 divided by the total number of epithelial cells of each histological lesion $\times$ 100. Each histologic subtype (i.e., intraductal papillary carcinoma, papilloma, epithelial hyperplasia, or fibrocystic change) was evaluated for cytoplasmic MAb DF3 reactivity, and the epithelial cells within each category were individually scored for MAb reactivity (Table 1). However, the score of the most severe histological category present in each patient was utilized for Table 1. For example, when papillary carcinoma, papilloma, and epithelial hyperplasia were found in the same specimen, the scoring of carcinoma was utilized for MAb DF3 reactivity. At least five fields, or more than 200 epithelial cells, of malignant or benign lesions were evaluated for the presence of intracellular cytoplasmic reddish-brown diaminobenzidine precipitate that was indicative of MAb DF3 binding. Cells with only luminal binding of MAb DF3, characteristic of the normal and benign epithelial cells of the breast, were not included.

RESULTS

Nineteen papillary carcinomas and 16 benign papillary lesions were analyzed for DF3 antigen expression on the basis of cytoplasmic reactivity of MAb DF3 by using formalin-fixed, paraffin-embedded sections. A percentage of cytoplasmic reactivity of MAb DF3 with each lesion from different individuals is summarized in Table 1. Luminal staining of MAb DF3 was observed in benign papillary lesions. However, because of results of

Table 1. Cytoplasmic DF3 Reactivity with Papillary Lesions of the Breast

Case No.	% of Cytoplasmic Reactivity with MAb DF3[a]			
	PAP CA[b]	PAP/CRIB CA[c]	PAP[d]	HTD[e]
Papillary carcinomas				
1	30		<5	5
2	50			
3	90			
4	0			0
5	85		15	20
6	5			0
7	<5		0	0
8	0			
9	10			
10	20			
11	40			10
12	90			
13	50		15	15
14	25		0	
15	10		0	0
16		40		0
17	70			<5
18		80		
19	5			
Benign papillary lesions				
1			0	<5
2			0	
3			0	1
4			0	1
5			0	
6			0	
7			1	1
8			0	0
9			1	
10			10	5
11			0[f]	
12			<5[f]	
13			<5	
14			10	
15			0	0
16			0	

[a]Scoring method for immunohistochemical reactivity is described in "Materials and Methods."
[b]PAP CA, intraductal papillary carcinoma.
[c]CRIB CA, intraductal cribriform carcinoma.
[d]PAP, intraductal papilloma.
[e]HTD, epithelial hyperplasia in terminal duct-locular unit.
[f]Nipple adenoma.

previous observations,[17,21] we did not score the luminal reactivity of MAb DF3 in this study.

Among the 19 papillary carcinomas examined, 17 showed cytoplasmic reactivity with MAb DF3, whereas the other two were nonreactive on the basis of cytoplasmic binding. Figure 1 shows cytoplasmic DF3 staining with papillary carcinoma. Reactivity of MAb DF3 with the cytoplasm, luminal surfaces, and extracellular-secreting components was characteristic for papillary carcinoma of the breast. All were diagnosed to be intraductal carcinoma on H&E stained slides, except two patients who had foci of invasive carcinomas. Benign papillary components, including papillomas (n=6) and epithelial hyperplasias in terminal duct-lobular units (n=10), adjacent to these carcinomas were also scored for cytoplasmic DF3 reactivity. All of the benign lesions were less reactive than the respective carcinoma lesions; three of six papillomas and five of ten epithelial hyperplasias were positive.

Benign papillary lesions (n=16) of noncancer patients, in general, demonstrated only luminal bindings to MAb DF3 (Table 1 and Figures 2 and 3). MAb DF3 weakly reacted with 6 of 16 benign papillary lesions. No benign tumors, however, demonstrated more than 10% cellular reactivity with MAb DF3. Histological subtypes of papillary lesions, i.e., intraductal papilloma (PAP) and epithelial hyperplasia (HTD) in terminal duct-lobular units, were individually evaluated for their cytoplasmic immunoreactivities to MAb DF3. MAb DF3 reacted with the luminal surfaces but did not react with the cytoplasm of epithelial and myoepithelial cells. Epithelial hyperplasias in terminal duct-lobular units were also scored for cytoplasmic DF3 reactivity. Figure 3 illustrates an example of epithelial hyperplasias with pleomorphic cell arrangement and a two-cell pattern. Although five of seven epithelial hyperplasias showed weak cytoplasmic reactivity with MAb DF3, only less than 5% of epithelial cells were reactive with MAb DF3 (Table 1).

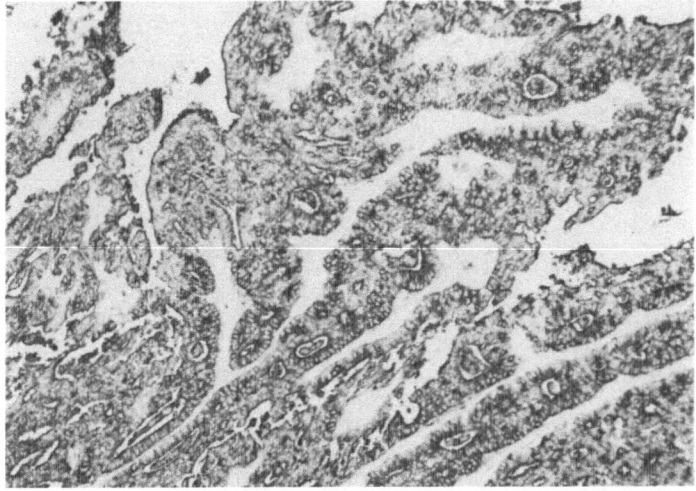

Fig. 1. Intraductal papillary carcinoma showing strong apical and cytoplasmic stainings for MAb DF3. This and the following photomicrographs are immunoperoxidase stainings with MAb DF3 and counterstained with hematoxylin. (×130)

187

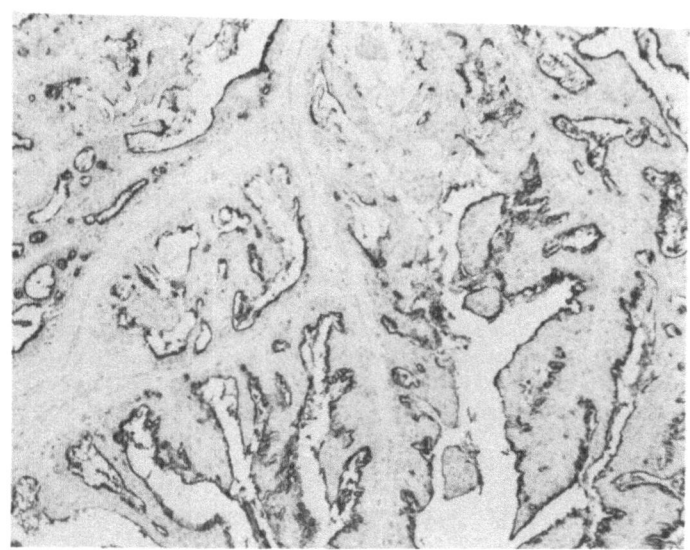

Fig. 2. Intraductal papilloma with prominent fibrovascular stalks, complex glandular patterns,
and well-preserved two-cell layers. MAb
reacts with the luminal surfaces but does
not react with the cytoplasm. (×170)

We have compared the percentage of cells with cytoplasmic reactivity
in papillary carcinomas and benign papillary lesions. There was a markedly
heterogeneous expression of DF3 antigen among the papillary carcinomas
examined, but 12 of 19 (63%) papillary carcinomas demonstrated more than
20% of carcinoma cells expressing this antigen, whereas none of the benign
lesions examined from noncancer patients demonstrated more than 10% of
reactive epithelial cells. This difference was statistically significant
($P < 0.01$) by Wilcoxon rank sum test for nonparametric methods.[26]

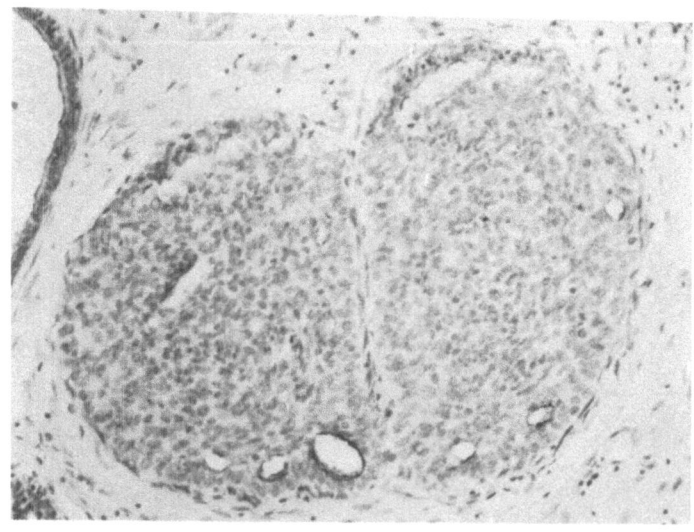

Fig. 3. Epithelial hyperplasia in the terminal duct-
lobular unit showing weak luminal staining
for MAb DF3. (×220)

As mentioned above, benign lesions were found in the specimens with
papillary carcinoma (Table 1). Two specimens containing a spectrum of
benign papillary lesions through atypia to papillary carcinoma were
observed (cases 5 and 13 of papillary carcinomas in Table 1). A focus of
such a spectrum is shown in Figure 4. Higher magnifications of this lesion
demonstrate that the area consisting of definitively benign epithelial
cells (Figure 4B) shows only luminal binding to MAb DF3, the area with
atypical cells and atypical structures (cribriform-like lumina) (Figure 4C)
shows luminal staining as well as cytoplasmic staining with MAb DF3, and
the area with definitive carcinoma cells shows strong cytoplasmic
reactivity to MAb DF3 (Figure 4D). This result shows that an increasing

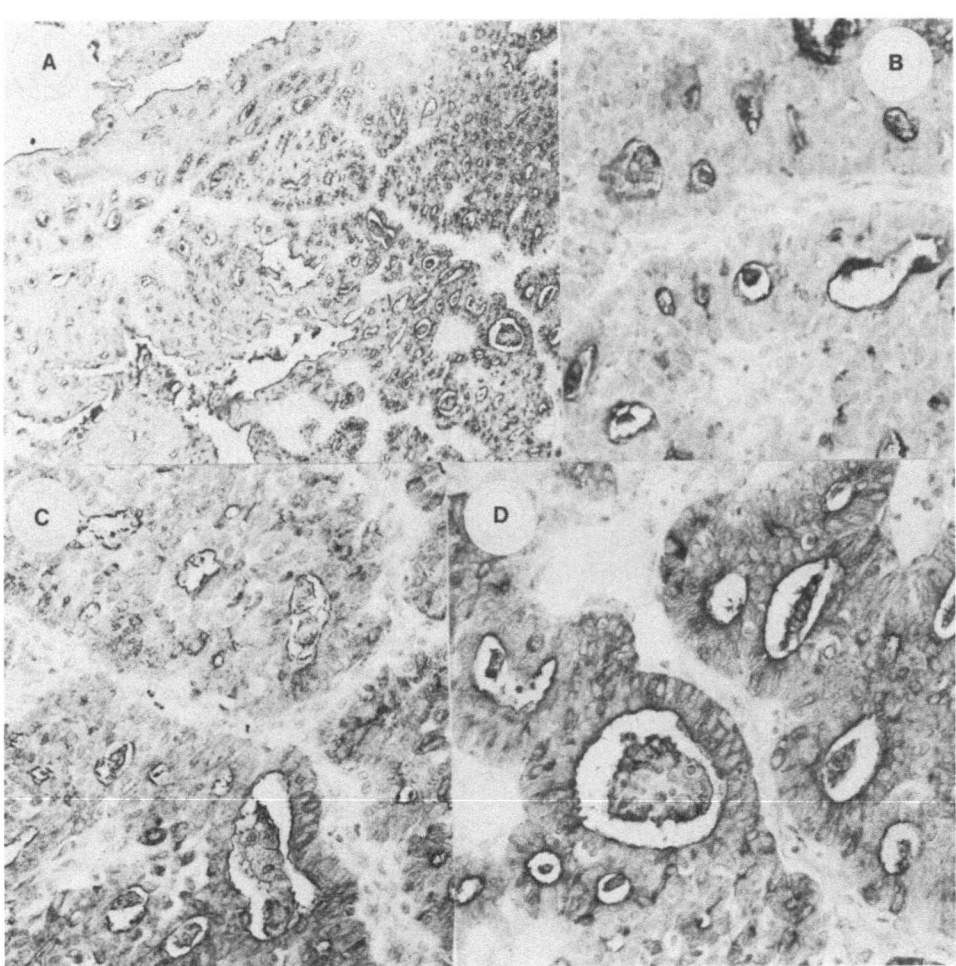

Fig. 4. (A) A transition from papilloma through atypical hyperplasia to
papillary carcinoma. (×130) (B) A higher magnification of area
showing apical reactivity of MAb DF3 with benign papilloma.
(×330) (C) A higher magnification of area that has a relative
monotonous change of epithelial cells and cribriform-like lumina
but lacks the complete criteria for the diagnosis of carcinoma.
Note that MAb DF3 reacts with the cytoplasm of atypical cells.
(×330) (D) A higher magnification of area showing obvious carcinoma. Note the strong cytoplasmic reactivity of MAb DF3. (×330)

DF3 antigen expression in the cytoplasm correlates with the transition from benign papillary lesion through atypical hyperplasia to carcinoma.

DISCUSSION

We have investigated DF3 antigen expression in benign and malignant papillary lesions of the breast to define whether any biological difference exists between these lesions. The data suggest that the DF3 antigen is expressed in the cytosol of intraductal papillary carcinomas but is rarely expressed in benign papillary lesions of the breast. Using immuno-histochemical methods, we have previously demonstrated an elevated DF3 antigen expression in the cytoplasm of in situ carcinomas as well as atypical hyperplasias of ductal and lobular types compared with hyper-plastic lesions without atypia and nonproliferative lesions.[21] In this study, atypical hyperplasias were not included except in the two cases that were suggestive of malignant transformation from papilloma through atypia to carcinoma. Instead, we focused our observations on the expression of DF3 antigen in benign and malignant papillary lesions to determine whether MAb DF3 distinguishes papillary carcinoma from benign papilloma. The results shown here indicate that MAb DF3 can help to differentiate malig-nant versus benign papillary lesions because DF3 preferentially stains malignant lesion cytoplasmically. This is potentially important because these lesions are sometimes difficult to distinguish.

DF3 antigen has been shown to be present on apical borders of secre-tory mammary epithelial cells and in the cytosol of less differentiated malignant cells.[17] This apical and cytoplasmic binding pattern has also been described using MAbs generated against human milk fat globule mem-brane[27] and breast carcinoma cells.[14,28] It may be speculated that the apical binding of MAb DF3 with secretory mammary epithelial cells is related to the DF3 antigen in human milk, and the cytoplasmic binding with carcinoma cells is related to the breast carcinoma-associated DF3 antigen.[18,20]

A spectrum of histologic changes from nonatypical hyperplasia through atypia (borderline lesion) to carcinoma within papillary lesions in the terminal duct-lobular unit has been demonstrated by a three-dimensional reconstruction study.[21] It is interesting to note that, in this study, specimens containing a similar spectrum showed increasing DF3 antigen expression in the cytoplasm with the transition to carcinoma. It is thus possible that the peripheral papilloma may have malignant potential as its transition to atypia and carcinoma demonstrates an enhanced level of cytoplasmic DF3 antigen.

To further define the biological implications of these findings, we suggest a larger series of papillary lesions "suggestive of malignant transformation" be stained with DF3 and analyzed for DF3 cytoplasmic staining.

REFERENCES

1. D. Carter, Intraductal papillary tumors of the breast, *Cancer* 39:1689 (1977).
2. W. D. Dupont and D. L. Page, Risk factors for breast cancer in women with proliferative breast disease, *N. Engl. J. Med.* 312:146 (1985).
3. N. Ohuchi, R. Abe, and M. Kasai, Possible cancerous change of intraductal papillomas of the breast: a 3-D reconstruction study, *Cancer* 54:605 (1984).

4. F. T. Kraus and R. D. Neubecker, The differential diagnosis of papillary tumors of the breast, *Cancer* 15:444 (1962).

5. J. G. Azzopardi, "Problems in Breast Pathology," W. B. Saunders, Philadelphia (1979), pp. 113-166.

6. R. W. McDivitt, F. W. Stewart, and J. W. Berg, "Tumors of the Breast: Atlas of Tumor Pathology," Second Series, Part 2, AFIP, Washington, DC (1968), pp. 29-49.

7. M. M. Black and A. B. Chabon, In situ carcinoma of the breast, *Pathol. Annu.* 4:185 (1969).

8. D. L. Page, W. D. Dupont, L. W. Rogers, and M. S. Rados, Atypical hyperplastic lesions of the female breast, *Cancer* 55:2698 (1985).

9. D. Colcher, P. Horan Hand, M. Nuti, and J. Schlom, A spectrum of monoclonal antibodies reactive with human mammary tumor cells, *Proc. Natl. Acad. Sci. USA* 78:3199 (1981).

10. J. Taylor-Papadimitriou, J. A. Peterson, J. Arklie, J. Burchell, R. L. Ceriani, and W. Bodmer, Monoclonal antibodies to epithelium-specific components of the human milk fat globule membrane: production and reaction with cells in culture, *Int. J. Cancer* 28:17 (1981).

11. K. C. Gatter, Z. Abdulazia, P. Beverley, J. F. R. Corvalan, C. Ford, F. B. Lane, M. Mota, J. R. G. Nash, K. Pulford, H. Stein, J. Taylor-Papadimitriou, C. Woodhouse, and D. Y. Mason, Use of monoclonal antibodies for the histological diagnosis of human malignancy, *J. Clin. Pathol.* 35:1253 (1982).

12. M. Nuti, Y. A. Teramoto, R. Mariani-Costantini, P. Horan Hand, D. Colcher, and J. Schlom, A monoclonal antibody (B72.3) defines patterns of distribution of a novel tumor associated antigen in human mammary carcinoma cell population, *Int. J. Cancer* 29:539 (1982).

13. C. H. Thompson, S. L. Jones, R. H. Whitehead, and I. F. C. Mckenzie, A human breast tissue associated antigen detected by a monoclonal antibody, *J. Natl. Cancer Inst.* 70:409 (1983).

14. L. A. Papsidero, G. A. Croghan, M. J. O'Connel, L. A. Valenzuella, T. Nemoto, and T. Ming Chu, Monoclonal antibodies (F36/22 and M7/105) to human breast carcinoma, *Cancer Res.* 43:1741 (1983).

15. S. A. Stacker, C. Thompson, C. Riglar, and I. F. C. Mckenzie, A new breast carcinoma antigen defined by a monoclonal antibody, *J. Natl. Cancer Inst.* 75:801 (1985).

16. S. Iacobelli, E. Arno, A. D'Orazio, and G. Coletti, Detection of antigens recognized by a novel monoclonal antibody in tissue and serum from patients with breast cancer, *Cancer Res.* 46:3005 (1986).

17. D. Kufe, G. Inghirami, M. Abe, D. Heyes, H. Justi-Wheeler, and J. Schlom, Differential reactivity of a novel monoclonal antibody (DF3) with human malignant versus benign breast tumors, *Hybridoma* 3:223 (1984).

18. H. Sekine, T. Ohno, and D. W. Kufe, Purification and characterization of high molecular weight glycoprotein detectable in human milk and breast carcinoma, *J. Immunol.* 135:3610 (1985).

19. D. F. Hayes, T. Ohno, M. Abe, H. Sekine, and D. W. Kufe, Detection of elevated plasma DF3 levels in breast cancer patients, *J. Clin. Invest.* 75:1671 (1985).

20. M. Gion, R. Mione, R. Dittadi, L. Griggio, G. Munegato, M. Valsecchi, O. D. Maschio, and G. Bruscagnin, Carcinoembryonic antigen, ferritin, tissue polypeptide antigen, and CA15/3 in breast cancer: relationship between carcinoma and normal tissue, *Int. J. Biol. Markers* 1:33 (1986).

21. N. Ohuchi, D. L. Page, M. Merino, M. J. Viglione, D. W. Kufe, and J. Schlom, Expression of tumor-associated antigen (DF3) in atypical hyperplasias and in situ carcinomas of the breast, *J. Natl. Cancer Inst.* 79:109 (1987).

22. N. Ohuchi, R. Abe, T. Takahashi, F. Tezuka, and M. Kyogoku, Three-dimensional atypical structure in intraductal carcinoma differentiating from papilloma and papillomatosis of the breast, *Breast Cancer Res. Treat.* 5:57 (1985).

23. N. Ohuchi, R. Abe, T. Takahashi, and F. Tezuka, Origin and extension of intraductal papillomas of the breast: a three-dimensional reconstruction study, *Breast Cancer Res. Treat.* 4:117 (1984).

24. S. R. Wellings, S. M. Jensen, and R. G. Marcum, An atlas of subgross pathology of the human breast with special reference to possible cancerous lesions, *J. Natl. Cancer Inst.* 55:231 (1975).

25. C. D. Haagensen, C. Bodian, and D. E. Haagensen, "Breast Carcinoma. Risk and Detection," W. B. Saunders, Philadelphia (1981), pp. 146-237.

26. R. D. Remington and M. A. Schork, "Statistics with Applications to the Biological and Health Sciences," Prentice-Hall, Inc., Englewood Cliffs, NJ (1970), pp. 313-315.

27. J. Arklie, J. Taylor-Papadimitriou, W. Bodmer, M. Egan, and R. Millis, Differential antigens expressed by epithelial cells in the lactating breast are also detectable in breast cancers, *Int. J. Cancer* 28:23 (1982).

28. G. A. Crogan, D. Lawrence, L. A. Papsidero, A. Luis, T. Nemoto, R. Penetrante, and T. Ming Chu, Tissue distribution of an epithelial and tumor-associated antigen recognized by monoclonal antibody F36/22, *Cancer Res.* 43:4980 (1983).

SESSION IV

POTENTIATION OF ANTI-TUMOR EFFICACY RESULTING FROM THE COMBINED ADMINISTRATION OF INTERFERON α AND OF AN ANTI-BREAST EPITHELIAL MONOCLONAL ANTIBODY IN THE TREATMENT OF BREAST CANCER XENOGRAFTS

Luciano Ozzello[1], Carolyn M. DeRosa[1], Edward W. Blank[2], Kari Cantell[3], David V. Habif[4], and Roberto L. Ceriani[2]

[1]Division of Surgical Pathology
Columbia-Presbyterian Medical Center, New York, NY 10032

[2]John Muir Cancer and Aging Research Institute
Walnut Creek, CA 94596

[3]National Public Health Institute, 00280 Helsinki
Finland

[4]Department of Surgery, Columbia-Presbyterian Medical
Center, New York, NY 10032

INTRODUCTION

It has been previously shown that natural interferons (nIFNS) -α and -γ delivered intralesionally (IL) to xenografts of human breast carcinomas in nude mice exerted a greater inhibitory effect than when they were administered systemically (1). Similarly, in patients with advanced malignant melanoma treated with IL injections of IFNα the local anti-tumor effects were found to be significantly greater than the systemic effects (2). These observations suggest that the success of IFN therapy may depend, at least in part, on the ability to concentrate the IFN in the target tissue. Unfortunately, to achieve high local concentrations of IFN without causing undesirable side effects is difficult because IFNs are rapidly eliminated. Therefore, it would be desirable to devise means by which IFNs could be selectively delivered to tumors and retained in them for long periods of time. This might be possible by coupling IFNs to monoclonal antibodies (MoAbs) directed against antigens specifically expressed by the tumor cells.

In support of this hypothesis are the in vitro studies of Alkan, et al. who observed an enhancement of the anti-viral and anti-proliferative effects of IFNs on cells carrying Epstein-Barr virus membrane antigens when the IFN was delivered coupled to MoAbs against those antigens (3). Furthermore, IFNs, by stimulating the antigenic expression of mammary carcinoma cells (4) may act synergistically with MoAbs to those antigens enhancing their anti-tumor effects (5). It has also been shown that anti-human milk fat globule MoAbs can exert a growth inhibitory effect on human breast cancer xenografts (6), and that this inhibitory effect is intensified when the MoAbs are conjugated to[131]I (7).

In the present study, we treated human breast cancer xenografts with nIFNα and an anti-human milk fat globule MoAb Mc5 delivered IL singly or in combination. The preliminary results of this study are described below and indicate that the growth inhibiting efficacy of these 2 agents is greater when they are administered together than when they are used alone.

MATERIALS AND METHODS

Natural human leukocyte interferon was produced (8), partially purified (9) and further purified by immunoadsorption on Sepharose containing mouse NK2 MoAb anti-human IFN-α (10). During the final purification step albumin was omitted from the elution buffer. The purified interferons were stored at -70°C. They had a specific activity of about 2×10^8 international units (IU) per mg of protein.

Murine MoAb Mc5 (11) detects an approximately 400 kilodaltons mucin-like molecule of the cell surface of human breast epithelial cells, both normal and neoplastic. MoAb Mc5 was purified by procedures already reported (7).

Conjugation of MoAb Mc5 and nIFNα was performed as described (12), where the reaction was performed at room temperature and stopped at 10 minutes at a final concentration of 1.45 mg per ml of MoAb Mc5 and 1.8 mg per ml of dimethyladipimate (DMA). Quenching of the reaction was introduced by glycine to a final concentration of 0.088 M. The conjugation procedure did not alter the antiviral activity of the IFN.

Xenografts of human mammary carcinoma cells MCF-7 were transplanted bilaterally in the subcutaneous (sc) tissue of the lateral thoracic regions of female BALB/c nude mice. Because of estrogen dependency of the tumors, a pellet of 17-β-estradiol (1.25 mg in cholesterol) was inserted sc prior to transplantation. IL injections were started when the tumors reached an average size of 75 mm^3. One tumor of each animal was injected while the opposite tumor was left undisturbed. Injections were carried out daily for 4 cycles of 5 days each separated by injection-free intervals of 2 days. The following experimental groups were used:

1. 20 mice received injections of nIFNα conjugated to Mc5. Each injection delivered 2×10^5 IU of nIFNα and 5 μg of Mc5 in PBS with 0.2 mg bovine serum albumin (BSA), 0.0066 mg DMA and 0.088 M glycine;

2. 10 mice were given separate injections of nIFNα (2×10^5 IU) and of Mc5 (5 μg) delivered concomitantly in PBS with 0.2 mg BSA and 0.088 M glycine.

    Control groups included:

    1. 20 mice treated with nIFNα (2×10^5 IU);

    2. 20 mice receiving injections of Mc5 (5 μg);

    3. 18 mice injected with PBS.

Each injection was given in PBS with 0.2 mg BSA. In addition, to test whether the glycine used in the conjugation procedure had any effects on the tumors, in half of the animals of each control group 0.088 M glycine was added to the PBS.

All animals were sacrificed 24 hours after the last injection. The therapeutic effects were assessed by determining the tumor volumes at the beginning of each treatment cycle and at the time of sacrifice with the formula:

$$V = \frac{\pi}{6} \cdot (d_1 \cdot d_2 \cdot d_3)$$

in which d_1, d_2, d_3 represent the 3 largest diameters. In addition, to provide a common term of comparison, the growth increment (GI) for a 10-day period was calculated for each tumor using the formula:

$$GI = \frac{V_2 / V_1}{T} \cdot 10$$

where V_1 and V_2 represent the tumor volumes at the beginning and at the end of a treatment period and T the duration of treatment in days.

The mean and standard error of the volumes and of the GI values of each group were used for comparative analyses. Since no statistically significant differences were found between the control mice that received 0.088 M glycine and those that did not, the values of all mice of each group were pooled. Statistical significance was checked using Student $\underline{t}$ test with a significance level of 0.05.

RESULTS

As in previous studies, the injected tumors were used to assess the local therapeutic effects, whereas the systemic effects were evaluated on the contralateral (noninjected) tumors (1,13). It should be pointed out that because of species specificity of IFNs, the human nIFNα used in these experiments could not affect the immunological system of the host; the anti-tumor effects, therefore, were due only to the direct action of the nIFNα on the tumor cells (13). The volumetric progression of the tumors is illustrated in Figs. 1 and 2. All injected tumors in the experimental and control groups continued to grow during therapy. No actual regression was observed in any of the tumors. However, the volumetric increase was significantly smaller in the groups treated with nIFNα and Mc5, whether conjugated or not, than in the other groups. A similar trend, but of lesser magnitude, was shown by the noninjected tumors.

These findings are corroborated by the observations on the GIs (Table 1). Considering first the injected tumors, it was found that, in comparison with the PBS controls, the mice treated with nIFNα conjugated to Mc5 had a much smaller GI, especially after 4 treatment cycles ($P \ll 0.0005$). The GI of mice treated with unconjugated nIFNα and Mc5 showed only a small and statistically insignificant difference with that of the PBS controls during the first 2 cycles, but a substantial lowering of the GI became manifest in the 3rd and 4th cycles ($P < 0.01$). Small, although statistically significant differences in GI were detected between mice treated with nIFNα alone and the PBS controls after 2 ($P < 0.025$) and 4 cycles ($P < 0.0005$). An even lesser effect was shown by the Mc5-treated mice, an effect that was noticeable only at the end of therapy ($P < 0.0025$). Comparing the group of mice treated with nIFNα conjugated to Mc5 with those receiving unconjugated nIFNα and Mc5 it can be seen that the latter had a significantly higher GI after 2 weeks of therapy ($P < 0.01$), whereas no difference between these 2 groups could be detected after 4 cycles. On the contrary, by the end of the 4th cycle of therapy, the GI of mice treated with nIFNα alone became much greater than that of mice receiving nIFNα and Mc5 conjugated ($P < 0.0025$) or unconjugated ($P < 0.005$). Noninjected tumors showed only minor differences in GI between the PBS control and the other groups. The differences widened

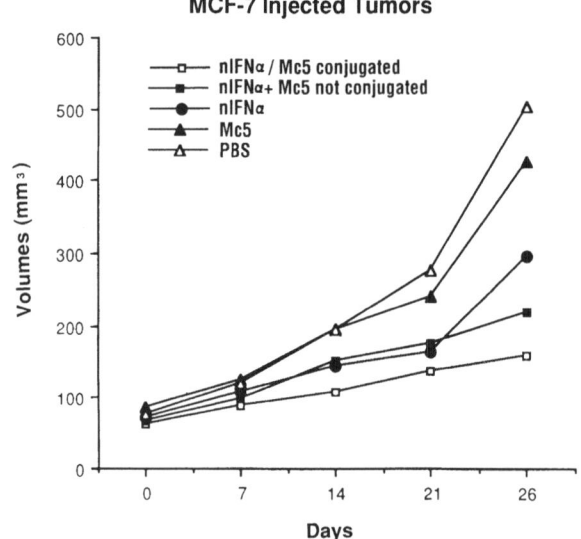

Fig. 1   Effects of 4 cycles of therapy on the mean volumes of MCF-7
tumors injected intralesionally.

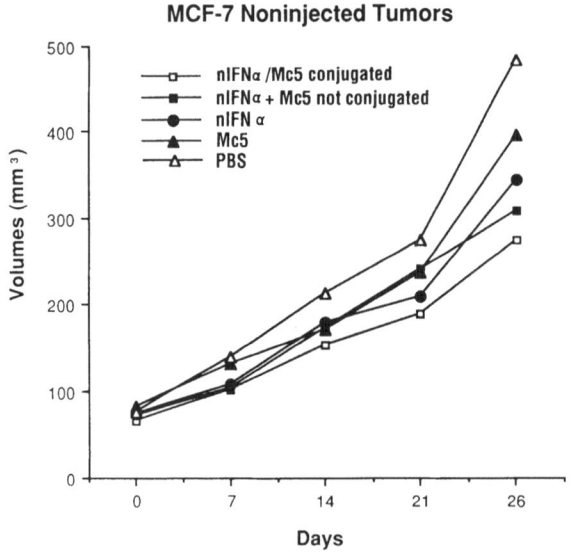

Fig. 2   Systemic effects of 4 cycles of therapy on the mean volumes
of MCF-7 tumors.

slightly and became statistically significant after 4 cycles of therapy, but they remained strikingly smaller than those shown by the corresponding injected tumors.

DISCUSSION

This study indicates that human nIFNα and MoAb Mc5 exerted a greater anti-tumor effect on MCF-7 xenografts when they were administered in combination than when they were given alone. Indeed, the injected tumors of animals treated with nIFNα alone showed only a moderate growth inhibitory effect which was comparable to that obtained in previous studies using the same dosage and treatment modalities (1,13). Even lesser effects were produced by Mc5 alone. This limited response was expected since in this study Mc5 was used at a much lower concentration than that previously found to cause pronounced inhibition of the growth of breast cancer xenografts including MCF-7 (6). Therefore, it would appear that the therapeutic response of our tumors to IL injections of nIFNα and Mc5 combined was greater than it would be expected from an additive action only, and that the 2 agents most likely acted through a synergistic process.

The synergistic effects were manifested mainly in the injected tumors, i.e. locally rather than systemically. It should be noted that in previous experiments in which nIFNα was used alone or in combination with nIFNγ the difference between the local and systemic effects was less striking (1,13). Such behavior is interesting, although unclear. It could be due, at least in part, to differences in molecular weight in the injected preparations. Natural leukocyte IFN is a small molecule as compared to the sizeable complex of nIFNα (MW ca. 20,000) and Mc5 (MW ca. 150,000) when conjugated in a 1:1 ratio. Therefore, it is possible that the complex remains longer than free IFN at the injected site.

The mechanism responsible for the potentiation of nIFNα and Mc5 in the present experiments is not yet understood. It could be due to targeting of the IFN by the MoAb, a mechanism that has been found to be operative in vitro using IFN coupled to a tumor-specific MoAb and by means of 2 cross-linked MoAbs, one specific for a cell antigen and the other for IFN (3,14). In our model, nIFNα covalently conjugated to Mc5 acted more rapidly than the 2 agents administered concomitantly by separate injections. In fact, during the first 2 weeks of therapy, the tumors injected with the conjugated preparation displayed a significantly lower GI than those treated with unconjugated nIFNα and Mc5. This suggests a greater synergistic interaction between the conjugated agents, presumably as a result of a targeting effect. At the end of the 4th treatment cycle, however, the difference in GI between the groups treated with the conjugated and unconjugated nIFNα and Mc5 was no longer apparent. Therefore, the possibility exists that some other mechanism played a role in producing the delayed effects of the unconjugated nIFNα and Mc5.

It is also possible that nIFNα stimulated the expression of antigens detectable by Mc5 thus making the carcinoma cells a better target for the tumoricidal action of the MoAb. This type of mechanism has been found to be effective on human colon cancer xenografts in which the expression of a tumor antigen was enhanced by the administration of recombinant IFNα thereby leading to an increased binding of a MoAb to the target cells (5). However, our results, especially the different early responses to conjugated and unconjugated nIFNα and Mc5, are difficult to explain solely on the basis of this mechanism. Furthermore, in previous experiments, the administration of natural and recombinant IFNα to MCF-7 xenografts over a period of 2 weeks did not result in any appreciable enhancement of immunostaining of the carcinoma cells by Mc5 (13).

The presently available evidence does not allow to draw definite conclusions, although it appears likely that more than 1 mechanism is responsible for the synergistic action of nIFNα and Mc5. The results described above are encouraging and indicate the need for further study in order to improve the effectiveness of this therapeutic approach and to elucidate the mechanism involved.

TABLE 1. GROWTH INCREMENT OF MCF-7 TUMORS TREATED IL WITH nIFNα and Mc5*

Treatment	N	Injected Tumors		Noninjected Tumors	
		2 cycles	4 cycles	2 cycles	4 cycles
nIFNα/Mc5 conjug.	20	1.2+0.08	1.0+0.1	1.7+0.1	1.7+0.1
nIFNα + Mc5 nonconj.	10	1.5+0.1	1.1+0.1	1.7+0.1	1.7+0.2
nIFNα	20	1.4+0.1	1.6+0.2	1.7+0.1	1.8+0.1
Mc5	20	1.6+0.1	1.9+0.1	1.5+0.1	1.9+0.1
PBS	18	1.8+0.1	2.5+0.2	2.0+0.2	2.5+0.2

* Mean ± Standard Error

ACKNOWLEDGEMENTS

Partial support was received from the Winfield Baird Foundation, William J. and Mary F. Cooper Research Fund, Jerome E. Goldman Cancer Research Fund, Margaret Milliken Hatch Foundation, Milstein Medical Research Foundation, Ambrose Monell Foundation, Mrs. Mary K. Monell, Mr. and Mrs. Anthony K. Moulton, Mr. and Mrs. George M. Shapiro, Theodore and Renée Weiler Foundation, and the Weissman Charitable and Educational Fund and NIH-NCI Grant R01-CA 39936. We are grateful to Hanna-Leena Kauppinen at The Finnish Red Cross Blood Transfusion Service for the purification of the interferon by immunoadsorption.

REFERENCES

1. L. Ozzello, D.V. Habif, C.M. DeRosa, and K. Cantell, Treatment of human breast cancer xenografts using natural interferons α and-γ injected singly or in combination, J. Interferon Res. 8:679 (1988).

2. P. von Wussow, B. Berthold, F. Hartmann, and H. Deicher, Intralesional interferon-alpha therapy in advanced malignant melanoma, Cancer 61:1071 (1988).

3. S.S. Alkan, S. Miescher-Granger, D.G. Braun, and H.K. Hochkeppel, Antiviral and antiproliferative effects of interferons delivered via monoclonal antibodies, J. Interferon Res. 4:355 (1984).

4. R. Tran, P. Horan Hand, J.W. Greiner, S. Pestka, and J. Schlom, Enhancement of surface antigen expression on human breast carcinoma cells by recombinant human interferons, J. Interferon Res. 8:75 (1988).

5. J.W. Greiner, F. Guadagni, P. Noguchi, S. Pestka, D. Colcher,P.B. Fisher, and J. Schlom, Recombinant interferon enhances monoclonal antibody-targeting of carcinoma lesions in vivo, Science 235:895 (1987).

6. R.L. Ceriani, E.W. Blank, and J.A. Peterson, Experimental immunotherapy of human breast carcinomas implanted in nude mice with a mixture of monoclonal antibodies against human milk fat globule components, Cancer Res. 47:532 (1987).

7. R.L. Ceriani, and E.W. Blank, Experimental therapy of human breast tumors with ^{131}I-labeled monoclonal antibodies against the human milk fat globule, Cancer Res. 48:4664 (1988).

8. K. Cantell, S. Hirvonen, H.-L. Kauppinen and G. Myllyla, Production of interferon in human leukocytes from normal donors with the use of Sendai virus, Methods Enzymol. 78:29 (1981).

9. K. Cantell, S. Hirvonen, and H.-L. Kauppinen, Production and partial purification of human immune interferon, Methods Enzymol. 119:54 (1986).

10. H.-L. Kauppinen, S. Hirvonen, and K. Cantell, Effect of purification procedures on the composition of human leukocyte interferon preparations, Methods Enzymol. 119:27 (1986).

11. R.L. Ceriani, J.A. Peterson, J.Y. Lee, R. Moncada, and E.W. Blank, Characterization of cell surface antigens of human mammary epithelial cells with monoclonal antibodies prepared against human milk fat globule. Som. Cell Gen. 9:415 (1983).

12. J.L. Dickerson, J.J. Kornuc, and D.C. Rees, Complex formation between Flavodoxin and Cytochrome c. J. Biol. Chem. 260:5175 (1985).

13. L. Ozzello, D.V. Habif, C.M. DeRosa, and K. Cantell, Effects of intralesional injections of interferons-α on xenografts of human mammary carcinoma cells (BT-20 and MCF-7), J. Interferon Res. 8:208 (1988).

14. S.S. Alkan, H. Towbin, and H.K. Hochkeppel, Enhanced antiproliferative action of interferon targeted by bispecific monoclonal antibodies, J. Interferon Res. 8:25 (1988).

IMMUNOLYMPHSCINTIGRAPHY WITH BCD-F9 MONOCLONAL ANTIBODY AND ITS $F(ab')_2$

FRAGMENTS FOR THE PREOPERATIVE STAGING OF BREAST CANCERS

Rosemonde Mandeville, Christian Schatten, Norbert Pateisky,
Marie-Josée Dicaire, Benoît Barbeau and Brigitte Grouix

Immunology Research Center
Institut Armand-Frappier
Laval-des-Rapides, Québec, Canada

First Department of Obstetrics and Gynecology
University of Vienna, Vienna, Austria

ABSTRACT

    In breast cancer, assessment of axillary lymph node status is
the most important prognostic factor for accurate staging, management
and follow-up of patients with primary tumors. Several studies suggest
that preoperative staging with techniques as direct breast lymphography,
ultrasound and CT-scan often fail to identify the extent of the metastatic involvement in the axilla. To this end, we have developed a
novel, simple, non-invasive and reliable immunolymphscintigraphic (ILS)
technique that allows the accurate preoperative diagnosis of lymph
node metastasis in patients with early stages of breast cancer[1-4].
In this article, we report on a consecutive series of thirty-nine breast
cancer patients undergoing preoperative staging by ILS using the BCD-F9
monoclonal antibody or its $F(ab')_2$ fragments. Each patient received
1 mg of a purified preparation containing 1 mCi of Iodine-123, by a
subcutaneous injection into the fingerwebs between the 2nd and 3rd
finger of both hands. Scans obtained 4, 8 and 12 hours after injection
demonstrated adequate tumor accumulation of radiolabeled antibody and
accurate tumor visualisation without any background substraction.
ILS results were always compared to the histopathological staging.
When intact immunoglobulin molecules were injected, 10 out of 11 patients
with breast cancer were true positives and 19 out of 21 were true nega-
tives. For the $F(ab')_2$ fragments, ILS results were positive in 3 out
of 3 patients with metastatic cancer and negative in 3 out of 4 patients
without metastatic involvement of the axilla. Most importantly to
our study, all of the 12 patients with benign breast disease studied
showed no positive imaging.

INTRODUCTION

Although the feasibility of radiolabeling antibodies and the demonstration by external scanning that such antibodies localize in target organs was demonstrated 40 years ago[5], it was undoubtedly the advent of the hybridoma technology and the development of monoclonal antibodies (MAbs) of well-defined specificity, low cross-reactivity, and high affinity to human tumor-associated antigens that has rekindled interest in immunoscintigraphy and allowed the development of a panel of potentially useful tumor markers. Actually, radioimmunodetection of tumors has become the subject of intense research efforts and clinical trials have demonstrated that MAbs can be administered quite safely and will localize specifically to carcinomas, melanomas and human lymphomas[6-12]. But immunoscintigraphy is still at an early developmental stage and it rarely discloses neoplasms of diameters smaller than 1.0 cm. Recent data have shown that this technique can complement more conventional radiologic techniques and can even detect, in some cases, occult distant metastasis[17].

We have focussed our studies on the BCD-F9 monoclonal antibody as it appears to meet all the criteria of a useful marker for the radioimmunodetection of axillary lymph node metastasis in breast cancer patients[13,14]. BCD-F9 is a murine IgG2a monoclonal antibody which was generated by the hyperimmunization of mice with a preparation of whole BT-20 breast carcinoma cells[15,16]. This antibody identifies a novel human breast associated cell surface antigen: gp39. Using fresh frozen human tissues, we have previously reported[4] that this antigen is present in 69% of the mammary adenocarcinomas studied and 51% of their metastatic tumors. In benign breast lesions, 75% of the fibrocystic diseases and the fibroadenomas studied were positive. In normal tissues, positive staining was mainly confined to the mammary cells, the only two exceptions being the smooth muscle cells surrounding blood vessels and basement membranes lining few epithelia. All the organs of the gastrointestinal, the respiratory, and the genitourinary systems studied were negative, except for a moderate to very low reactivity with the glandular epithelium of the oesophagus and the larynx. Of the 34 non-mammary human neoplasms of epithelial origin studied, only hepatocarcinomas (4/4) were strongly positive while ovarian adenocarcinomas (3/4) were focally positive. Unlike another anti-breast cancer MAb already described[15], BCD-F9 does not bind to any subset of circulating lymphocytes, leucocytes, erythrocytes or any sarcomas and lymphomas.

We have selected Iodine-123 as the radionuclide to test the feasibility of using our MAb for radioimaging mainly because we believe that I-123 is the best gamma-emitting radioisotope presently available. Its energy of 129 keV is perfectly suited for imaging with a gamma camera[1-4,16-19]. Although its half-life of 13 hours is quite short, I-123 represents an optimal tracer especially when it is coupled to the smaller F(ab) or F(ab')$_2$ antibody fragments which penetrate more easily into the tumor and are rapidly cleared from the circulation[18,20-22]. In this paper we present results obtained when I-123 labeled-BCD-F9 was administered subcutaneously to 39 patients with a suspected diagnosis of breast cancer. We also compare the use of F(ab')$_2$ fragments to the intact antibody molecule.

PATIENTS AND METHODS

Patients

A series of 39 patients with either suspected malignant or benign breast lesions were investigated by immunolymphscintigraphy (ILS) a

204

few days before surgery. Twenty-seven had clinical, radiological or cytological evidence of breast cancers, while twelve had benign lesions. All patients gave their informed consent to participate in this trial and were included in a previously ongoing program for the preoperative staging of breast cancer at the First Department of Obstetrics and Gynecology, University of Vienna, Vienna, Austria. In case of malignant tumors, a modified radical mastectomy with axillary lymph nodes dissection was performed. For benign lesions, only a simple tumorectomy was required. All surgical materials from both the primary lesions and the axillary dissection were subjected to conventional histopathological examinations. In each patient, the thyroid was blocked pharmaceutically, and hypersensitivity against murine immunoglobulin tested by a subcutaneous injection of 10 μl of normal mouse IgG. Seven patients were given the F(ab')$_2$ fragments of the BCD-F9 MAb, while thirty-two received the intact immunoglobulin molecule. None of these patients showed any sign of discomfort during or after the injection of the radiolabeled BCD-F9 or its F(ab')$_2$ fragments. No allergies to the injected antibodies were noted.

Monoclonal antibodies

The monoclonal antibody BCD-F9 is a murine IgG2a directed against a 39 Kd glycoprotein present on the cell surface membrane of breast epithelial cells of normal and malignant origin. The immunization procedure, cell fusion protocols, MAb production techniques and specificity tests of BCD-F9 have been described elsewhere[13,14]. Ascites were collected after the i.p. inoculation of 10^7 BCD-F9 hybridoma cells in Pristane-primed BALB/c mice. The immunoglobulin in the ascitic fluid was precipitated by three sequential ammonium sulphate treatments and F(ab')$_2$ fragments prepared by pepsin digestion of the IgG molecule as already described[3]. Briefly, a purified preparation of BCD-F9 IgG at 0.6 mg/ml in 0.1 M citrate buffer (pH 4.2) was incubated for 3 hours at 37°C with pepsin (Sigma Chemical Co.) at 75 μg/ml. The digest was rapidly neutralized by the addition of 1.0 M Tris base to a final pH of 7.5 to 8.0 and then dialyzed. Its purity was determined by SDS-PAGE electrophoresis. Both IgG and F(ab')$_2$ fragment preparations were filtered and all end lots were tested for freedom from contamination with Mycoplasma and adventitious viruses, for pyrogenicity, sterility, and general safety.

Immediately prior to their subcutaneous injection, the intact antibody molecule or its fragments were labeled with Iodine-123 using the Iodogen method as already described[1]. A Sephadex G-10 column was used to separate protein-bound and free I-123 after completion of the reaction. Before and after iodination, immune reactivity was tested in an RIA assay using either BT-20 or MCF-7 cells as both of these mammary carcinoma cell lines express the gp39 antigen. More than 90% of the antibody remained immunoreactive after radiolabeling and there was no immunoglobulin aggregates after the iodination procedure as tested by HPLC profiles.

In vivo imaging

For radioimaging, approximately 1 mg of I-123-labeled intact IgG or its F(ab')$_2$ fragment with an activity of approximately 1 mCi per mg of protein, were injected subcutaneously between the 2nd and 3rd finger of both hands. Three static scintigrams of both axillary regions were recorded at predefined intervals, i.e. 4, 8 and 12 hours after injection of the radiolabeled MAb preparations. Criteria for scan interpretation were based on previous experimental data comparing both the healthy and the tumor-bearing site[1-4]. The accumulation of hot

Table 1. Correlations of ILS results with histopathological findings

BCD-F9	Total Nb of patients tested	True Positive[a] (TP)	True Negative[b] (TN)
Intact antibody	32	10/11	19/21
F(ab')$_2$ fragments	7	3/3	3/4

[a] True positive (TP) value = Nb of positive results as confirmed by conventional histopathology divided by the total number of positive ILS results.
[b] True negative (TN) value = Nb of negative results by histopathology divided by the total number of negative ILS results.

spots of radioactive material was judged to be suggestive of metastatic involvement only when the activity deposited in the ipsilateral axilla remained throughout the whole length of the scanning procedure, and when the observed count-rate of hot spots was significantly different than that of the non-affected side. To verify our results we applied a special statistical program by means of "regions of interest technique", i.e.; regions in both the tumor and normal tissues of the same size were compared for the absolute amount of MAb uptake. Gauss-curves were then plotted where the sum of counts corresponds to the maximum of the curve and the square root of the standard deviation. When the overlay of both curves was less than 1%, hot spots were identified as metastatic lesions and uptake of radiolabeled BCD-F9 in the axillary lymph nodes was judged to be specific. Image interpretation was performed without knowledge of any other investigation results, namely mammography and/or circulating tumor markers.

RESULTS AND DISCUSSION

BCD-F9 immunoglobulin is of the IgG2a isotype and peptic digestion of the molecules regularly yielded 60% of F(ab')$_2$ fragments. Both intact Ig molecules and F(ab')$_2$ fragments were satisfactorily iodinated and after radiolabeling 90% iodinated intact IgG molecules and F(ab')$_2$ fragments with an activity of 1 mCi per mg of protein could be recovered. Tables 1 and 2 summarize data on a consecutive series of 39 patients studied up to August 1988: In thirty-two patients we administered the whole IgG molecule of BCD-F9 and in seven patients its F(ab')$_2$ fragment. Both MAb preparations had been previously labeled with I-123. Scintigraphic images with both the MAb and its fragments were perfectly clear and allowed tumor visualisation in the affected axilla without any background substraction. Fig. 1 illustrates a representative scan 8 hours post injection where 3 different axillary ganglia are visible and where the blood pool radioactivity is reduced to a very low degree; accumulation of radiolabeled antibody was mainly confined to the spleen. We have also observed another difference in scintigraphic images between the F(ab')$_2$ fragments and the intact antibody concerning the clearance rate, i.e.; a more rapid decrease in blood radioactivity was demonstrated.

Table 2. Validation of the ILS technique using the intact BCD-F9 monoclonal antibody or its F(ab')$_2$ fragments

ILS Results			Intact Antibody	F(ab')$_2$ Fragments	Overall Results
Sensitivity	=	$\dfrac{TP}{TP + FN}$	91%	100%	93%
Specificity	=	$\dfrac{TN}{TN + FP}$	90%	75%	88%
Accuracy	=	$\dfrac{TP + TN}{\text{Total Nb of Pts}}$	91%	86%	90%
Positive Predictive Value	=	$\dfrac{TP}{TP + FP}$	83%	75%	81%
Negative Predictive Value	=	$\dfrac{TN}{TN + FN}$	95%	100%	96%

TP = True Positive; FP = False Positive
TN = True Negative; FN = False Negative
Pts = patients

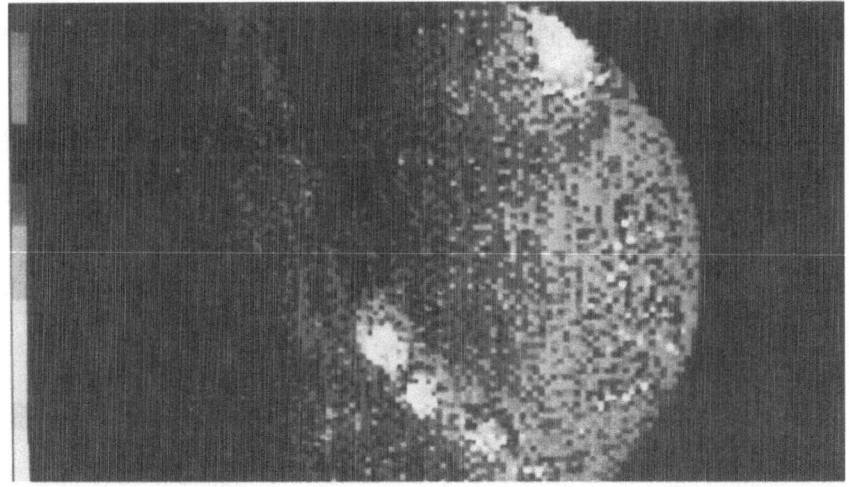

Fig. 1. Photograph of scintigram (anterior view of left axillary
region) of representative breast cancer 8 hours post injection
of radiolabeled BCD-F9. Three hot spots are visualized demonstrating
high antibody uptake due to axillary involvement (apex of the
axilla too). Note the low background reactivity in blood stream
and the accumulation of radioactive material in the spleen.

The image in Fig. 1 does not prove specificity of binding; one might argue[24-26] that non-specific uptake of antibodies might be greater in hyperplastic nodes than in a normal nodes. We demonstrated specificity by simultaneously using specific and nonspecific radiolabeled MAbs of the same isotype (IgG2a). In this double-labeling technique 123-I-BCD-F9 and 125-I-F(ab')$_2$ fragments of a monoclonal antibody, 4C4, specific for Hepatitis B surface antigen (graciously supplied by SORIN BIOMEDICA) were used in a limited number of patients. No positive scans were obtained in any of the 5 control patients injected with the non specific 4C4 antibody.

In our hands, delivery via the lymphocytics proved to be very useful in the visualisation of axillary lymph node metastasis of breast cancer patients. Weinstein et al.[24,25] had previously reported that compared to the i.v. route, delivery via the lymphatics, provided a more efficient means for localizing antibody in lymph nodes. Our results tend to prove this point and reveal that the ILS technique, using BCD-F9 is quite efficient[1-4]. The overall sensitivity of this technique was 93%, the specificity 88%, and the accuracy 90% (Table 2). We have also employed fragmented MAbs, because Larson et al.[8,20,21,26] had suggested that the Fc region of the molecule is the portion most likely to trigger allergic responses. Several authors have also demonstrated[18,22,23] a marked improvement in the immunoscintigraphic techniques when F(ab')$_2$ fragments were labeled with I-123. In this study, we noticed a marked decrease in background activity in the blood vessels and a more rapid clearance when F(ab')$_2$ fragments were used instead of the intact MAb (Fig. 1). However, a slight increase in the specificity was also noted (Table 2).

We used the Theory of Bayes[27] as modified by Leclerc and Douville[28], to calculate both the positive predictive values and the negative predictive values of our ILS technique (Table 2). For the intact antibody it was 81% and 96%, respectively. With the F(ab')$_2$ fragments the positive predictive value was raised to 75% while the negative predictive value dropped to 100%. We rather think that these differences between results obtained with the intact IgG and the F(ab')$_2$ fragments (Tables 1 and 2) are not very significant, principally because of the small number of patients investigated to date with the BCD-F9 F(ab')$_2$ fragments. We also believe that these promissing results need to be confirmed by a larger prospective controlled clinical trial, in order to test the benefits of the ILS and to establish if this exciting new technology can become a precise, reliable tool for clinical decision making.

ACKNOWLEDGEMENTS

The authors wish to thank Dr. C. Hours of the Quality Control Center and Dr. J. Lecomte from the Hybridoma Service at Institut Armand-Frappier. Special thanks to Dr. Mary Clare Walker for kindly reviewing this article and Miss Sylvia Girardon for expert advice during the preparation of the manuscript.

REFERENCES

1. R. Mandeville, N. Pateisky, K. Philipp, E. Kubista, F. Dumas and B. Grouix, Immunoscintigraphy of axillary lymph node metastasis in breast cancer patients using monoclonal antibodies: First clinical findings, Anticancer Research 6:1257 (1986).
2. N. Pateisky, C. Schatten, H. Enzelsberger, J. Burchell and R. Mandeville, Immunlymphszintigraphie: Ein neues Verfahren für nicht-invasives Lymphknoten-Staging, dargestellt am Beispiel des Mammakarzinoms, Dtsch. Med. Wschr., 113:250 (1987).

3. C. Schatten, N. Pateisky, H. Enzelsberger, B. Grouix and R. Mandeville, Clinical value of immunolymphscintigraphy in patients with breast cancer, In Vivo, in press (1988).

4. R. Mandeville, N. Pateisky, C. Schatten, A. Amarouch, M. Zelechowska, S. Sidrac-Ghali, L. Giroux and B. Grouix, Axillary lymphscintigraphy with 123-I-labeled monoclonal antibody for the preoperative detection of lymph node metastasis in breast cancer patients, in "Monoclonal Antibodies in Clinical Oncology", J.Y. Douillard and R.A. Carrano, eds., Marcel Deckker Publisher, N.Y., in press (1989).

5. D. Pressman and G. Keighley, The zone of activity of antibodies as determined by the use of radioactive tracers. The zone of activity of nephrotoxic antikidney serum, J. Immunol. 59:141 (1948).

6. J.-P. Mach, F. Buchegger, M. Forni, J. Ritschard, C. Berche, J.-D. Lumbroso, M. Schreyer, C. Girardet, R.S. Accolla and S. Carrel, Use of radiolabeled monoclonal anti-CEA antibodies for the detection of human carcinoma by external photoscanning and tomoscintigraphy, Immunol. Today 2:239 (1981).

7. T. Ghose, S.T. Norwell, J. Aquino, P. Belitsky, J. Tai, A. Guclu and A.H. Blair, Localization of 131-I-labeled antibodies in human renal cell carcinomas and in a mouse hepatoma and correlation with tumor detection by photoscanning, Cancer Res. 40:3018 (1980).

8. S.M. Larson, J.P. Brown, P.W. Wright, J.A. Carrasquillo, I. Hellstrøm, K.-E. Hellstrøm, Imaging of melanoma with I-131-labeled monoclonal antibodies, J. Nuclear Med. 24:123 (1983).

9. H.M. Smedley, P. Finan, E.S. Lennox, A. Ritson, F. Takei, P. Wraight and K. Sikora, Localisation of metastatic carcinoma by a radiolabelled monoclonal antibody, Br. J. Cancer 47:253 (1983).

10. J. Bubenik, J. Kieler, P. Perlmann, S. Paulie, H. Koho, et al., Monoclonal antibody against human urinary bladder carcinomas. Selectivity and utilization for gamma scintigraphy, Eur. J. Cancer Clin. Oncol. 21:701 (1985).

11. A.H. Zimmer, S.T. Rosen, S.M. Spies, M.R. Palovina, J.D. Minna, W.C. Spies and E.A. Silverstein, Radioimmunoimaging of human small cell lung carcinomas with I-131 tumor specific monoclonal antibody, Hybridoma 4:1 (1985).

12. P.A. Bunn, J.A. Carrasquillo, A.M. Keeman, et. al., Imaging of T-cell lymphoma by radiolabelled monoclonal antibodies, Lancet ii:1219 (1984).

13. R. Mandeville, J. Lecomte, F.-M. Sombo, J.P. Chausseau and L. Giroux, Production, purification and biochemical characterization of monoclonal antibodies reacting with breast carcinoma cells, in "Monoclonal Antibodies: Diagnostic and Therapeutic Applications in Tumor and Transplantation", S.N. Chaterjee, ed., PBS Publishing Compagny Inc., Littleton, Mass. (1985): 63.

14. R. Mandeville, L. Giroux, J. Lecomte, J.-P. Chausseau, F. Dumas, I. Ajdukovic, D. Vidal and F. Boury, Production and characterization of monoclonal antibodies showing a different spectrum of reactivity to human breast tissue, Cancer Detection and Prevention 10:89 (1987).

15. D.F. Hayes, M.R. Zalutsky, W. Kaplan, M. Noska, A. Thor, D. Colcher and D.W. Kufe, Pharmacokinetics of radiolabeled monoclonal antibody B6.2 in patients with metastatic cancer, Cancer Res. 46:3157 (1986).

16. N. Pateisky, K. Philipp, W.D. Skodler, K. Czerwenka, G. Hamilton and J. Burchell, Radioimmunodetection in patients with suspected ovarian cancer, J. Nucl. Med. 26:1369 (1985).

17. G.L. Buraggi, L. Callegaro, A. Turrin, N. Cascinelli, et al., Immunoscintigraphy with ^{123}I, ^{99m}Tc and ^{111}In-labelled F(ab')$_2$ fragments of monoclonal antibodies to a human high molecular weight-melanoma associated antigen, J. Nucl. Med. 28:283 (1984).

18. B. Delaloye, A. Bischof-Delaloye, F. Buchegger, V. vonFliedner, J.-P. Grob, J.-C. Volant, J. Pettavel and J.-P. Mach, Detection of colorectal carcinoma by emission-computerized tomography after injection of ^{123}I-labeled Fab or F(ab')$_2$ fragments from monoclonal anti-carcinoembryonic antigen antibodies, J. Clin. Invest. 77:301 (1986).

19. A.A. Epenetos, D. Snook, H. Durbin, P.M. Johnson and J. Taylor-Papadimitriou, Limitations of radiolabeled monoclonal antibodies for localization of human neoplasms, Cancer Res. 46:3183 (1986).

20. S.M. Larson, J.A. Carrasquillo, K.A. Krohn, R.W. McGuffin, D.L. Williams, I. Hellstrøm, K.-E. Hellstrøm and D. Lyster, Diagnostic imaging of malignant melanoma with radiolabeled antitumor antibodies, JAMA 249:811 (1983).

21. S.M. Larson, J.A. Carrasquillo and J.C. Reynolds, Radioimmunodetection and radioimmunotherapy, Cancer Invest. 2(5):363 (1984).

22. F. Buchegger, C.M. Haskell, M. Schreyer, B.R. Scazziga, R. Randin, S. Carrel and J.-P. Mach, Radiolabeled fragments of monoclonal anti-CEA antibodies for localization of human colon carcinoma grafted into nude mice, J. Exp. Med. 158:413 (1983).

23. S.E. Halpern, F. Buchegger, H. Schreyer and J.-P. Mach, Effect of size of radiolabeled antibody and fragments on tumor uptake and distribution in nephrectomized mice, J. Nucl. Med. 25:p112 (1984).

24. J.N. Weinstein, M.A. Steller, A.M. Keeman, D.G. Covell, M.E. Key, S.M. Sieber, R.K. Oldham, K.M. Hwang and R.J. Parker, Monoclonal antibodies in the lymphatics: Selective delivery to lymph node metastases of a solid tumor, Science 222:423 (1983).

25. M.A. Steller, R.J. Parker, D.G. Covell, O.D. Holton III, A.M. Keeman, S.M. Sieber and J.N. Weinstein, Optimization of monoclonal antibody delivery via the lymphatics: the dose dependence, Cancer Res. 46:1830 (1986).

26. S.M. Larson, Radiolabeled monoclonal anti-tumor antibodies in diagnosis and therapy, J. Nucl. Med. 26:538 (1985).

27. T. Bayes, An essay toward solving a problem in the doctrine of chance, Philos. Trans. R. Soc. London 53:370 (1763).

28. P. Leclerc and P. Douville, Probabilité et théorème de Bayes, Ann. Biochim. Clin. Qué. 24(4):149 (1985).

REACTION OF ANTIBODIES TO HUMAN MILK FAT GLOBULE (HMFG) WITH SYNTHETIC

PEPTIDES

Pei X. Xing, Kerry Reynolds, Joe J. Tjandra, Xi L. Tang,
Damian F.J. Purcell and Ian F.C. McKenzie

Research Centre for Cancer and Transplantion
Department of Pathology
The University of Melbourne
Parkville, Victoria, 3052, Australia

Introduction

In the last decade many efforts have been made to produce monoclonal antibodies which react specifically with breast cancer, but not with normal tissue. Most of the antibodies selected appear to react with mammary mucins - whether immunizations were done with fresh breast cancer tissue or metastases, cell lines, or with crude or purified extracts of human milk fat globule (HMFG). These antibodies share many characteristics, such as a preferential reaction with mammary tumours and weak reaction with normal tissue; almost all react with adenocarcinomas of other origin, e.g. pancreas, colon and lung; and most react with high molecular weight mucins (Mr>200,000), although reactions with lower molecular weight components (e.g. 70,000) have also been found on sodium dodecyl sulfate-polyacrylamide gel electrophoresis (SDS-PAGE) analysis [1-6].

HMFG, when purified with monoclonal antibodies, consists mostly of O-linked sugars with a central core protein Mr 70,000-140,000 - the value of 70,000 being obtained on material "stripped" using hydrogen fluoride [7]. Of the antibodies which react with whole HMFG, some react with carbohydrate epitopes and others with the central core protein [7].

Recently, using monoclonal antibodies, several laboratories have obtained partial length cDNAs coding for the core protein [8,9,10]. It was of interest to find that the cDNA clones contained a 60 base pair nucleotide repeating unit, coding for a 20 amino acid protein, and indeed it is likely that this repeating unit was responsible for the reaction of the monoclonal antibodies with procaryotic expression libraries in the λgt11 vector. Using the amino acid sequence obtained from these clones (PDTRPAPGSTAPPAHGVTSA) we have synthesized peptides of varying lengths to determine the reactivity of three anti-HMFG antibodies (BC1, BC2 and BC3), produced in our laboratory[11]. The studies indicated that the three antibodies reacted with a 5-mer peptide - APDTR - which is the smallest epitope which we could detect.

Materials and Methods

The antibodies BC1, BC2 and BC3 have been described elsewhere[11]. Briefly, they were produced by immunizing mice with HMFG and testing after fusion on HMFG by an enzyme-linked immunosorbent assay (ELISA) procedure and subsequently characterized by the immunoperoxidase staining of tissue sections and by SDS-PAGE. All react with breast cancer tissue, give a weak reaction on normal tissue and react with components of Mr approx. 230-280,000; however, they can be distinguished by their different pattern of reactivity on tissue sections[11]. An antibody to colon carcinoma was also used, 5C1, which reacts with a mucin but not with HMFG (unpublished finding).

Peptides (Table 1) were synthesized in our laboratory using the Merryfield solid phase synthesis method with an Applied Biosystems model 430A automated peptide synthesizer (Foster City, CA, USA)[12]. Peptides were named according to the first and last amino acids with reference to the 24-mer peptide in Table 1. Longer peptides (p1-24, p1-15, p16-24) were purified on reverse phase HPLC; shorter peptides were not purified. As a control for antibody binding the T4N1 peptide was synthesized, this is the N-terminus of mouse CD4. It does not react with the antibodies.

Table 1. Synthetic peptides

p1-24	PDTRPAPGSTAPPAHGVTSAPDTR
p21-24	PDTR
p20-24	APDTR
p19-24	SAPDTR
p18-24	TSAPDTR
p17-24	VTSAPDTR
p16-24	GVTSAPDTR
p15-24	HGVTSAPDTR
p14-24	AHGVTSAPDTR
p14-23	AHGVTSAPDT
p1-15	PDTRPAPGSTAPPAH
PA+p1-15	APDTRPAPGSTAPPAH
T4N1	KTLVLGKEQESAELPCECY

The antibodies were tested on the peptides by three methods; the first two involving the peptides in solid phase, the last in liquid phase. In the first method, peptides were coated in 96 well plates at 20µg/ml in 0.05M carbonate buffer, pH9.6, for 2 hrs at 37°C, washed and non-specific binding sites then blocked with 2% bovine serum albumin (BSA). Plates were then washed in phosphate buffered saline (PBS) 0.5% Tween 20. Secondly, peptides were conjugated to BSA using the glutaraldehyde coupling method[13] and examined in a direct binding assay. The conjugation was to ensure efficient binding of peptide to the plate and also to reproduce adjacent repeating units as found in the native HMFG. Using either peptide alone or BSA-peptide coated onto plates, purified antibody was added to wells and incubated at room temperature for two hours, washed and sheep anti-mouse immunoglobulin labelled with horse radish peroxidase added and incubated for one hour at room temperature, washed and ABTS [2, 2'-azino-di-(3-ethyl-benzthiazoline sulfonate)] substrate added[11]. In some cases binding to HMFG was also measured, where HMFG at 10μg/ml was bound onto the plates. In the third assay, peptides were examined in liquid phase by incubating antibody with dilutions of peptide $(0.4 \times 10^{-3}$ - 0.8mM) or with HMFG (0.4μg/ml - 800μg/ml) for 1 hour at room temperature prior to adding to plates which were coated with 10μg/ml of HMFG. Then inhibition of antibody binding to HMFG was quantitated with sheep anti-mouse immunoglobulin labelled with horse radish peroxidase.

Results

We had previously shown that antibodies BC1, BC2 and BC3 reacted with HMFG [11] (Fig. 1). We were also able to show that the antibody reacted with "stripped" HMFG core protein[11]. Therefore it remained to determine whether the antibodies reacted with the peptides and with which segment of the peptide sequence.

Reaction of antibodies with p1-24: All three antibodies reacted with p1-24 peptides, indicating that their reaction with HMFG could totally or partially be explained by reaction with the peptide sequence found in the tandem repeat. It was noted that the three antibodies gave different reactions with BC3 >BC2 > BC1 (Fig. 1).

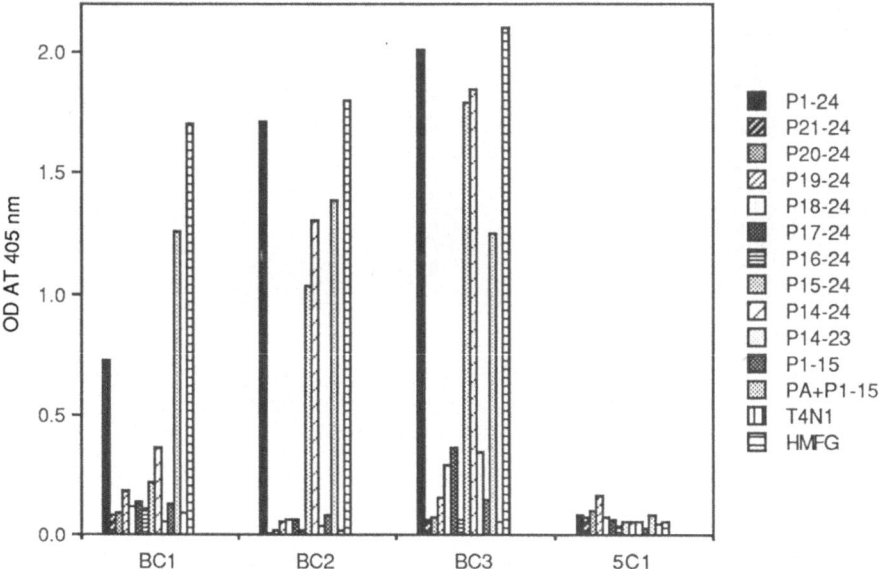

Figure 1   Binding of antibodies BC1, BC2, BC3 and negative control antibody 5CI at concentration of 75μg/ml to the synthetic peptides, negative control peptide T4N1 and HMFG bound directly to the ELISA plate.

Reactions with p1-15, p15-24, p16-24: Reactions with these peptides are shown in Figures 1, 2, 3. It was clear that all three antibodies reacted with p16-24; whereas none reacted with p1-15. However, the reaction with p15-24 and p16-24 (GVTSAPDTR) did not occur in direct binding assay, but the BSA-peptide reacted with the monoclonal antibodies in the direct binding ELISA and strongly in the inhibition test (Fig. 1,2,3). Differences among the three antibodies were noted in that BC1 showed virtually no reaction with p15-24, BC2 reacted moderately, while BC3 gave a very strong reaction - almost as strong as the reaction obtained on HMFG itself or on the peptide p1-24 (Fig. 1). Thus, the reactive epitope appeared to be in the "right" ten amino acids (HGVTSAPDTR) but not in the "left" 15 amino acids (PDTRPAPGSTAPPAH). It was noted that in these two sequences (from the left and right hand sides) PDTR is the common sequence and as p15-24 reacts and p1-15 does not, we conclude that PDTR itself is not a reactive epitope for these antibodies. However, the difference between the left and right hand amino acids, with regard to PDTR, is that p15-24 has alanine (A) in front of the PDTR, whereas p1-15 does not. A new peptide was synthesized with A on the N-terminal end of p1-15 - this peptide reacted with the three antibodies in each of the three assays (Fig. 1,2,3), indicating that APDTR may well be the reactive determinant. Further tests were performed to confirm this finding.

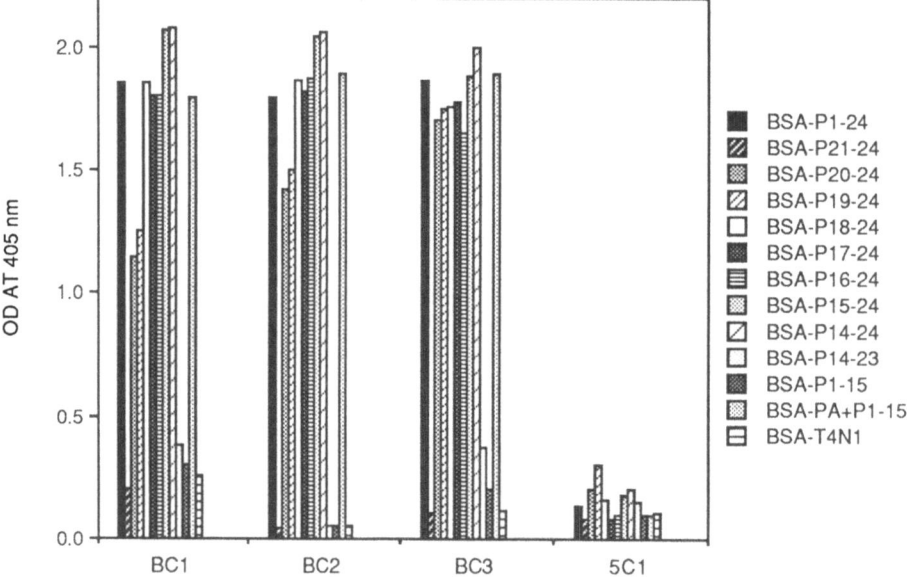

Figure 2   Binding of antibodies BC1, BC2, BC3 and control antibody 5C1 at a concentration of 33μg/ml to the BSA-conjugated peptides and negative control BSA-T4N1 peptide bound directly to the ELISA plate.

Reaction of antibodies with short synthetic peptides: Peptides were synthesized on a backbone of PDTR by adding a single amino acid at a time, removing some of the resin and testing the peptide in all three assays. Thus PDTR, APDTR ,etc were made, the additions being made up to AHGVTSAPDTR which was previously shown to be reactive. The results showed that PDTR was non-reactive with the three antibodies used in each of the three assays. By contrast, APDTR was able to react provided it was bound to BSA or used in the liquid phase inhibition assay (Fig. 1,2,3). We therefore concluded that APDTR is the reactive epitope for the three antibodies, although it was noted from the results that the reactions of the three antibodies differed.

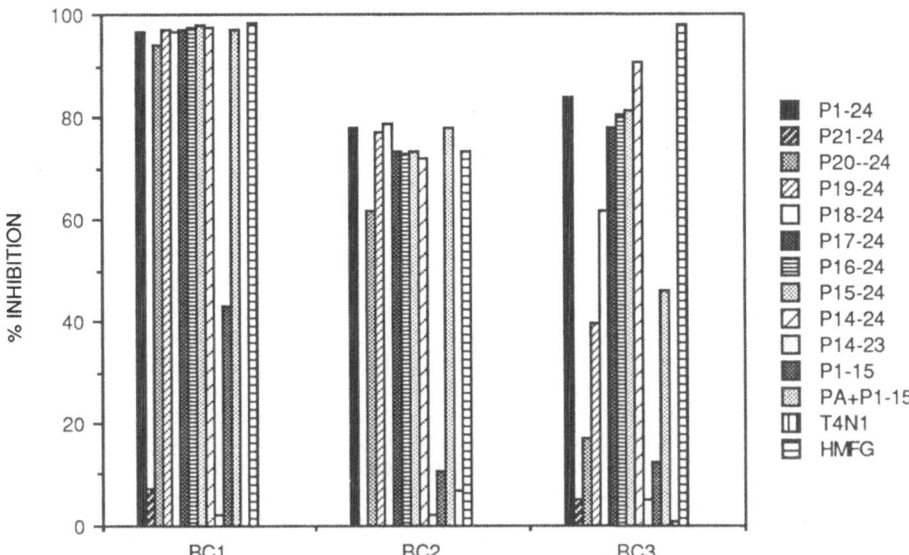

Figure 3   Inhibition of the binding of antibodies BC1, BC2, BC3 and control
antibody 5C1 to HMFG using peptides at concentration of 0.4mM and
HMFG at 400µg/ml.

Importance of R (arginine) in APDTR: A new peptide p14-23 was synthesized which
lacked arginine from the C-terminal end. This peptide was non-reactive and we
therefore concluded that arginine is required at the C-terminal end for reactivity of
the antibodies (Fig. 1,2,3).

Discussion

The studies described herein demonstrate that three antibodies, of different Ig
classes, produced to HMFG all react with the synthetic peptide APDTR. They are
unable to react with the correct peptides ($\leq$ 9 amino acids) when they were bound
directly onto plates, but clearly react when the peptides were conjugated to BSA, or
when used in an inhibition assay when the peptides were in liquid phase. While it is
possible to suggest that the reactions to these antibodies were purely with peptide,
we are unable to exclude an additional role of carbohydrate in the epitope as we have
not produced APDTR with carbohydrate attached to the threonine (or serine in longer
peptides) and indeed would not know which carbohydrate to attach at these points. We
noted that the reactions with HMFG were much stronger than with the synthetic
peptides, and suspect that carbohydrate may play some role in this epitope.

The difference in reactions of the peptide in the solid phase and liquid phase is of
interest and may indicate that the conformation of the 5-mer peptide is important in
the reactivities, however it cannot be excluded that the 5-mer itself binds poorly to
the plate and requires intermediate coupling to the BSA or other carriers to obtain
sufficient concentration on plates for reactivity.

It was of further interest to find that the three antibodies reacted with what must be
the same epitope, whereas previous studies have indicated they block each other
poorly or partially when tested on HMFG, leading us to conclude originally that they
reacted with different epitopes[11]. What can be the explanation for this apparent
difference in results? Firstly, BC3 is an IgM and may have a different spectrum of

reactivity because of its size - as indicated by the differing reactions in direct binding and inhibition tests to BC1 and BC2. Secondly the antibodies could be of differing affinity which could explain these results. The affinity of BC1 and BC2 were measured: BC1 is approximately $1.7 \times 10^9 M^{-1}$, BC2 is $1.7 \times 10^{10} M^{-1}$, i.e. BC2 had a ten fold higher affinity for HMFG[14] and this could explain the apparent difference in reactions on HMFG. However, it is also possible that APDTR forms a major part of an epitope but additional peptides or carbohydrates make up the whole epitope detected by the individual antibodies.

These studies are of interest, demonstrating that at least some of the anti-mucin antibodies to breast cancer react with peptides and that APDTR is immunogenic, at least when found in HMFG. In preliminary studies we have not yet been able to demonstrate that APDTR is itself immunogenic in mice and we are still trying to make antibodies to p1-24 peptide. However, it could be that these anti-peptide antibodies could be more sensitive in serum assays to measure circulating mucins in cancer (as opposed to normal subjects) and we are currently designing a serum test to determine this. Secondly, for the same reason, if the antibodies are more specific for breast cancers than say anti-carbohydrate antibodies, they could be more useful in imaging and for therapy. However, this remains to be seen. It has also been suggested that the core protein of HMFG is hidden in a carbohydrate coating in normal subjects, and that this is exposed in patients with cancer. If this is the case, then subjects may not be immunologically tolerant to this core protein and patients with cancer, with the exposed core protein, could well have antibodies to the core protein or synthetic peptides. If this is so, and we are currently testing this, then the peptides of the core protein could form the basis for a vaccine for immunization against breast cancer.

Summary

The mammary mucin presented by HMFG contains a core protein, cDNAs of which have recently been isolated. Using the nucleotide sequence from these cDNA clones the peptide sequence for a 20 amino acid repeating unit was obtained (PDTRPAPGSTAPPAHGVTSA) and synthetic peptides made from this sequence. Three of our anti-HMFG antibodies (BC1, BC2, BC3) were tested on this and on shorter synthetic peptides, and demonstrated that the major reactivity was with the peptide in the right hand side of the p1-24 peptide. When small synthetic peptides were produced the predominant reaction was with those containing the sequence APDTR. The presence of amino acid in the position of alanine is essential for when this is removed (PDTR) there is no reactivity; similarly when R is removed there is also no reactivity. Thus the 5-mer peptide APDTR is an immunogenic epitope in HMFG .

References

1.   J. Taylor-Papadimitriou, J. Peterson, J. Arklie, J. Burchell, R.L. Ceriani and W.F. Bodmer, Monoclonal antibodies to epithelium - specific components of human milk fat globule membrane: production and reaction with cells in culture. Int. J. Cancer 28:17 (1981).

2.   J. Hilkens, F. Buijs, J. Hilgers, Ph. Hageman, J. Calafat, A. Sonnenberg, and M. van der Valk, Monoclonal antibodies agaisnt human milk-fat globule membranes detecting differentiation antigens of the mammary gland and its tumours. Int. J. Cancer, 34:197 (1984).

3.   D. Kufe, G. Inghirami, M. Abe, D. Hayes, H. Justi-Wheeler and J. Schlom, Differential reactivity of a novel monoclonal antibody (DF3) with human malignant versus benign breast tumours. Hybridoma, 3:223 (1984).

4.   R.L. Ceriani, J.A. Peterson, J.Y. Lee, R. Moncada and E.W. Blank, Characterization of cell surface antigens of human mammary epithelial cells with monoclonal antibodies prepared against human milk fat globule. Somatic Cell Genetics, 9:415 (1983).

5.   I.O. Ellis, C.P. Hinton, J. MacNay, C.W. Elston, A. Robins, A.A.R.S. Owainati, R.W. Blamey, R.W. Baldwin and B. Ferry, Immunocytochemical staining of breast carcinoma with the monoclonal antibody NCRC11: A new prognostic indicator. Br. Med. J., 290:881 (1985).

6.   S.A. Stacker, C.H. Thompson, C. Riglar and I.F.C. McKenzie, A new breast carcinoma antigen defined by a monoclonal antibody. J. Natl. Cancer Inst., 75:801 (1985).

7.   J.Burchell, S. Genlder, J. Taylor-Papadimitriou, A. Girling, R. Millis and D. Lamport, Development and characterization of breast cancer reactive monoclonal antibodies directed to the core protein of the human milk mucin. Cancer Res. 47:5476 (1987).

8.   S.J. Gendler, J.M. Burchell, T. Duhig, D. Lamport, R. White, M. Parker and J. Taylor-Papadimitriou, Cloning of partial cDNA encoding differentiation and tumour-associated mucin glycoproteins expressed by human mammary epithelium. Proc. Natl. Acad. Sci. USA. 84:6060 (1987).

9.   J. Siddiqui, M. Abe, D. Hayes, E. Shani, E. Yunis and D. Kufe, Isolation and sequencing of a cDNA coding for the human DF3 breast carcinoma - associated antigen. Proc. Natl. Acad. Sci. USA. 85:2320 (1988).

10.   S. Gendler, J. Taylor-Papadimitriou, T. Duhig, J. Rothbard and J. Burchell, A highly immunogenic region of a human polymorphic epithelial mucin expressed by carcinomas is made up of tandem repeats. J. Biol. Chem. 263:12820 (1988).

11.   P.X. Xing, J.J. Tjandra, S.A. Stacker, J.G. Teh, C.H. Thompson, P.J. McLaughlin, and I.F.C. McKenzie, Monoclonal antibodies reactive with mucin expressed in breast cancer. Immunol. Cell Biol. (in press) (1988).

12.   R.S. Hodges and R.B. Merrifield, Monitoring of solid phase peptide synthesis by an automated spectrophotometric picrate method. Anal. Biochem. 65:241 (1975).

13.   J.P. Briand, S. Muller, and M.H.V. Van Regenmortel, Synthetic peptides as antigens: Pitfalls of conjugation methods. J. Immunol. Methods, 78:59 (1985).

14.   P.X. Xing, J.J. Tjandra, K. Reynolds, P.J. McLaughlin, D.F.J. Purcell and I.F.C. McKenzie, The reactivity of Anti-HMFG (Human Milk Fat Globule) Antibodies with synthetic peptides. J. Immunol. (in press) (1988).

INDIVIDUALLY SPECIFIED DRUG IMMUNOCONJUGATES

IN CANCER TREATMENT

Robert K. Oldham, Shuen-Kuei Liao,
John R. Ogden and William H. Hubbard

Biotherapeutics, Inc.
347 Riverside Drive, P.O. Box 1676
Franklin, TN 37065

ABSTRACT

Forty-three patients, including 13 patients with metastatic breast cancer, each received an individually-specified combination of either Adriamycin (24 patients) or mitomycin-C (19 patients) conjugated murine monoclonal antibodies. Tumors were typed using a panel of antibodies with both immunohistochemistry and flow cytometry. Cocktails composed of 2-6 antibodies were selected based on binding greater than 80% of the malignant cells in the biopsy specimen. These monoclonal antibody cocktails were drug conjugated and administered intravenously.

Seventeen out of twenty-four patients had reactions (fever, chills, pruritis and skin rash) to the administration of Adriamycin immunoconjugates, but these were tolerable in all but two patients. In several patients it was demonstrated that there was limited antigenic drift among various biopsies within the same patient over time. Up to 1 gram of Adriamycin and up to 5 grams of monoclonal antibody were administered. Two patients with breast carcinoma had definite improvement in ulcerating skin lesions. The limiting factor appeared to be a variable dissociation of active Adriamycin from the antibody which unpredictably caused hemopoietic depression.

Similar findings were noted in 19 patients with mitomycin-C conjugates. Thrombocytopenia at a 60mg dose of mitomycin-C in this schedule was dose limiting. Preliminary serological evidence suggests that the development of an IgM antibody which is specific against the mouse monoclonal antibody has the specificity and sensitivity to predict clinical reactions. These antibodies were quantitatively less in mitomycin-C than Adriamycin treated patients.

INTRODUCTION

This paper describes patients treated with specifically
tailored monoclonal antibody combinations combined with
Adriamycin or mitomycin-C. The hypothesis that an
individually specified immunoconjugate would be necessary to
cover virtually all cancer cells in a variety of sites
dominated this research. Single monoclonal antibodies
localize in areas of malignancy and to individual malignant
cells (1,2). Antigens can vary within patients in clusters
of tumor cells both by location and over time
(microheterogeneity). Tumor associated antigens may also
vary during phases of tumor cell maturation. We have typed
tumors from more than 150 patients and quantitative
differences are the rule. No two have demonstrated precisely
the same typing pattern (macroheterogeneity). Thus, an
attempt was made to identify combinations of antibodies which
could potentially recognize all of the malignant cells within
a variety of primary and metastatic sites. This was done by
making a large number of monoclonal antibodies against
freshly dispersed tumor cells, xenograft cells or cell lines
recently derived from tumor biopsies. The panel was then
used to type the individual patient's tumor biopsy.
Cocktails were specified to bind greater than 80% of the
cells within the tumor. To that end, preparation of as many
as six antibodies were administered to patients following
drug conjugation.

These antibodies were usually greater than 95% pure,
maintained immunoreactivity after conjugation and were tested
for safety in a variety of systems prior to administration to
patients (Fig. 1). We demonstrated the feasibility of
treating patients with mixtures of monoclonal
immunoconjugates and addressed technical considerations
involved in the process.

MATERIALS AND METHODS

Patient Selection

Twenty males and twenty-three females participated in
this trial. A variety of other cancer types were included as
shown in Table 1.

Patient characteristics and entry proceudres are further
described elsewhere (3). After a determination of
suitability for the study and informed consent, tissue
samples were obtained by biopsy. All typing was done on
frozen tissue, either directly on the biopsy or on tissue
which had been expanded by a xenograft in nude mice or by
tissue culture propagation. Antibody selection was by
immunoperoxidase and flow cytometry as described in detail
elsewhere (3,4).

Antibody Selection and Preparation

Immunization of mice and preparation of hybridomas are
described elsewhere (3,4). Over 100 antibodies were
available for tissue typing and we selected 28 for the
standard panel with 19 used for this study. Seven of these

were acquired elsewhere and 21 were produced in the Biotherapeutics' laboratory. Five of these originated from immunization with breast cancers, eleven from melanomas, three from adenocarcinomas of the kidney, two from an islet cell carcinoma of the pancreas, and seven from colon carcinomas (3). The majority of the antibodies were IgG_1 with the exception of two IgG_2's (melanoma) and five IgG_3's (colon carcinomas).

Frozen tissue specimens (from fresh or cryopreserved primary or metastatic tumors) were assessed for binding of 19 murine monoclonal antibodies from our panel. Out of the 43 patients (one breast cancer patient received one course of Adriamycin and another of mitomycin-C immunoconjugate) included in the subject study, flow cytometry analysis was performed on tumor biopsy cells from 23 of the patients (53%). The agreement between the two techniques was approximately 90%. Interaction of different antibodies was determined on flow cytometry by measurement of the above-described parameters on cells exposed to two or more of the antibodies simultaneously, or sequentially to determine the degree to which the antibodies interacted, either additively or subtractively.

Preparation and Testing of Drug Immunoconjugates

After selection of appropriate monoclonal antibodies, production was scaled up in ascites, and these antibodies were purified in gram amounts and chemically conjugated with Adriamycin (cis-aconitate linker) or mitomycin-C (glutanic acid linker) as is fully described elsewhere (5).

Adriamycin was tightly associated with antibody, but the exact nature of the linkage is unknown (5). A significant percentage of Adriamycin (30-40%) was covalently linked; the remaining drug was tightly but non-covalently associated with antibody. These preparations were stable for at least 6 months in phosphate buffered saline. Mitomycin-C monoclonal antibody molar ratios reproducibly range from 4 to 15, but differed amongst various antibodies. Free mitomycin-C was removed by tangential flow ultrafiltration (Minitan) and the conjugate mixed with mannitol and stored in the dark at 10° centigrade.

The mitomycin-C and Adriamycin immunoconjugates underwent endotoxin analysis (chromagenic LAL test), sterility testing (trypticase soy broth (aerobes, fastidious), thioglycolate broth (anaerobes, aerobes), Sabourad's dextrose agar (fungi), general safety testing (in guinea pigs and mice), and, when cells were available, in vitro cytotoxicity testing ^{3}H-thymidine or ^{75}Se-selenomethionine uptake using the patients own tumor as target and non-tumor cells) and in vivo anti-tumor testing (nude mouse xenograft) prior to administration (5).

Analysis by flow cytometry indicated that these immunoconjugates retained immunoreactivity after conjugation. Conjugates prepared in this manner exhibited antibody specific in vitro cell-killing properties. Animal studies indicated 5-15-fold lower non-specific lethal toxicity from the conjugate when compared with free drug. These conjugates failed to produce soft tissue necrosis when injected intradermally at drug levels, which in an unconjugated state cause severe damage.

Flow cytometric analysis of Adriamycin and MMC conjugates indicated that the breadth of tumor cell coverage remains similar with only a small decrease in the intensity of the binding following conjugation (5). The Adriamycin conjugates were very stable in vitro but the deconjugation half-time of the Br-1-MMC immunoconjugate was found to be one day at 37° centigrade and 21 days at 10° centigrade. In vivo xenograft studies with Me-7 and Br-1 have demonstrated both comparable anti-tumor activity and diminished cytotoxicity of the immunoconjugate to free drug. These preclinical results with mitomycin-C conjugates are fully described elsewhere (6).

Clinical Monitoring

Testing of serum samples for human anti-mouse immunoglobulin was done with a particle concentration fluorescent immunoassay (7). Patient biopsies were tested for the presence (in vivo targeting) of murine antibody by immunoperoxidase histochemistry or by flow cytometry using goat anti-mouse antibodies as the developing agent.

RESULTS

For this report, 43 patients including 13 patients with breast cancer were treated. All antibodies for breast cancer were against membrane determinants of tumor cells. No significant changes were seen in total serum complement, immunoglobulins or lymphocyte subsets (data not shown).

Heterogeneity and Antibody Selection

Table 2 represents 5 patients with breast carcinoma and their typing pattern with 9 monoclonal antibodiesand controls. The variability of tissue typing of breast carcinomas is apparent with monoclonal antibody Br-1 typing positive for all the breast carcinomas, but never with 100% of the cells in any tumor. In order to insure typing and saturation, a panel of monoclonal antibodies was needed.

We have examined biopsies, cell lines and xenografts for antigenic expression and stability over time (Tables 3 and 4). Reasonable concordance between biopsy and xenograft was seen but antigenic drift over time is characteristic of tumor derived cell lines. The histological evaluation for selection of antibodies was complemented by flow cytometry of viable tumor cell suspensions reacted with the monoclonal antibodies. In Table 5, two examples are shown demonstrating both an additive effect and a negative effect of mixing other antibodies.

Localization and Saturation Studies

Table 6 shows localization of antibodies after immunoconjugate infusion in 5 patients with breast cancer.

Localization of the antibody cocktail was consistently seen
(19/24; 83%). Saturation was seen in 9 instances.
Localization was demonstrated on cancer cells as early as 4
days after starting treatment and as long as 10 days after
the last infusion.

Saturation was seen at 1.65 gram antibody in one case
and in 5 cases at over 2 grams cumulative dose antibody.
This suggests high doses of antibody (over 2 grams) are
necessary to saturate the various epitopes on carcinoma
cells.

Similar data for mitomycin-C conjugates are summarized
for 4 patients with breast cancer (Table 7). Saturation was
seen in 4/13 patients generally at antibody doses of 2 grams
or more.

Toxicities

In general, the most frequent toxicities were rash,
fever, and chills (Table 8).

Serological responses with evidence for development of
anti-mouse immunoglobulins are summarized elsewhere (8).
Twelve patients had toxic reactions out of 21 tested. Of the
twelve remaining patients who had toxic reactions, ten of the
twelve had a specific IgM directed against their monoclonal
antibody cocktails. Six severe allergic reactions requiring
epinephrine were seen in 4 patients. All of these patients
had circulating IgM against mouse antibody. Three had
previously received mouse antibody and two were treated with
immunoconjugates (using epinephrine.

Anti-Tumor Activity

Five minor responses were seen with Adriamycin
conjugates. No responses were seen with mitomycin-C although
several patients had less tumor related pain after treatment.
Two patients with breast carcinoma had isolated improvements
in skin ulcerations. Three additional patients with other
types of cancer had minor responses. None of these minor
responses were sufficient to reach a partial response (50%
reduction in mean tumor diameter) by protocol criteria (9).

DISCUSSION

The data presented here demonstrate the feasibility of
using a panel of monoclonal antibodies in order to type all
tumor cells in a biopsy. Tumor typing can be done from
relatively small samples of tumor. We have successfully
typed tumor cells from sputum of patients with lung carcinoma
and from ascites and pleural fluid of patients with breast
cancer. Although it is conceivable that one antibody might
eventually be found which would react an entire population of
tumor cells, we have not seen this phenomenon in over 150
patients. Indeed, the evidence is overwhelming that there is
a heterogeneity in the membrane antigenic array. Our data
suggests that this is not infinite. Reasonable coverage of
the antigenic array can be achieved with 3-6 antibodies for
any one tumor. Our data demonstrate that it is feasible to

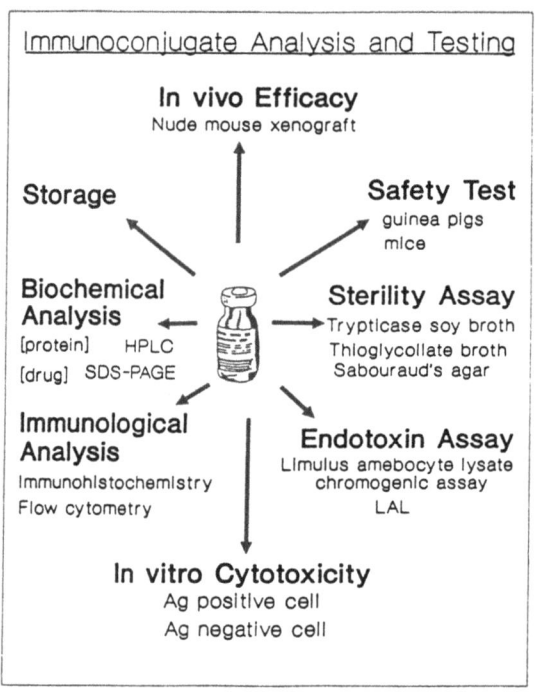

Figure 1.

TABLE 1. DISEASE CATEGORIES

Tumor Type	No. patients treated with Adriamycin immunoconjugates	No. patients treated with Mitomycin-C immunoconjugates	Total
Breast CA	10[a]	4[a]	14[a]
Carcinosarcoma	0	1	1
Cholangiosarcoma	1	0	1
Colo-rectum CA	2	3	5
Hepatoma	0	1	1
Islet Cell CA	1	0	1
Leiomyosarcoma	1	1	2
Lung CA	2	1	3
Lymphoma (CLL)	1	0	1
Ovarian	1	2	3
Parotid	1	0	1
Prostate CA	1	2	3
Renal Cell CA	1	1	2
Schwannoma	0	1	1
Squamous Cell CA (tongue, mouth, penis)	3	2	4
	24	19	43

[a] Note that one patient with breast infiltrating ductal carcinoma was first received Adriamycin immunoconjugate and six months later Mitomycin-C immunoconjugate therapy. Thus, the total number of different patients with breast carcinoma is 13 instead of 14.

TABLE 2. HETEROGENEOUS EXPRESSION OF ANTIGENS
IN BREAST TUMOR BIOPSIES AS REVEALED
IN IMMUNOHISTOCHEMICAL TYPING

MoAb	Breast carcinoma of patient				
	BLO	JAK	RUB	PAR	GIB
Anti-tumor	+	2+	4+	+	4+
BA-Br-1	3+	−	3+	3+	3+
BA-Br-3	−	−	4+	+	−
BT-Co-1	−	2+	3+	−	2+
BT-Co-4	2+	3+	2+	2+	+
BT-Co-6	+	3+	2+	+	4+
BA-Me-4	3+	−	−	2+	+
BA-Me-5	−	−	−	+−	−
BT-Me-7	−	−	+	+−	2+
Control					
Anti HLA-ABC	3+	4+	2+	4+	4+
Mouse IgG	−	−	−	−	−
PBS	−	−	−	−	−

TABLE 3. COMPARISON OF ANTIBODY REACTIVITY IN
BIOPSY AND XENOGRAFT DERIVED CELL LINES,
BRXBR1

Antibody	Cell Line	
	Biopsy	Xenograft
W6-32	3	2
EMA	3	3
BaBR1	3	2
BaBR3	1	1
BaBR5	0	0
BaBR6	2	1
BaBR7	2	3
BaBR8	1	1
BTCo1	1	0
BTCo7	1	1
Cytokeratin	3	2

Reactivity on a scale of 0-4

TABLE 4. REACTIVITY OF ANTIBODIES WITH PASSAGE OR
BRXBR6X BREAST CARCINOMA CELL LINE

| Antibody | Biopsy | Cell Line | |
		Passage 3	Passage 7
BR-1	+	W+	–
3	+	+	+
4	+	+	ND
5	–	–	–
Co-1	+	W+	–
2	+	W+	–
3	+	W+	ND
4	+	ND	+
5	+	W+	–
Me-4	+	–	–
5	+	W+	W+
7	W+	W+	W+
8	W+	W+	W+

TABLE 5. FLOW CYTOMETRIC ANALYSIS OF MONOCLONAL
ANTIBODY BINDING TO TUMOR CELLS

TEST TARGET	ANTIBODY	% CELLS POSITIVE	PEAK MEAN CHANNEL	TYPE OF INTERACTION
Ovarian	Br-1	80	97	
Carcinoma	Br-3	74	104	
	Co-6	80	95	
	Br-1+Br-3+Co-6	126	126	Additive
Carcinoma-Sarcoma Cells	Br-1	82	121	
	Br-3	37	87	
	Br-5	12	53	
	Br-1+Br-3+Br-5	59	10	Subtractive

TABLE 6. IN VITRO AND IN VIVO REACTIVITY OF MOABS WITH TUMOR CELLS IN SURGICALLY REMOVED BREAST CANCER LESIONS DURING AND AFTER ADRIAMYCIN–MOAB IMMUNOCONJUGATE THERAPY

Patient (Tumor Type)	MoAb Cocktail	Type of Specimen	Cumulative Dose of MoAb (mg) Before Biopsy	Cumulative Days Past Initial Treatment Before Biopsy	Number of Days Past Last Treatment Before Biopsy	Immunoperoxidase Reactivity of MoAb Cocktail Score [a]		Comments	
						In vitro	In vivo	Localization	Saturation
WEN	BR-1 Br-3	Pleural effusion	75	4	4	4+	1+	Yes	No
	BR-4	Pleural effusion	150	15	2	3+	0	No	
		Pleural	500	27	3	4+	1+	Yes	No
DAV	Br-1 Br-5	Skin	1750	9	2	4+	3+	Yes	No
	Br-4	Skin	2700	20	1	4+	4+	Yes	Yes
HAG	Br-1 Br-2 Br-3	Pleural effusion	375	17	1	4+	1+	Yes	No
	Br-4	Skin	850	18	1	4+	2+	Yes	No
	Me-4	Pleural effusion	1100	28	8	4+	3+	Yes	No
		Pleural effusion	1100	30	10	4+	1+	Yes	No
NELS	Br-1 Br-3	Pleural effusion	1550	7	1	1+	1+	Yes	Yes
	Co-1	Lymp node effusion	1650	7	1	3+	2+	Yes	No
		Pleural effusion	4200	41	23	1+	0	No	
HUB	Br-1	Skin	8041	11	1	3+	2+	Yes	No

[a] See Table 8 footnote for details

TABLE 7. IN VITRO AND IN VIVO REACTIVITY OF MOABS WITH BREAST CANCER CELLS IN SURGICALLY REMOVED LESIONS DURING AND AFTER MITOMYCIN–C MOAB IMMUNOCONJUGATE THERAPY

Patient (Tumor Type)	MoAb Cocktail	Type of Specimen	Cumulative Dose of MoAb (mg) Before Biopsy	Cumulative Days Past Initial Treatment Before Biopsy	Number of Days Past Last Treatment Before Biopsy	Immunoperoxidase Reactivity of MoAb Cocktail Score [a]		Comments	
						In vitro	In vivo	Localization	Saturation
BUL	Br-1 (90%) Co-1 (10%)	Chest skin met. (3/11/88	1674	7	2	2+	1+	Yes	No
RUB	Br-1 (12%) Br-3 (65%) Br-6 (9%)	Peri- cardial effusion (3/12/88)	985	3	1	4+	4+	Yes	Yes
		Chest wall module	2573	9	2	3+	1+	Yes	No
MOR	Br-1 (48%) Br-3 (21%) Co-6 (100%)	Chest skin nodule (6/9/88)	2198	8	1	2+	1+	Yes	No
GER	Br-1 (26%) Br-3 (21%) Br-5 (25%) Co-6 (28%)	Pleural effusion (6/30/88)	2317	8	1	3+	2+	Yes	No

[a] See Table 8 footnote for details

TABLE 8. SIDE EFFECTS

Rash, Chills, Fever (> 102° F)	11
Neutropenia (<1,000) Thrombocytopenia (<50,000)	8
Rash Alone	19
Periorbital Edema	1
Dyspnea or Chest Tightness	3
Nausea or Emesis	15
Hives or Pruritis	13
Abdominal Pain and Arthralgia	1
Symptoms Requiring Epinephrine	6

treat patients, observe localization and saturation of the tumor with monoclonal antibodies. Patients can be retreated using appropriate precautions.

Our major problem with the use of the monoclonal antibody immunoconjugates is the difficulty in effectively binding chemotherapeutic agents to them. As discussed in detail elsewhere (6-9) the major technical problem in the conjugation of Adriamycin was instability in serum and for mitomycin-C, it was rapid dissociation at 37° centigrade (6). In patients, a variable amount of drug release was observed which caused unpredictable toxicity especially with the "RDF" stabilized Adriamycin preparation. Thus, the cisaconitic method used for conjugation of Adriamycin to monoclonal antibodies needs further improvement.

Other investigators have continued to test unconjugated antibodies in therapeutic trials with limited success (10, 11). Increasingly, investigators are looking to immunoconjugates using isotopes and toxins to increase the killing capacity and differential toxicity of these antibody preparations (12-15). Most of these investigators have used a single antibody and a few are now attempting to use fixed ratio antibody combinations. However, the macro and microheterogeneity illustrated by studies would seem to mitigate against the ultimate success of these approaches. It is possible that radio-immunoconjugates may circumvent heterogeneity but radio-toxicity to other organs and limited tumor radiosensitivity may severely limit this approach of the common solid tumors.

The thesis that targeting and perhaps internalization of the monoclonal antibody into the cell may obviate cellular resistance patterns for drugs, prevent generalized drug toxicity and increase sensitivity of tumor cells to the agent must be further tested in humans. To that extent, we are now exploring the use of this technology with mitomycin-C, Daunorubicin, Adriamycin and ricin conjugated antibodies. Other investigators are exploring the use of radioisotopes. These endeavors should prove to be an exciting area of cancer biotherapy as the science expands (16,17).

REFERENCES

1. Bernhard, M.I., Hwang, K.M., Foon, K.A., et al.: Localization of Indium and Iodine-Labeled Monoclonal Antibodies in Guinea Pigs Bearing Line 10 Hepatocarcino-ma Tumors. Cancer Research 43:4429-4433, 1983.
2. Goldenberg, D.M., DeLand, F.H.: History and Status of Tumor Imaging and Radiolabeled Antibodies: J. Biol. Resp. Modif. 1:121-136, 1982.
3. Avner, B.P., Liao, S.K., Avner, B., et al.: Therapeutic Murine Monoclonal Antibodies Developed for Individual Cancer Patients. J. Biol. Resp. Modif. (In Press), 1988.
4. Liao, S.K., Meranda, C., Avner, B.P., et al.: Immuno-histochemical Phenotyping of Human Solid Tumors with Monoclonal Antibodies in Devising Biotherapeutic Strategies. Cancer Immunol. and Immunother. (In Press) 1989.
5. Ogden, J.R., Leung, K. Kunda, S.A., Telander, M.W., Avner, B.P., Liao, S.K., Thurman, G.B., Oldham, R.K.: Immunoconjugates of Doxorubicin and Murine Anti-Human Breast Carcinoma Monoclonal Antibodies Prepared via an N-Hydroxysuccinimide Active Ester Intermediate of Cisaconityl Doxorubicin: Preparation and In Vivo Cytoxicity. Molecular Biotherapy (In Press), 1988.
6. Orr, D.W., Oldham, R.K., and Lewis, M.: Phase I Trial of Mitomycin-C Immunoconjugates. (In Preparation), 1988.
7. Avner, B.P., Gaydos, B., Liao, S.K., Thurman, G.B., Oldham, R.K.: Characterization of a Method Using Viable Human Target Cells as the Solid Phase in a Cell Concentration Fluorescent Immunoassay (CCFIA) for Screening of Monoclonal Antibodies and Hybridoma Supernatants. J. Immunol. Meth. 113:123-135, 1988.
8. Avner, B., Swindell, L., Sharp, E., Liao, S.K., Avner, B.P., Oldham, R.K.: Monitoring of Patient Immune Reponses to Intravenous Therapy with Murine Monoclonal Antibodies Conjugated to Adriamycin: Relevance to Clinical Events. Cancer Research (Submitted), 1988.
9. Oldham, R.K., Lewis, M., Orr, D.W., Avner, B.P., Liao, S.K., Ogden, J., Avner, B., and Birch, R.: Adriamycin Custom-Tailored Immunoconjugates in the Treatment of Human Malignancies. Molecular Biotherapy (In Press), 1988.
10. Houghton, A., Mintzer, D., Cordon-Cardo, C., et al: Mouse Monoclonal IgG-3 Antibody Detecting GD-3 Ganglioside: A Phase I Trial in Patients with Malignant Melanoma. Proc. Natl. Acad. Sci. (USA), 82:1242-1246, 1985.
11. Oldham, R., Foon, K., Morgan, C., et al.: Monoclonal Antibody Therapy of Malignant Melanoma: In Vivo Locatlization and Cutaneous Metastases After Intravenous Administration. J. Clin. Oncol. 2:1235-1244, 1984.

12. DeNardo, S., DeNardo, G., O'Grady, L., et al: Pilot Studies of Radioimmunotherapy of B-Cell Lymphoma and Leukemia Using I-131 Lym-1 Monoclonal Antibody: Antibod. Immunoconj. Radiopharm. 1(1):17-33, 1988.

13. Rosen, S., Zimmer, A., Goldman-Leikin, R., et al: Radio-immunodetection and Radioimmunotherapy of Cutaneous T-Cell Lymphomas Using I-311 - Labeled Monoclonal Antibody: An Illinois Cancer Counsel Study. J. Clinical Oncology 5(4):562-73, 1987.

14. Epenetos, A., Monroe, A., Stewart, S., et al: Antibody-Guided Radiation of Advanced Ovarian Cancer with Intraperitoneally Administered Radiolabeled Monoclonal Antibodies. J. Clin. Oncol. 5(12):1890-1899, 1987.

15. Spitler, L., DelRio, M., Khentizan, A., et al: Therapy of Patients with Malignant Melanoma Using a Monoclonal Anti-Melanoma Antibody-Ricin A Chain Immunotoxin: Cancer Research 47:1717-1723, 1987.

16. Oldham, R.K.: Monoclonal Antibodies - Does Sufficient Selectivity to Cancer Cells Exist for Therapeutic Application? J. Biol. Resp. Modif. 6:277-284, 1987.

17. Oldham, R.K.: Immunoconjugates - Drugs and Toxins. In: Oldham, R.K. (Ed.) Principles of Cancer Biotherapy. Raven Press, New York, pp. 319-335, 1987.

A PHASE I STUDY OF THE ANTI-BREAST CANCER IMMUNOTOXIN 260F9

MAB-rRA GIVEN BY INTRAVENOUS CONTINUOUS INFUSION

Bruce J. Gould,[1]   Michael J. Borowitz,[2]
Eric S. Groves,[3] and Arthur E. Frankel,[1,4]

[1]Department of Hematology/Oncology
Duke University Medical Center
Durham, NC 27710

[2]Department of Pathology
Duke University Medical Center
Durham, NC 27710

[3]Cetus Corporation
1400 Fifty-Third Street
Emeryville, CA 94608

[4]To whom requests for
reprints should be
addressed

INTRODUCTION

Immunotoxins (IT) are biologically derived compounds that are under development as anti-neoplastic agents (1). An immunotoxin consists of a carrier protein that guides a covalently linked toxin to a tumor cell. Monoclonal antibodies which have specificity for tumor cell. Monoclonal antibodies serve as carrier molecules. Plant or bacteria derived toxins such as ricin, pseudomonas exotoxin, and diphtheria toxin are commonly used cellular poisons (2).

Ideally, the IT attaches to the tumor cell surface through the monoclonal antibody's interaction with its epitope. Afterwards, the surface bound IT enters the cell by receptor mediated endocytosis. Inside the cell, the toxin splits from the monoclonal antibody and inhibits protein synthesis. Ricin inactivates 60s ribosomes while pseudomonas exotoxin and diphtheria toxin inactivate elongation factor 2 (3).

The IT 260F9 MAB-rRA, was developed for the treatment of breast cancer. The 260F9 MAB-rRA (monoclonal antibody) binds to a poorly defined 55 kd antigen that is present on 50% of the breast cancer cell lines. When tested against a panel of normal tissues, the antibody bound to esophagus, kidney, stomach, tonsils, liver, skin, uterus, bladder, and breast. The 260F9 MAB did not bind to lung, colon, brain, heart, ovary, bone marrow, and blood cells.

The toxin portion of the 260F9 MAB-rRA is derived form ricin, a protein synthesized by castor bean seeds. Ricin is composed of two chains that are joined by a disulfide bond: the B chain binds to beta-pyranosyl galactoside residues on cell surfaces and facilitates toxin entry into cell while the A chain (RTA) inhibits protein synthesis by enzymatically cleaving a critical adenosine base from the 60s submit of ribosomes (4). One molecule of RTA can inhibit the entire protein synthesis within a cell.

The ricin A chain gene was cloned and expressed in Escherichia coli ant the resultant recombinant RTA (rRA) was found to be as potent as the native molecule at inhibiting protein synthesis. Because the rRA lacks a cell binding domain, it is not cytoxic unless it is linked to a ligand.

In order to link 260F9 MAB and rRA, a reactive thiol group was added to the 260F9 MAB incubating it with 2-iminothiolane and DTNB (5,5' dithio-bis(2-nitrobenzoic acid). When rRA, which has a constituent thiol group, was mixed with the derivatized antibody, the compounds became joined by a disulfide bond. The resultant IT, 2609F9 MAB-rRA, was found to be a potent IT with a IC50 of < 1 nM for 3 of 4 breast cancer cell lines (5).

Studies of nude mice that have been transplanted with human breast cancer showed that the IT was effective at inhibiting tumor growth. Afterwards, monkeys were treated with ten daily boluses of the IT and only malaise, anorexia, and hypoalbuminemia were observed (6). These promising preclinical studies lead to the initiation of a Phase I study.

CLINICAL RESULTS

Five patients with biopsy proven metastatic breast carcinomas that had failed standard therapies were selected for treatment. The patients were treated at Duke University Medical Center from June 1987 through August 1987. Four patients received a single, 8 day course of treatment while the fifth received 6 days of therapy. The immunoconjugate was administered by continuous infusion through a central venous catheter. Three patients received 50 ug/kg/day of the immunotoxin for total daily doses of 2.8, 3.0, and 3.02 mg. Two others received 100 ug/kg/day for total daily doses of 6.8 and 7.5 mg. Two patients underwent chest wall tumor biopsies within 48 hours after completing therapy for IT penetration analyses.

The 260F9 MAB-rRA shared many adverse effects observed with other ITs. All the patients suffered fevers > 38.4C, anorexia, malaise, fluid, retention, and arthralgias and myalgias. Although several patients complained of dyspnea, none had chest X-ray evidence of congestive heart failure. Moderate dose diuretics (Lasix 60 mg) failed to reverse the fluid retention, but the fluid gain did resolve with discontinuation of the IT in three patients. Nausea and discontinuation of the IT in three patients. Nausea and diarrhea were transient problems for only one patient. Another patient had her therapy stopped on day 6 when she developed evidence of allergic reaction that was manifest as an erythematous-vesicular rash, finger arthritis, and eosinophilia. All the aforementioned side effects except the fluid retention resolved with discontinuation of therapy.

Two patients required hospitalizations 5 and 7 days after treatment of pulmonary edema and symptomatic peripheral edema that was unassociated with acute cardiac diseases. These patients' fluid overload responded quickly and completely to moderate dose diuretics and they had no further volume problems.

One patient who had advanced pulmonary disease prior to therapy died during the initial hospitalization. She died of progressive cardiopulmonary failure that was precipitated by Staphylococcus sepsis. The contribution of the IT to the patient's death is unclear.

Several laboratory abnormalities developed during the course of the infusion in each patient. Two notable abnormalities were the falls in the serum albumin to 3.0 gram kd and serum sodium levels to 126 meg/L and 120 meg/L in two patients (although neither of these patients manifested mental status changes). No proteinuria was found to explain the hypoalbuminemia: urine sodium studies were not done. Minor elevations of the liver transaminase, serum glucose, and serum triglycerides also developed in several patients. All the abnormal laboratory values returned to normal within 72 hours of completing the infusions.

Debilitating plexopathies and neuropathies occurred in three patients, two at the 50 ug/kg/d dose and one at the 100 ug/kg/d dose. The neurologic symptoms began as a plexopathy on the side of previous chest wall radiation about two weeks after the completion of the infusion. Over the ensuing two weeks the patients developed typical sensory-motor neuropathies of the other three extremities. The diagnosis were confirmed by neurologic examinations and nerve conduction studies in the three cases. The neuropathies were most severe at 2-3 months after treatment and resulted in a decline in Karnofsky status from 80% (normal activity with effort) to 40% (incapable of self care). During the following six months, the patients had complete recovery of their motor function, but they continued to suffer from paresthesia of their hands and feet.

A sural nerve biopsy was done in one patient during the period of profound neuropathic disturbance which showed marked axonal loss and segmental demyelination. No inflammatory infiltrates or other abnormalities were found on microscopic examination. The biopsy failed to reveal any bound IT or 260F9 MAB; however, immunoperoxidase studies showed that the 260F9 antigen was present on the nerve in a distribution consistent with either Schwann cells or myelin.

A clinical responses were followed by radiologic studies

and by serial measurements of chest wall lesions. There were no findings suggestive of tumor stabilization, tumor regression, a mixed response or symptomatic improvement in any patient. Three patients died within nine months following treatment and a fourth patient has progressive disease one year later. Immunoperoxidase analyses were done on chest was biopsies from two patients and neither the immunotoxin nor its components could be detected. The breast cancer cells within both biopsies bound 260F9 MAB in vitro.

The 260F9 MAB-rRA serum levels were determined by immunoradiometric assay. The steady state IT concentration was reached at 24 hours for the group. Once steady states were reached, the IT concentrations remained constant for a week in four patients. One patient's level remained steady for 3 days; afterwards, it dropped by one-third and remained constant until the end of the infusion. Assuming an immunotoxin distribution limited to a 3-liter plasma volume, an immunotoxin half-line between 4-6 hours was calculated for each patient.

tHE LEVELS OF ANTI-rRA AND ANTI-260F9 MAB antibodies were assayed by an immunoradiometric assay which does not distinguish between IgG and IgM. All patients except one developed anti-IT antibodies by day 9. Four patients developed anti-rRA antibodies and three generated anti-260F9 MAB antibodies. Only the patient with sepsis and who was the most heavily pretreated did not form antibodies to either component of the IT.

DISCUSSION

This was the first trial in which an IT was administered by a continuous infusion. Four patients maintained steady state levels for eight days while one patient had a 33% drop in her levels. The fall in her steady state levels may have been caused by anti-IT antibodies. The calculated half-life of 4-6 hours is substantially longer than the 43 minute half-life for T101-RTA, the only other IT in which human half-life data is published (7). Animal studies have shown that RTA immunoconjugates are quickly cleared from the circulation by the liver (8). This clearance is partially mediated by the binding of mannose residues on RTA to oligosaccharide receptors on Kupffer cells. Therefore the absence of glycosylated moieties on rRA may have accounted for the prolonged half-life of 260F9 MAB-rRA conjugate.

No tumor regression was seen in this study, however, only low doses were used because of toxicities. Although blood levels of the IT were maintained for one week in four patients, it is unlikely that the levels were high enough to cause diffusion into the tumor bed. The absence of IT in the tumor and the presence of the 260F9 antigen in two biopsies suggests that tumor penetration was more of a problem than resistant cells.

Despite observations from animal trials suggesting that the IT would be well tolerated, moderate acute and severe subacute toxicities were seen. Fevers, malaise, myalgias, peripheral edema, weight gain, and hypoalbuminemia were toxicities common to all patients and have been reported with other IT trials (9, 10). However, this is the first trial to report a targeted toxicity. Three patients developed a debilitating neuropathy 2-3 weeks after treatment. The debilitation was maximal two months later after which the patients gradually recovered. The time course of the neuropathy was suggestive of a single toxic injury that was temporally related to the IT administration. The 260F9 MAB was further implicated when in vitro immunoperoxidase studies found intense staining of the nerve sheath by the antibody. The immunoperoxidase studies and the clinical course of the neuropathy provided good evidence that the 260F9 MAB-rRA played a role in the university.

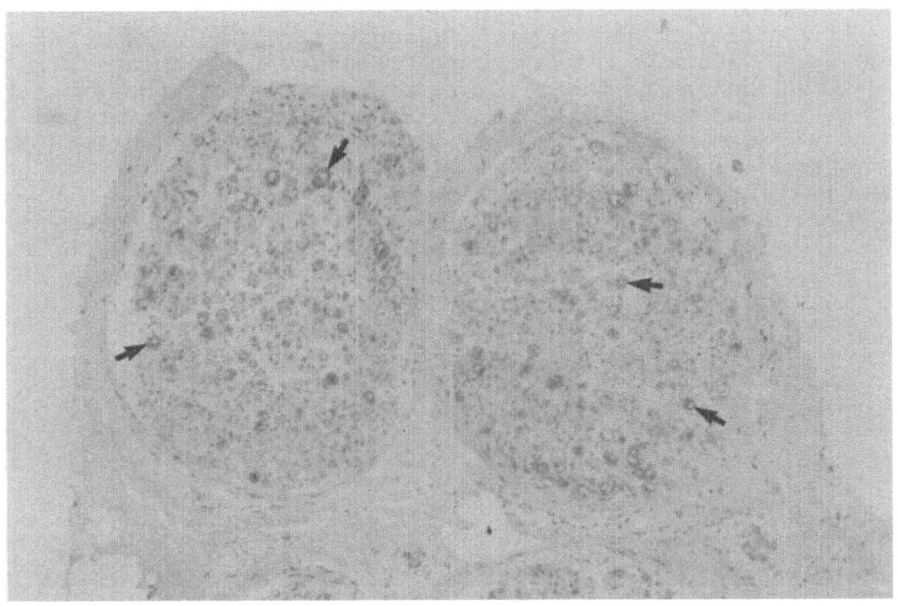

Figure 1 A microphotograph of a patient's nerve which shows immunoperoxidase staining (arrows) after in vitro pretreatment with 260F9 MAB. The staining Pattern is suggestive of 260F9 MAB binding to either the myelin sheaths or Schwann cells.

REFERENCES

1. Frankel A, Houston L, Issell, B. Prospects for immunotoxin therapy in cancer. Ann. Rev. Med. 37:125-142 1986.
2. Pastan I, Willingham M, Fitzgerald J. Immunotoxins. Cell 47:641-648 1986.

3. Olnes S, Sandvig K. How protein toxins enter and kill cells. In: Immunotoxins. A. E. Frankel, ed. Kluwer Academic Pub., Norwell, MA 39-74 1988.
4. Robertus J. D. Toxin structure. In: Immunotoxins. A. E. Frankel, ed. Kluwer Academic Pub., Norwell, MA 11-24 1988.
5. Bjorn M, Ring D, Frankel A. Evaluation of monoclonal antibodies for the development of breast cancer immunotoxins. Cancer Res. 45: 1214-1221 1985.
6. Data on file at the Cetus Corporation.
7. Hertler A, Schlossman D, Borowitz M, Blythnman H, Caselas P, Frankel A. Anti-CD5 immunotoxin for chronic lymphocytic leukemia: enhancement of cytotoxicity with human serum albumin-monensin. Inter. J. of Cancer 43:215-219.
8. Blakey D, Thorpe P. Prevention of carbohydrate-mediated clearance of ricin-containing immunotoxins by the liver. In:Immunotoxins. A. E. Frankel, ed. Kluwer Academic Pub., Norwell, MA 457-474 1988.
9. Spitler L, del Rio M, Khentigan A, Wedel N, Brophy N, Miller L, Harkonen W, Rosendorf L, Lee H, Mischak R, Kawahata R, Stoudemire J, Fradkin L, Bautista E, Scannon P. Therapy of patients with malignant melanoma using a monoclonal antimelanoma antibody-ricin A chain immunotoxin. Cancer Res. 47: 1717-1723 1987.
10. Hertler A, Schlossman D, Borowitz M, Laurent G, Jansen F, Schmidt C, Frankel A. A phase I study of T101 ricin A chain immunotoxin in refractory chronic lymphocytic leukemia J. of Biological Response Modifiers 7:97-113 1988.

IN VIVO STUDIES OF RADIOLABELED MONOCLONAL ANTIBODIES Mc5

AND KC4 IN HUMAN BREAST CANCER

Paul A. Bunn, Jr.[1], David G. Dienhart[1],
Raymond F. Schmelter[2], James L. Lear[2], Gary Miller[3],
Duane C. Bloedow[4], Cliff Longley[5], Philip Furmanski[5],
Roberto L. Ceriani[6]

From the Division of Medical Oncology[1], Department of
Medicine[1], Department of Radiology[2], Department of
Pathology[3] and School of Pharmacy[4] at the University of
Colorado Health Sciences Center; AMC Cancer Research
Center[5]; University of Colorado Cancer Center[1-5]; and the
John Muir Cancer and Aging Research Institute[6]

INTRODUCTION

Breast cancer is the most common malignancy in women in the United States, with over 130,000 new cases developing annually (1). Despite improved methods for early detection and treatment, the death rate from breast cancer in the United States has not changed over the past 25 years. Nearly all patients who die from breast cancer do so as a result of widespread systemic metastases. Metastatic breast cancer is difficult to detect early and impossible to cure with currently available treatment modalities.

The development of the hybridoma technology by Kohler and Milstein allowed for production of large quantities of monoclonal antibodies. Using mammary epithelial antigens or human malignant cells as immunogens, polyclonal and murine monoclonal antibodies were developed which react with the vast majority of human breast cancers (2-4). In the late 1970s Ceriani and co-workers described a breast specific antigen system which they called human mammary epithelial antigens (HME) which were initially prepared from human milk fat globule membranes (HMFG) (2,5,6). A series of monoclonal antibodies were developed which recognized various components of the HMFG (5,6). These monoclonal antibodies, which reacted with antigens on normal breast epithelium, lactating breast epithelium and malignant breast cancer cells, were used to detect circulating breast cancer antigens in the serum of nude mice bearing human tumor xenografts and in humans with breast cancer (7). The antigens recognized by these antibodies were shown to be glycoproteins. The antigens recognized by the HMFG and Mc5 antibodies were shown to have a molecular weight in excess of 400,000 daltons (5).

Using malignant human adenocarcinomas as immunogens, Hofeinz *et al* developed a series of KC murine monoclonal antibodies which also recognized differentiation antigens in normal and malignant epithelial cells (4). One antibody, termed KC4G3, was shown to be an IgG3 antibody which recognized a 438 Kd cell surface and 490 Kd cytoplasmic antigen. Blocking studies suggested that KC4G3 and Mc5 recognized the same high molecular weight antigen (unpublished results, RC).

We have performed a number of *in vivo* studies in nude mice bearing human breast adenocarcinoma cell lines and in human breast cancer patients to explore the potential clinical utility of these antibodies for imaging and therapy. These studies are summarized in this manuscript.

METHODS AND MATERIALS

Monoclonal Antibodies

KC4G3 is an IgG3 murine monoclonal antibody produced and provided by Coulter Immunology (Hialeah, FL) in affinity purified sterile form. Mc5 is an IgG1 murine monoclonal antibody produced and affinity purified by one of the authors (RLC).

For radioconjugate studies a KC4G3-DTPA chelate was prepared. Indium-111 (5 mCi) was then mixed with 1 mg of KC4G3 for 20 minutes at room temperature. Mc5 was radiolabeled with 131-Iodine by the Chloramine T method (8) with 2 mg of antibody, 400 μCi of ^{131}I, 5 μl of chloramine T (50 μg/ml H_2O), a 10 second reaction time, and termination by 5μl $Na_2S_2O_5$ (100 μg/ml H_2O). The labeled protein was separated from free iodide by passage through a Sephadex G-25 column. The immunoreactivity of each radiolabeled antibody was determined using a linear extrapolation method at infinite antigen (on coated beads) excess (9). The immunoreactivity of the iodinated Mc5 averaged 85% and the 111-In labeled KC4 reactivity averaged 60%.

Human Tumor Cell Lines: The human breast adenocarcinoma cell line ZR-75 was obtained from the ATCC. The MX-1 human breast adenocarcinoma tumor line was maintained in the laboratory of one of the authors (RLC). The BALL-1 cell line is a human B cell lymphocytic leukemia cell line obtained from Ikuro Kimura from the Cancer Institute Division of Pathology, Okayama, Japan.

Athymic Nude Mice

BALB/c nude mice were purchased from Life Sciences or raised in the John Muir colony and housed in sterile conditions. The mice were approximately 6 weeks of age when 10^7 cells were innoculated subcutaneously in the flank under sterile conditions.

Patients

Eleven patients were studied; all had histologically confirmed adenocarcinoma of the breast. Immunostaining of their tumor tissue showed reactivity with KC4 prior to antibody administration. These 11 patients had 47 sites of disease detected clinically by other means including physical examination, chest and other x-rays, bone and other radionuclide scans, and CT scans. All patients had adequate renal, pulmonary, cardiac, hepatic, and marrow function. All gave written informed consent for the study which was approved by the University of Colorado Institutional Review Board.

Antibody Administration

Radiolabeled antibody was administered intravenously to mice via the tail vein. For human studies radiolabeled KC4 was given intravenously over 1-5 hours. The total antibody dose was 1 mg (1 patient), 100 mg (4 patients), 250 mg (4 patients) and 500 mg (2 patients). The antibody preparation was achieved by mixing 0, 99, 249 or 499 mg of unlabeled KC4G3 with 1 mg of antibody labeled with 5 mCi 111-In.

Gamma Camera Imaging

Images were obtained with a GE 400 at (General Electric, Milwaukee, WI) gamma camera and the data were stored and processed in a DEC Scintigraphic Data Analyzer (Digital Electronics, Maynard, MN). For human studies, region-of-interest views were obtained from the skull, anterior and posterior chest, abdomen and extremities. Scans were obtained 48 or 72 hours after antibody administration with counting for 7 minutes and no background subtraction. Nude mice were imaged with a gamma camera using a pinhole collimator.

Pharmacokinetics

Blood collections from humans were obtained at 1, 2, 4, 8, 12, 24, 48, 72 and 96 hours postinfusion. For murine studies, serial blood collections were obtained via orbital collections at the indicated time points. The volume of distribution, clearance rate and t 1/2 times were determined by computer modeling with the ESTRIP program (10). Statistical determination of the number of exponentials to describe the data and refinement of the slopes and intercepts was performed with the computer program PCNONLIN (Statistical Consultants , Lexington, KY) (11). Urinary clearance of radioactivity was performed by gamma counting of aliquots collected over 5 days in humans and 2 weeks in mice. Tissue distribution in mice was determined by sacrificing the mice at specified time points, weighing and counting the dissected organ or tumor.

Serum Antibody Levels

Antibody levels were determined by competition assay using iodinated KC4G3 tracer and cold KC4G3 antibody. KC4 antigen coated beads were incubated with patient serum and I-125 labeled KC4G3. The beads were washed, centrifuged and counted to calculate the amount of bound antibody.

Serum Antigen Levels

Serum antigen levels were determined before antibody administration by a sandwich radioimmunoassay using KC4G3 coated beads and serial dilutions of patient sera. After overnight incubation I-125 KC4G3 was added and the beads were washed, centrifuged and counted to quantitate free serum antigen.

Immunohistochemistry

Immunoperoxidase staining of tumor tissues was performed using a modified avidin-biotin complex procedure. Tissues were scored by the percentage of positive cells (0 = negative, 1+ = 1-25%, 2+ = 26-50%, 3+ = 51-75%, 4+ = >75%), by staining intensity (0-4+), and by cellular distribution (apical, cytoplasmic, membrane).

Tumor Measurement

Bidimensional tumor measurements were made in nude mouse xenografts at the time points indicated. Tumor volume was calculated using the formula $V = 4/3 \pi r^3$ where the radius was determined from the average of the bidimensional measurement.

RESULTS

Nude Mouse Imaging and Biodistribution

Gamma camera images obtained within 24 hours of antibody administration showed most of the antibody in the blood pool. Excellent tumor images were obtained at 48 or 72 hours when the blood pool activity had diminished and the tumor uptake was maximal (Figure 1). Tumor activity declined slowly after this time, while the blood pool decayed more rapidly. Nonspecific hepatic uptake was noted at all times, however. Tumor images were not dependent on dose over the range of 10-1000 µg. The tumor images were specific as demonstrated by the administration of the same doses of 111-In-KC4G3 to nude mice bearing human tumors with no antigen (Figure 1) and by the administration of an irrelevant antibody to ZR-75 adenocarcinoma bearing mice (data not shown). Image quality could be improved by the subtraction method using an 131-I labeled irrelevant antibody (data not shown).

The normal organ and tumor biodistributions of the 111-In-KC4G3 at 72 and 336 hours in nude mice bearing the ZR-75 breast adenocarcinomas and the control BALL-1 tumors are shown in Figure 2. At all time points there was more uptake in the ZR-75 tumors

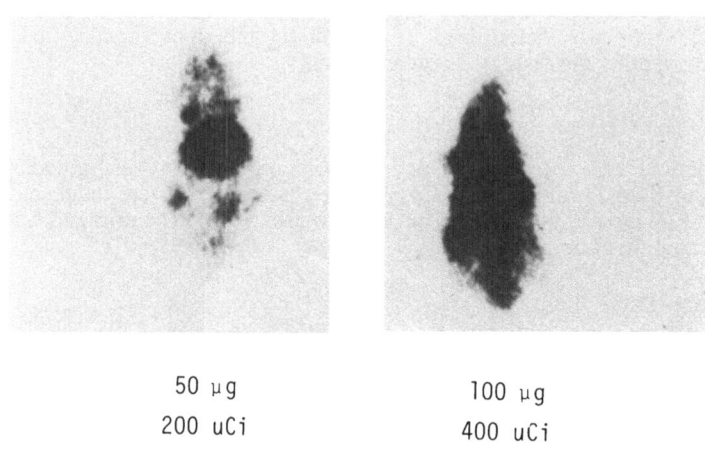

50 μg
200 uCi

100 μg
400 uCi

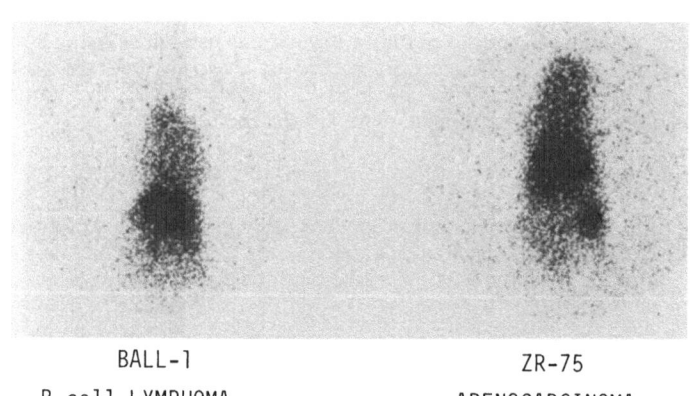

BALL-1
B-cell LYMPHOMA

ZR-75
ADENOCARCINOMA

Figure 1.   Results of imaging athymic nude mice bearing ZR-75 human breast adenocarcimonas or non-antigenic BALL-1 tumors with ^{111}In-KC4G3. In the upper two panels the images showed exellent tumor uptake in the left flank tumor, which was similar in mice given two different doses. In the lower two panels the control BALL-1 right flank tumor showed no uptake whereas the right flank ZR-75 tumor showed excellent uptake after administration of ^{111}In-KC4G3(50 μg).

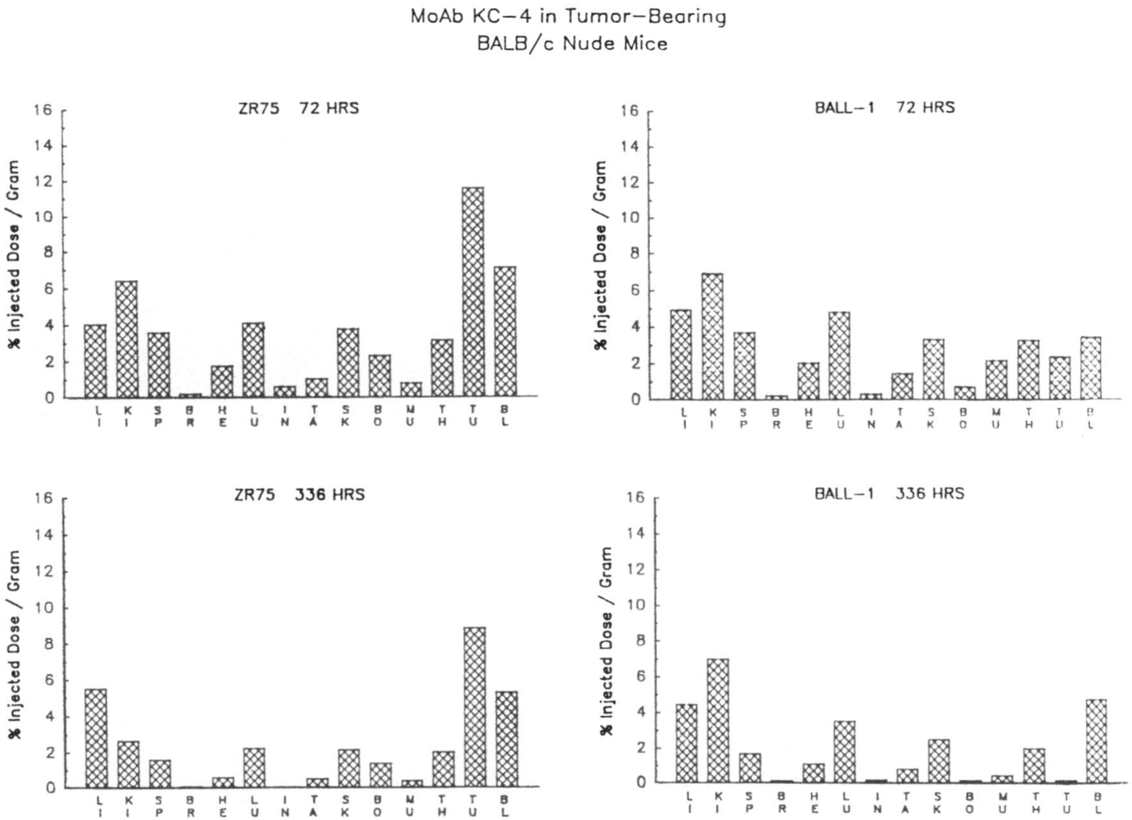

MoAb KC-4 in Tumor-Bearing
BALB/c Nude Mice

Figure 2. Biodistribution of 111-In-KC4G3 in athymic nude mice bearing ZR-75 breast adenocarcinoma or non-antigenic BALL-1 tumors at 72 and 336 hours after 111-In-KC4G3 antibody administration (100 µg KC4G3, 11 µCi 111-In). The tissues were: LI = liver, KI = kidney, SP = spleen, BR = brain, HE = heart, LU = lung, IN = intestine, TA = tail, SK = skin, BO = bone, MU = muscle, TH = thyroid, TU = tumor, BL = blood.

241

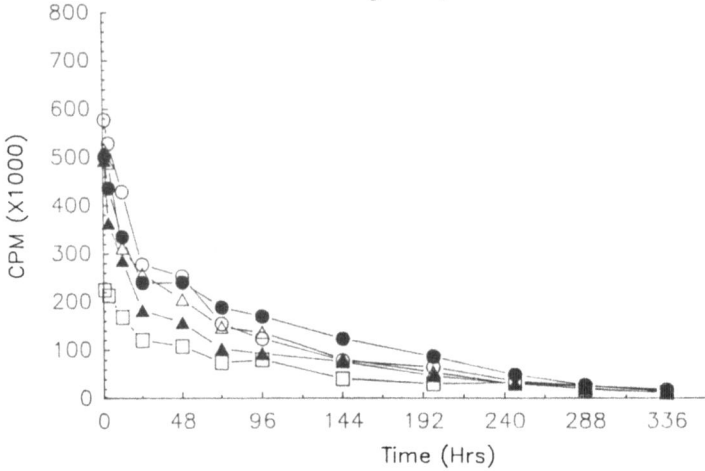

Serum Clearance of MoAb KC−4 in ZR75
Tumor−Bearing BALB/c Nude Mice

Figure 3.   Serum clearance of 111-In-KC4G3 in athymic nude mice bearing ZR-75
                tumors. The curves show a biphasic decay with an initial rapid phase and
                a slower secondary phase. The doses shown in the curves were 10μg ▭;
                50 μg ▲ ; 100 μg △ ; 500 μg ● ; and 1000 μg ○ . Quantitative aspects
                of these curves are shown in Table 1.

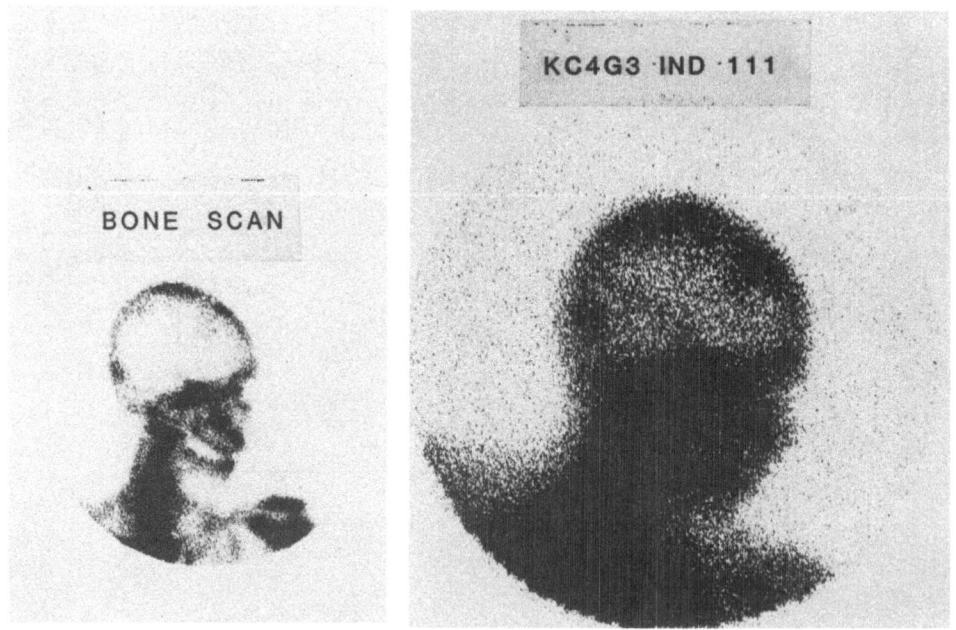

Figure 4.   Results of a radionuclide bone scan (left panel) and the gamma camera
                image at 72 hours after 111-In-KC4G3 administration (5 mCi, 250 mg;
                right panel). Both the bone scan and the KC4G3 scan show identical skull
                lesions.

242

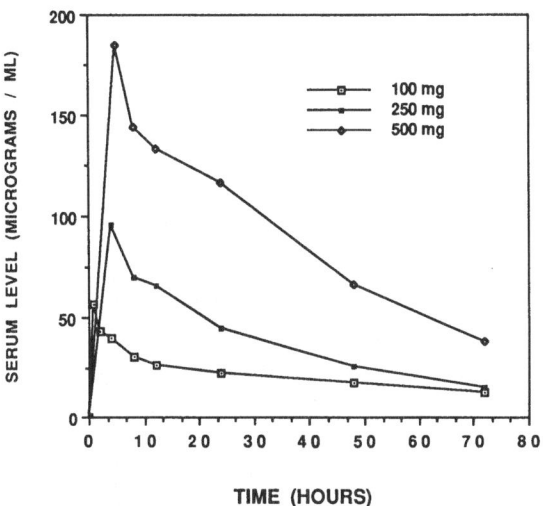

Figure 5.   Serum clearance of immunoreactive KC4G3 in doses from 100-500 mg in
              human patients with breast cancer. Quantitative aspects of these curves
              are shown in Table 3.

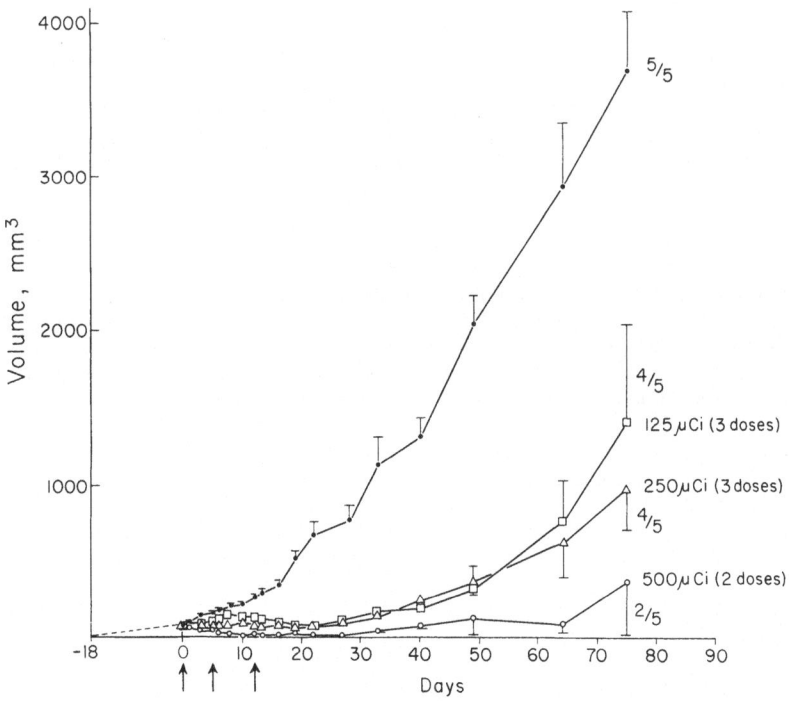

Figure 6.   Results of 131-I-Mc5 in athymic nude mice bearing established
              transplanted human breast cancers. Antibody doses were administered at
              the times indicated by the arrows. Means and Standard errors are
              indicated by the bars.

tumors than in normal tissues and the tumor activity decayed more slowly over time than the normal tissue activity. The ZR-75 tumor uptake was specific whereas the normal tissue uptake was not, as demonstrated by the biodistribution of the same dose of KC4G3 in the control mice. In this case there was little tumor uptake, whereas normal tissue distribution was similar to that of mice bearing ZR-75 tumors.

The serum clearance of various doses of 111-In-KC4G3 in nude mice bearing the human ZR-75 tumor xenografts is shown in Figure 3. There was no apparent difference in the rate of clearance based on antibody dose. The urinary clearance was less than 20% over 14 days at all dose levels, with the majority of this occurring within the first 96 hours. The volume of distribution, t 1/2, and clearance rates in nude mice without tumors and nude mice bearing ZR-75 tumors are shown in Table 1. The volume of distribution was considerably larger in the nude mice bearing the tumors showing that the antibody is distributed in this space. The serum clearance, the T 1/2 alpha and T 1/2 beta were similar in the tumor and non-tumor bearing animals as might be expected. The long half-life for this murine monoclonal antibody in a mouse is similar to other murine studies but considerably longer than the half-life in humans (see below).

Human Tumor Imaging and Clearance

As in the murine model, images obtained within 24 hours of antibody administration showed considerable blood pool activity. Tumor activity increased through 48-72 hours and then declined at a slow rate. Excellent images could be obtained at 72 hours because the blood pool activity had diminished markedly by that time point. An example of an image obtained at 72 hours, compared to a normal bone scan, is shown in Figure 4. In this case the skull lesions are easily visualized by both scans. The sensitivity of detecting sites of breast cancer was not strictly dose related, as lesions were imaged successfully at all doses. Table 2 shows the results of imaging in 11 patients given doses from 1-500 mg. Primary lesions were successfully imaged in 2/2 instances whereas a minority of metastatic lesions were successfully imaged. Imaging of metastatic sites was related to the size of the lesion. The majority of large lesions were imaged whereas a minority of small lesions were successfully imaged. The radiolabeled antibody was able to reach the tumor sites as shown by post-administration biopsy as well as by the images. The biopsies were weighed and counted for radioactivity and analyzed for immunoreactive antibody by immunohistochemistry and flow cytometry. Antibody was present in the biopsy specimens by these methods, though the antigen saturation was higher at higher doses.

The serum clearance of the antibody by dose is shown in Figure 5. The rate of clearance was similar over the 3 doses. ELISA assay for immunoreactive antibody and absolute counts showed that the higher antibody doses gave higher serum levels. In fact, an antibody dose of 500 mg gave serum levels in excess of 40 µg/ml for more than 72 hours. Thus, for therapy studies, antibody administration twice or three times weekly would maintain persistently high antibody levels. The urinary clearance showed less than 20% excretion of the injected dose over 96 hours at all dose levels.

The pharmacokinetic analysis of these data determined by either serial radioimmuno-assay for immunoreactive antibody or by gamma counting is shown in Table 3. The data are similar by either method with a volume of distribution of 2.8 liters. The serum t 1/2 of 26.5 to 35.6 hours is considerably shorter than in the nude mouse, but similar to that reported for other murine monoclonal antibodies in humans.

Therapeutic Results of Radiolabeled Antibody in Nude Mice Bearing Human Breast Cancers

We elected to study 131-I-Mc5 as a therapeutic agent because KC4G3 loses much of its immunoreactivity when iodinated by the chloramine T method. The therapeutic results of varying doses of 131-I-Mc5 in nude mice with MX-1 mammary tumors is shown in Figure 6. There was a clear dose response relationship over doses of 125 µCi to 500 µCi. The latter dose completely eliminated all palpable tumors, and histologic examination showed only necrosis without viable tumor. Single antibody doses produced tumor growth inhibition but not total reduction. Administration of labeled irrelevant antibody or 131-I alone showed little or no growth inhibition (data not shown). Unlabeled Mc5 alone also showed little or no growth inhibition.

DISCUSSION

The potential utility of antibodies and radiolabeled antibodies in human tumor imaging and therapy has been recognized for many years. The development of the hybridoma technology for mass producing monoclonal antibodies led to the ability to test this potential in human cancer patients. The ubiquitous distribution of human mammary epithelial antigens (HME-ag) also referred to as human milk fat globule antigens or MAM (mammary) antigens on normal lactating breast and human breast cancers was described in the late 1970s and early 1980s (2,3,5,6). Monoclonal antibodies to these antigens were developed and described during this period (4-6). We have evaluated the utility of two such antibodies in imaging and treating human breast cancers xenografted into nude mice and in imaging human breast cancer patients.

In athymic nude mice bearing human breast cancer xenografts, 111-In labeled KC4G3 showed excellent and specific tumor imaging. Tumor images were not affected by dose over a wide range (10-1000 µg). Images were best obtained at 3 days after administration since earlier images showed excess blood pool and later images were affected by decay of the 111-In label. The pharmacokinetic and biodistribution data showed that the plasma clearance had an initial rapid (10 hour) half-life followed by a long (100 hours) second half-life. These results are similar to those reported for other murine antibodies and suggested that the antibody was not severely damaged by the production, purification or radiolabeling process. The biodistribution showed excellent tumor to normal tissue ratios and excellent tumor uptake (10-20% of injected dose per gram). The tumor to normal tissue ratios improved over time as the blood pool cleared more rapidly than tumor. There was some non-specific hepatic uptake with both specific and irrelevant antibody.

The ability to target tumors in imaging studies of nude mice xenografts has progressed to successful therapeutic utility for 131-I labelled antibodies. There was a specific dose and schedule related growth inhibition of human breast cancer xenografts by the 131-I-Mc5 antibody. These encouraging results suggest that human trials should be actively pursued.

Our human data show that there are considerably more problems in humans. For imaging studies, metastatic deposits are often small and often overlie areas of nonspecific uptake in normal organs including the liver and bone marrow. Thus, the overall sensitivity is lower than in nude mice. The nonspecific clearance of the murine protein is greater in humans which leads to a shorter half-life and a lower percent of injected dose per gram of tumor in humans. Another potential problem in humans is the development of human anti-murine antibodies (HAMA). This develops in the majority of solid tumor patients given these and other antibodies. The development of HAMA will potentially limit the number of antibody doses that can be given to humans. Nonetheless, we have shown that radiolabeled KC4G3 can be given safely to patients over a wide dose range and that it can reach tumor in tissue sites. Although not all lesions can be successfully imaged, we expect the radiolabeled antibody is distributed to all tumor sites. The HME antigens are expressed on a variety of human epithelial malignancies. Other investigators have evaluated the ability of other radiolabeled antibodies, recognizing the same or similar antigens as Mc5 and KC4, to image metastatic human cancers (12-17). In general, the results of these studies are similar to those reported here with nonspecific antibody uptake limiting overall sensitivity.

There are few data using high doses of these radiolabled antibodies as therapy in human breast cancer patients. Other radiolabeled antibodies have been used in other tumors with some limited success (18,19). Our mouse data suggest that the growth of human breast adenocarcinomas in nude mice can be inhibited by doses which are potentially achievable in humans. It remains to be determined whether uptake and toxicity

TABLE 1. Pharmacokinetic Analysis of KC4G3 in Athymic Nude Mice

Parameter	Normal (No Tumor)	Breast Adenocarcinoma (ZR-75)
Volume of Distribution (initial) (ml)	2.0	5.1
Blood Clearance (ml/hr)	0.035	0.078
T 1/2 (alpha/beta) (hr)	10/94	8/102

TABLE 2. IMAGING BREAST CANCER WITH KC4G3-IN-111

	NO. SITES IMAGED/ TOTAL KNOWN	PER CENT
SITE: PRIMARY	2/2	100
METASTASES	16/45	36
SIZE: > 3 CM	10/16	63
1.5 - 3 CM	7/22	32
< 1.5 CM	1/9	11
DOSE: 1	2/6	33
100	4/7	57
190*	3/6	50
250	8/23	35
500	1/5	20

* INFUSION STOPPED EARLY DUE TO ACUTE DYSPNEA; SCH¹ ULED 250 MG.

TABLE 3. PHARMACOKINETIC ANALYSIS OF KC4G3 AND IN-111 LABEL IN BREAST CANCER PATIENTS

PARAMETER	KC4G3 (RIA)	IN-111 LABEL
VOLUME OF DISTRIBUTION	2.8 L +/- 0.4	2.8 L +/- 1.3
SERUM CLEARANCE	1.1 ml/min +/- 0.5	1.3 ml/min +/- 0.5
ELIMINATION CONSTANT	0.02 hr^{-1} +/- 0.01	0.03 hr^{-1} +/- 0.01
T 1/2	35.6 hr +/- 15.5	26.5 hr +/- 7.5

MEAN +/- SD

to normal organs will limit the dose of radiolabeled antibody which can be given safely to humans. We are about to institute a dose escalating Phase I study of 131-I-Mc5 in human breast cancer patients to answer this question.

ACKNOWLEDGEMENTS

This research was supported in part by Public Health Services research grant RR00051 from the Division of Research Resources, National Cancer Institute grants #1 P30 CA46934-01 and #PO1 CA42767-01A2, Coulter Immunology and The Cancer League of Colorado.

ADDRESS REPRINT REQUESTS TO

Paul A. Bunn, Jr., M.D.
Division of Medical Oncology - Box B171
University of Colorado Health Sciences Center
4200 East 9th Avenue
Denver,CO 80262 USA

REFERENCES

1. E. Silverberg and J. A. Lubera, Cancer statistics, Ca - A Journal for Clinicians. 38:5-22 (1988).
2. R.L. Ceriani, K.E. Thompson, J.A. Peterson, and S. Abrahm, Surface differentiation antigens of human mammary epithelial cells carried on the human milk fat globule. Proc. Natl. Acad. Sci (USA) 74:582-586 (1977).
3. J. Arklie, J. Taylor-Papadimitriou, W. F. Bodner, M. Eagan, and R. Mills, Differentiation antigens expressed by epithelial cells in the lactating breast are also detectable in breast cancer, Int. J. Cancer 28:23-29 (1981).
4. D. Hofheinz, D. Dienhart, G. Miller, et al., Monoclonal antibody, KC4G3, recognizes a novel, widely expresssed antigen on human epithelial cancers, Proc. Am. Assoc. Cancer. Res. 28:1552 (1987).
5. R. L. Ceriani, J. A. Peterson, L. Y. Lee, F. R. Moncada, and E. W. Blank, Characterization of cell surface antigens of human mammary epithelial cells with monoclonal antibodies prepared against human milk fat globule, Som. Cell Genet. 9:415-527 (1983).

6. J. Taylor-Papadimitriou, J. A. Peterson, J. Arklie, J. Burchell, R. L. Ceriani, and W. F. Bodner, Monoclonal antibodies to epithelium-specific components of human milk fat globule membrane production and reaction with cells in culture, Int. J. Cancer. 28:17-24 (1981).

7. R. L. Ceriani, E.H. Rosenbaum, M. Chandler, T.T. Trujillo, B. Myers and M. Sakada, Role of circulating human mammary epithelial antigens (HME-Ags) as serum markers for breast cancer. In "Tumor markers and their significance in the management of breast cancer." IP, C., ed., A.R. Liss, ed., 1986, pp.3-19.

8. F. C. Greenwood, W. M. Hunter and J.S. Glover, The preparation of 131-I-labeled human growth hormone of high specific activity, Biochem J. 89:114-119 (1963).

9. T. Lindmo, E. Boven, F. Cuttitta, J. Fedorko, and P.A. Bunn Jr., Determination of the immunoreactive fraction of radiolabeled monoclonal antibodies by linear extrapolation to binding at infinite antigen excess, J. Immunol. Methods. 72:77-86 (1984).

10. R. D. Brown and J. E. Manno, ESTRIP, a BASIC computer program for obtaining initial polyexponential parameter estimations in pharmacokinetics, J. Pharm. Sci. 67:1687-1691 (1979).

11. H. G. Boxenbaum, S. Riegelman, and R. M. Elashoff, Statistical estimations in pharmacokinetics, J. Pharmacokinet. Biopharmaceut. 2:123-148 (1974).

12. A. H. Epenetos, S. Mather, M. Granowska, et al., Targeting of iodine-123-labeled tumor-associated monoclonal antibodies to ovarian, breast, and gastrointestinal tumors, Lancet 2:99-1006 (1982).

13. R. M. Rainsbury, J. H. Westwood, R. C. Coomlees, and A. M. Neville, Location of metastatic breast carcinoma by a monoclonal antibody chelate labeled with indium-111, Lancet 2:934-938 (1983).

14. H. P. Kalofonos, G. B. Sivolopenko, N. I. Courteney-Luck, et al., Antibody guided targeting of non-small cell lung cancer using 111-In-labeled HMFG1 F(ab')$_2$ fragments, Cancer Res 48:1977-1984 (1988).

15. A. A. Epenetos, D. Snook, H. Durbin, P. M. Johnson, and J. Taylor-Papadimitriou, Limitation of radiolabeled monoclonal antibodies for localization of human neoplasms, Cancer Res. 46:3183-3191 (1986).

16. M. Granowska, K. E. Britton, J. H. Shepherd, et al., A prospective study of 123I-labeled monoclonal antibody imaging in ovarian cancer, J. Clin. Oncol. 4:730-736 (1986).

17. D. Dienhart, R. Schmelter, J. Lear, et al., Imaging and treatment of non-small cell lung cancer with monoclonal antibody KC4G3, Proc. Am. Soc. Clin. Oncol. 6:184 (1987).

18. S. T. Rosen, A. M. Zimmer, R. Goldman, et al., Radioimmunodetection and radioimmunotherapy of cutaneous T cell lymphomas using 131-I labeled monoclonal antibody: An Illinois Cancer Council study, J. Clin. Oncol. 5:562-573 (1987).

19. S. E. Order, G. B. Stillwagon, J. L. Klein, et al., Iodine 131 antiferritin, a new treatment modality in hepatoma: A radiation therapy oncology group study, J. Clin. Oncol. 3:1573-1582 (1985).

CONTRIBUTORS

M. Abe, Laboratory of Clinical Pharmacology, Dana Farber Cancer
Institute, Boston, MA   02115

M. Akimoto, Second Department of Surgery, Tohoku University School
of Medicine, Sendai 980, Japan

P.H. Aldenderfer, Department of Pediatrics, Medical University of
South Carolina, Charleston, SC   29425

B. Barbeau, Immunology Research Center, Institut Armand-Frappier,
Laval-des-Rapides, Québec, Canada; First Department of Obstetrics
and Gynecology, University of Vienna, Vienna, Austria

H. Battifora, Division of Pathology, Department of Anatomic
Pathology, City of Hope National Medical Center, 1500 East Duarte
Road, Duarte, CA   91010-0269

E.W. Blank, John Muir Cancer and Aging Research Institute, 2055
North Broadway, Walnut Creek, CA   94596

D.C. Bloedow, School of Pharmacy, University of Colorado Cancer
Center

M.J. Borowitz, Department of Pathology, Duke University Medical
Center, Durham, NC   27710

M. Boshell, Imperial Cancer Research Fund, P.O. Box 123, Lincoln's
Inn Fields, London WC2A 3PX, U.K.

P.A. Bunn, Jr., Division of Medical Oncology, Department of
Medicine, University of Colorado Cancer Center

J. Burchell, Imperial Cancer Research Fund, P.O. Box 123, Lincoln's
Inn Fields, London WC2A 3PX, U.K.

R.L. Ceriani, John Muir Cancer & Aging Research Institute, 2055
North Broadway, Walnut Creek, CA   94596

W. Caminiti, Abbott Laboratories, Department 90C, R1B, North
Chicago, Il 60064

K. Cantell, National Public Health Institute, 00280 Helsinki, Finland

R. D. Cardiff, Department of Pathology, University of California
School of Medicine, Davis, California 95616

K.L. Carraway, Department of Anatomy & Cell Biology, University of Miami School of Medicine, Miami, FL 33101

D. Carter, Department of Pathology, Yale University School of Medicine, New Haven, CT 06510

R.L. Ceriani, John Muir Cancer and Aging Research Institute, 2055 North Broadway, Walnut Creek, CA 94596

S. Chaitchik, Department of Oncology, Tel Aviv Medical Center, Sackler School of Medicine, Tel Aviv University

D. Corbin, Departments of Pharmacology, Surgery, and Medicine, School of Medicine, The Oregon Health Sciences University, Portland, Oregon

E. Cox, Department of Duke University, Durham, N.C.

C. M. DeRosa, Division of Surgical Pathology, Columbia-Presbyterian Medical Center, New York, NY 10032

M.J. Dicaire, Immunology Research Center, Institut Armand-Frappier, Laval-des-Rapides, Québec, Canada; First Department of Obstetrics and Gynecology, University of Vienna, Vienna, Austria

D.G. Dienhart, Division of Medical Oncology, Department of Medicine, University of Colorado Cancer Center

T. Duhig, Imperial Cancer Research Fund, P.O. Box 123, Lincoln's Inn Fields, London WC2A 3PX, U.K.

S. Enloe, John Muir Cancer and Aging Research Institute, 2055 North Broadway, Walnut Creek, CA 94596

A.E. Frankel, Department of Hematology/Oncology, Duke University Medical Center, Durham, NC 27710

P. Fung, Department of Immunology, University of Alberta; Biomira, Inc., Edmonton, Alberta, Canada

P. Furmanski, University of Colorado Health Sciences Center; AMC Cancer Research Center, University of Colorado Cancer Center

S. Gendler, Imperial Cancer Research Fund, P.O. Box 123, Lincoln's Inn Fields, London WC2A 3PX, U.K.

P. Gilna, The Ben May Institute, The University of Chicago, Illinois 60637

B.J. Gould, Department of Hematology/Oncology, Duke University Medical Center, Durham, NC 27710

G.L. Greene, The Ben May Institute, The University of Chicago, Illinois 60637

G. Greene, University of Chicago, Abbott Laboratories, Chicago, IL

B. Grouix, Immunology Research Center, Institut Armand-Frappier, Laval-des-Rapides, Québec, Canada; First Department of Obstetrics and Gynecology, University of Vienna, Vienna, Austria

E.S. Groves, Cetus Corporation, 1400 Fifty-Third Street, Emeryville, CA 94608

D. V. Habif, Department of Surgery, Columbia-Presbyterian Medical Center, New York, NY 10032

M. Hareuveni, Department of Microbiology, the George S. Wise Faculty of Life Sciences, Tel Aviv University, Tel Aviv, Israel

D.F. Hayes, Laboratory of Clinical Pharmacology, Dana Farber Cancer Institute, Boston, MA 02115

D. He, Department of Pathology, University of California School of Medicine, Davis, California 95616

C. Henningsson, Department of Immunology, Edmonton, Alberta, Canada

A. Hizi, Department of Histology and Cell Biology, Sackler School of Medicine, Tel Aviv University

J. Horev, Department of Microbiology, the George S. Wise Faculty of Life Sciences, Tel Aviv University, Tel Aviv, Israel

W.H. Hubbard, Biotherapeutics, Inc., 347 Riverside Drive, P.O. Box 1676, Franklin, TN 37065

S. Hull, Department of Anatomy & Cell Biology, University of Miami School of Medicine, Miami, FL 33101

A. Jolivet, INSERM U. 135 "Hormones et Reproduction", Faculté de Médecine Paris Sud, 94275 Le Kremlin-Bicêtre Cedex, France

I. Kafer, Abbott Laboratories, Department 90C, R1B, North Chicago, Il 60064

E.J. Keenan, Departments of Pharmacology, Surgery, and Medicine, School of Medicine, The Oregon Health Sciences University, Portland, Oregon

S. Kennedy, Laboratory of Pathology, National Cancer Institute, National Institutes of Health, Bethesda, MD 20892

I. Keydar, Department of Microbiology, the George S. Wise Faculty of Life Sciences, Tel Aviv University, Tel Aviv, Israel

P. Kiene, University of Hamburg

R. Kinders, Abbott Laboratories, Department 90C, R1B, North Chicago, IL 60064

L. Kinsel, Duke University, Durham, N.C.

R. Koganty, Biomira, Inc., Edmonton, Alberta, Canada

J. Konrath, University of Chicago, Abbott Laboratories, Chicago, IL

M.H. Kraus, Laboratory of Cellular and Molecular Biology, National Cancer Institute, Bethesda, Maryland

D.W. Kufe, Laboratory of Clinical Pharmacology, Dana Farber Cancer Institute, Boston, MA 02115

P. Kushner, Metabolic Research Unit, University of California, San Francisco, California 94143

J.L. Lear, Department of Radiology, University of Colorado Cancer Center

G. Leight, Duke University, Durham, N.C.

S.K. Liao, Biotherapeutics, Inc., 347 Riverside Drive, P.O. Box 1676, Franklin, TN 37065

M. Longenecker, Department of Immunology, University of Alberta; Biomira, Inc., Edmonton, Alberta, Canada

C. Longley, University of Colorado Health Sciences Center; AMC Cancer Research Center, University of Colorado Cancer Center

F. Lorenzo, INSERM U. 135 "Hormones et Reproduction", Faculté de Médecine Paris Sud, 94275 Le Kremlin-Bicêtre Cedex, France

M.J. Merino, Laboratory of Pathology, National Cancer Institute, National Institutes of Health, Bethesda, MD 20892

S. Mori, Second Department of Surgery, Tohoku University School of Medicine, Sendai 980, Japan

E. Milgrom, INSERM U. 135 "Hormones et Reproduction", Faculté de Médecine Paris Sud, 94275 Le Kremlin-Bicêtre Cedex, France

K.S. McCarty, Sr., Department of Duke University, Durham, N.C.

K. McCarty, Jr., Department of Duke University, Durham, N.C.

G. Manderino, Abbott Laboratories, Department 90C, R1B, North Chicago, IL 60064

G. MacLean, Department of Medicine, Cross Cancer Institute; Department of Medicine, Edmonton, Alberta, Canada

A. McEwan, Department of Nuclear Medicine, Cross Cancer Institute, Edmonton, Alberta, Canada

E. Mackie, Department of Immunology, University of Alberta; Biomira, Inc., Edmonton, Alberta, Canada

M. Madej, Biomira, Inc., Edmonton, Alberta, Canada

A. Noujaim, Faculty of Medicine and Faculty of Pharmacy, University of Alberta; Biomira, Inc., Edmonton, Alberta, Canada

J. Patrick, Abbott Laboratories, Department 90C, R1B, North Chicago, Il 60064

C. Plate, Abbott Laboratories, Department 90C, R1B, North Chicago, Il 60064

H. Rittenhouse, Abbott Laboratories, Department 90C, R1B, North Chicago, Il 60064

J. Spielman, Department of Anatomy & Cell Biology, University of Miami School of Medicine, Miami, FL 33101

J. Taylor-Papadimitriou, Imperial Cancer Research Fund, P.O. Box 123, Lincoln's Inn Fields, London WC2A 3PX, U.K.

M. Perrot-Applanat, INSERM U. 135 "Hormones et Reproduction", Faculté de Médecine Paris Sud, 94275 Le Kremlin-Bicêtre Cedex, France

J.F. Prud'homme, INSERM U. 135 "Hormones et Reproduction", Faculté de Médecine Paris Sud, 94275 Le Kremlin-Bicêtre Cedex, France

M.T. Vu Hai, INSERM U. 135 "Hormones et Reproduction", Faculté de Médecine Paris Sud, 94275 Le Kremlin-Bicêtre Cedex, France

N. Ohuchi, Second Department of Surgery, Tohoku University School of Medicine, Sendai 980, Japan

J. Schlom, Laboratory of Tumor Immunology and Biology, NCI, NIH, MD 20892

N. Ohuchi, Laboratory of Tumor Immunology and Biology, National Cancer Institute, National Institutes of Health, Bethesda, MD 20892

J.F. Simpson, Laboratory of Tumor Immunology and Biology, National Cancer Institute, National Institutes of Health, Bethesda, MD 20892

J. Schlom, Laboratory of Tumor Immunology and Biology, National Cancer Institute, National Institutes of Health, Bethesda, MD 20892

R. Mandeville, Immunology Research Center, Institut Armand-Frappier, Laval-des-Rapides, Québec, Canada; First Department of Obstetrics and Gynecology, University of Vienna, Vienna, Austria

C. Schatten, Immunology Research Center, Institut Armand-Frappier, Laval-des-Rapides, Québec, Canada; First Department of Obstetrics and Gynecology, University of Vienna, Vienna, Austria

N. Pateisky, Immunology Research Center, Institut Armand-Frappier, Laval-des-Rapides, Québec, Canada; First Department of Obstetrics and Gynecology, University of Vienna, Vienna, Austria

R.K. Oldham, Biotherapeutics, Inc., 347 Riverside Drive, P.O. Box 1676, Franklin, TN 37065

J.R. Ogden, Biotherapeutics, Inc., 347 Riverside Drive, P.O. Box 1676, Franklin, TN 37065

G. Miller, Department of Pathology, University of Colorado Cancer Center

P.X. Xing, Research Centre for Cancer and Transplantion, Department of Pathology, The University of Melbourne, Parkville, Victoria, 3052, Australia

K. Reynolds, Research Centre for Cancer and Transplantion, Department of Pathology, The University of Melbourne, Parkville, Victoria, 3052, Australia

J.J. Tjandra, Research Centre for Cancer and Transplantion, Department of Pathology, The University of Melbourne, Parkville, Victoria, 3052, Australia

X.L. Tang, Research Centre for Cancer and Transplantion, Department of Pathology, The University of Melbourne, Parkville, Victoria, 3052, Australia

D.F.J. Purcell, Research Centre for Cancer and Transplantion, Department of Pathology, The University of Melbourne, Parkville, Victoria, 3052, Australia

I.F.C. McKenzie, Research Centre for Cancer and Transplantion, Department of Pathology, The University of Melbourne, Parkville, Victoria, 3052, Australia

I. Tsarfaty, Department of Microbiology, the George S. Wise Faculty of Life Sciences, Tel Aviv University, Tel Aviv, Israel

D.H. Wreschner, Department of Microbiology, the George S. Wise Faculty of Life Sciences, Tel Aviv University, Tel Aviv, Israel

J.A. Peterson, John Muir Cancer and Aging Research Institute, 2055 North Broadway, Walnut Creek, CA 94596

C. Zoellner, John Muir Cancer and Aging Research Institute, 2055 North Broadway, Walnut Creek, CA 94596

G. Walkup, John Muir Cancer and Aging Research Institute, 2055 North Broadway, Walnut Creek, CA 94596

L. Ozzello, Division of Surgical Pathology, Columbia-Presbyterian Medical Center, New York, NY 10032

R.F. Schmelter, Department of Radiology, University of Colorado Cancer Center

T. Sykes, Biomira, Inc., Edmonton, Alberta, Canada

S. Taniuchi, Department of Pathology, University of California School of Medicine, Davis, California 95616

A.J. Strelkauskas, Department of Pediatrics, Medical University of South Carolina, Charleston, SC 29425

J. Siddiqui, Laboratory of Clinical Pharmacology, Dana Farber Cancer Institute, Boston, MA 02115

C. Tondini, Laboratory of Clinical Pharmacology, Dana Farber Cancer Institute, Boston, MA 02115

J. Slota, Abbott Laboratories, Department 90C, R1B, North Chicago, Il 60064

INDEX

Anti-tumor effect, 199
Anti-human IFN-α, 196
Antigen, 33, 55
    CA 19-9, 33
    CA125, 33
    class I, II, III, IV, V, 19
    cryptic antigen in sera, 55
    DF3 antigen, 190
    oncofetal, 19
    serum antigen, 34
    T antigen, 75
    T cell-dependent, 8
    target antigen, 4
    TFα-KLH, 8
    TFα
    tumor specific, 19
Antigen purification, MoAb
        6052, 38
Axillary lymph node status, 203

Benign breast disease, 58,
        183, 184
Breast cancer cell lines, 34
    MCF-7, 13, 14, 15, 34
    SKBr3, 34
    SW527, 34
    T47D, 34, 161, 162
    ZR-75, 244
Breast epithelial surface
        antigens, 95
Breast lymphography, 203
Breast mucin complex, 96, 97

cDNA, 120, 132, 161, 167
    cDNA clones, 83, 84
    cDNA coding, 50
    cDNA libraries, 41
    fusion proteins, 51, 96, 97
    gene coding, 161
    hybridizing mRNA, 167
Cancer,
    EGF receptor
    gene amplification, 106,
            107, 114

mucin secreting, 10
overexpression erbB-2, 106,
        107, 108, 114
primary mammary tumors, 108
protein, 114
receptor alternations, 114
tissue distribution, MoAb
        Mc5, 22
tissue distribution, MoAb
        Mc10, 23
Carcinoma in situ, 184
CEA levels, 46
Cell heterogeneity, 95
Cell lines,
    A431, 15
    Bris-8, 21
    Hela, HT-29, 21
    WI-38, 21
Cell proliferation, 119
Cisaconitic method, 229
Cloning,
    gene, 41
Chemotherapy,
    CMF 142
    alkeran, 142
    tamoxifen, 142
Core Protein, 81, 82, 84, 89,
        213, 216
    cDNAs, 216
    epitopes, 81, 85, 89

DNA enhancer elements, 119
    amplified DNA sequence, 106
Delayed type hypersensitivity
        (DTH) reaction, 9
Desmosomes, 16
Ductal carcinoma antigen, 57

Effect of estrogen replacement
        therapy, 154
    cytosolic progesterone
        receptor, 154
    on levels of cytosolic PR, 155

EGF-R overexpression, 108, 112
    protein, 114
    receptor, 114
    receptor alternations, 114
Epidermal growth factor (EGF)
            receptor, 105, 106
Epiglycanin, 9, 10
Epitope, 216
    mapping, 132
erbB proto-oncogene family, 105
    erbB-2, 106, 110, 114
    NIH/3T3 cells, 110, 112
        normal coding sequence,
        114
    v-erbB oncogene, 105
    v-erbB, 106
ESTRIP, 239
Estrogen, 119, 131
    estrogen agonists and
            antagonists, 119
    estrogen-induced protein, 137
Estrogen receptor, (ER), 119,
        120, 133
    DNA-binding domain, 121
    expression in heterologous
            cells, 123
    properties, 120
    structure, 120
    transcriptional activation,
        121
Experimental immunotherapy, 20

Fenestrated epitheliosis, 185
Flow cytometric analysis, 21,
            25, 26, 97, 100, 221
Fusion protein, 51, 96, 97

Gamma camera imaging, 238
    ^{111}In. 170.H.82, 7
Genomic DNA, 50
Genomic libraries, 168
Glycophorin, 3
Glycoprotein antigen 35-40,000
        daltons, 41
Golgi functions, 73
    monensin, 73
Growth factor receptor gene
            amplification and
            overexpression, 115

Heat shock protein hsp90, 120
Hematoporphyrin, 16
Hemopoietic depression, 219
Heterogeneity, 95
    among patients, 95
    antigenic, 33
    cell-to-cell, 95
Heterogeneity of DF3 antigen
            expression, 48
Heterogeneity of expression, 46
High molecular weight
            glycoprotein, 45

Histopathological findings, 206
Hormonal regulation, 119
Hormone binding, mechanism 120
Hormone response elements
            (HREs), 119
HSCORE, 143
Human anti-murine antibodies,
        222, 245
Human hybridomas, 33
Human milk fat globule, 56, 86,
        161, 211, 237, 245
    membranes, 96, 237
^{131}I-labeled MoAb therapy, 101

Imaging,
    human tumor, 244, 245
    imaging and biodistribution,
        239
    saturation studies, 222
    tumor, 245
Immunoassay, 46, 150,152
    antigens in sera H23, 161
    benign breast disease, 15
    breast cancer, 15
    breast cancer mucin assay, 61
    circulating antigen, 46
    circulating mucins, 55, 66
    clinical complete response, 65
    cryptic tumor antigen, 58
    cytosolic estrogen
        receptor, 152
    EIA, 46, 152, 154
    SBA, 152, 154
    ELISA, 86, 162, 165
    endocrine therapy, 131
    enzyme linked immunoassay, 46
    enzyme-linked, 152
    estrogen receptor, 150, 151
        ER levels, 151, 153
    immunoradiometric assay, 14
    IRMAK 18, 14, 15
    JDB1 serum antigen titre, 37
    normal women, 58
    partial response, 65
    progesterone receptor, 150,
        151
Immunoconjugate therapy, 231
    continuous infusion, 232
    patient selection, 220
    toxicities, 223, 233
Immunocytochemical analysis, 143
    evaluation, 146
    H222, 146
    JZB39, 146
Immunohistochemical reactivity,
        177
    B72.3, 177
    BT-20, 179
    DF3, 177
    LS-174, 179
Immunolymphscintigraphic
        technique, 203, 204

preoperative diagnosis of
        lymph node meta-
        stasis, 203
Immunoperoxidase technique,
        13, 46, 162, 173
    staining, 21, 135, 239
    test, 161
    IT 260F9 MAB-rRA, 231, 232
Immunostaining of progesterone
        receptor, 133
Immunotherapy,
    active specific immunotherapy
        (ASI), 4
    effect of antigen content, 101
    maximum tolerable dose (MTD),
        27
    neuropathy, 235
    percent inhibition of growth
        (%IG), 27, 28
    selection of MoAbs, 28
    therapy with ^{131}I-labeled
        MoAb, 101
Immunotoxin 260F9, 231
    clinical results, 232
    MAB-rRA, 231, 232
        serum levels, 234
Individually specified drug
        immunoconjugates,
        219, 221
Interferon, 195
Intracavitary immunotherapy, 20
Intraductal carcinoma, 185

Keratin,
    breast cancer, 15
    circulating, 14
    epithelial, 13
    extracellular, 13
    shed, 14
    urine, 15

Lambda gt11, 50, 84
    cDNA, 96
    clones, 96

MX-1, 25
Mammary mucins, also mucin
        complex, 211, 216
    anti-mucin, 216
    carbohydrate epitopes, 211
    cDNAs, 211
    circulating mucins, 216
    core protein, 211
    λgt11, 211
    mucin, 19, 45, 55, 71, 96,
        97, 161, 171, 183,
        211, 213, 237
        tandem repeat, 51, 213
    mucin complex, 46, 81, 82,
        84, 87, 89
        breast, 46, 96, 97
        cervical, 84

colonic, 84
core protein, 50, 87
gastic, 81
lung, 84
oligosaccharide side
        chains, 89
ovarian, 84
polymorphism, 48, 49, 51,
        83
O-linked sugars, 211
Maximal tolerable dose (MTD), 27
Molecular weight glycoproteins,
        81
Monoclonal Antibodies, 95, 131,
        132, 161, 163, 165, 229
B72.3, 171
BCD-F9, 203, 204, 206
biodistribution of ^{125}I-label-
        ed MoAb Mc5, 26
BrE1, 19, 21, 23, 24, 25, 26
CA15-3, 171, 173, 174
CA72-4, 173, 174
characteristics of MoAb Mc5,
        23
characteristics of MoAb BrE-1,
        24
cocktails, 20, 219
conjugates, 28
    adriamycin, 219, 221
    immunotoxin, 231
    mitomycin-C, 219, 221
DF3, 45, 171, 183
DUPAN-2, 172
EJ24, 15
F(ab)'$_2$ fragments, 203, 206
F36/22, 56, 57
H222, 141
H23, 161, 163, 165
histopathological distribution
        of human, 33
internalization, 229
JDB1, 34, 37, 38
JZB39, 141
KC4, 20, 245
KC4G3, 237
    antibody levels, 239
    biodistribution
        111-In-KC4G3, 239
    DTPA, 238
    serum antigen levels,
        174, 239
localization, 229
M85/34, 56, 57
Mc5, 19, 20, 21, 25, 196,
        199, 200, 245
MCF7, 168, 196
Mc5 and BrE-1 blood and
        tissue distribution, 27
Mc5 and BrE-1 maximum
        tolerable dose, 27

neoplastic tissue distribu-
        tion of MoAb Mc5, 22
OC125, 172
panel monoclonal antibodies,
        223
radiolabeled Mc5, 27, 28
ricin-A chain conjugated
        MoAb, 20
saturation, 229
steroid receptors, 131
steroid-induced proteins,
        131
tagged with^{131}I, 20
UCD/PR 10.11, 13
unconjugated MoAbs, 20
155H.7, 4, 6
170H.82, 4
^{131}I-anti-milk fat globule,
        20
    MoAbs Mc5 and BrE-1, 21
    neoplastic tissue distri-
        bution, 24
^{90}Y-Mc5, 27
^{125}I-Mc5, 27
^{131}I-Mc5, 27, 28, 244, 248
^{131}I-BrE-1, 27, 28
^{90}Y-BrE-1, 27
6052, 34, 37, 38
19-9, 172
115D-8, 171
UCD/AB 6.01, 14, 15, 16
UCD/AB 6.11, 14
UCD/PR 10.11, 14
Murine adenocarcinoma TA3-HA,
        10

Neuraminidase, 57, 66
    neuraminidase digestion, 58
nIFNα, 196, 199, 200
Nonpenetrating glycoprotein or
        NPGP, 21 (also see
        Mucin complex)
Normal breast epithelial
        antigens, 95
    tissue or cell-type
        specificity, 95
Nude mice, 100, 237
    transplanted breast tumor,
        100

Oligosaccharides, 72, 75
    cell surface, 72
    O-serine linkage, 3
    O-theronine linkages, 3

Papillary carcinomas, 183, 184
Pilloma, 183, 185
Papillomatosis (epitheliosis),
        183
Pemphigus, 16
Peptides synthetic, 212, 215

Percent inhibition of growth
        (%IG), 27, 28
PCNONLIN, 239
Pharmacokinetics, 239, 245
    biodistribution, 245
Phosphorylation, 120
Photosensitizer, 16
Polymorphic epithelial mucin, 81
Polymorphism, 48, 49, 83
Progesterone receptors, 119,
        125, 127, 132, 133,
        135
    antiestrogens, 127
    composition, 125
    heterogeneous, 135
    immunostaining, 135
    regulation of expression, 127
    structure, 125
Prognostic significance, 141
    disease-free interval, 141,
        146
    ERBIO, 142
    ER, 141
    ER-ICA, 142, 146
    ER positive, 141
    indicator of survival, 146
    (PgR), 141, 142, 146
    survival, 141, 166
    survival in human breast
        cancer, 146
    ten year survival patterns,
        141
Protooncogenes, 106

Rabbit reticulocyte system, 41
Radio-immunoconjugates, 229
Radioimmunoguided surgery, 33
Radioimmunoimaging studies, 3
    bone, 6
    breast tumor, 5, 203, 237,
        244
    colon, 5
    endometrium, 5
    imaging, 4
    111-Indium, 5
    131-Iodine, 5
    lung, 5, 6
    lymph nodes, 6
    ovary, 5
    radioimmunoimaging, 4, 203
Radioimmunotherapy (RIT), 19,
        21, 25
Rate of phenotypic variability,
        96
Regions of interest technique,
        206
Ribi adjuvant, 8
Ricin, 231, 232
    ricin A chain, 232
RNA analysis, 163
    poly-A RNA, 163

SV40/erbB-2 transfectants, 111
Serum clearance of antibody, 244
Sialomucin, 71
  cell surface, 71
Single cell heterogeneity, 100
SPECT, 5, 7
Steroid receptor analyses, 143
  binding assay, 149
  immunoassay, 149
Streptavidin-HPO, 36
Stripped HMFG, 213
Surface antigens, 84
Surface-cytoplasmic antigenic distribution, 98
Synergistic action, 200

Tamoxifen treatment, ER immunoassay, 155
Terminal duct hyperplasias, 185
Thomsen Friedenreich (TF), 3, 71
  antigen, 46
  TN antigens, 71
Tomographic camera, 5
Transitional cell carcinoma of the urinary bladder, 15
Transplantable human breast tumor MX-1, 21
Tumor-associated glycoconjugates (S-TAGs), 3
Tumor heterogeneity, 131, 222
  estrogen, 131
  estrogen-induced proteins, 131
    messenger RNA, 131
  mucin complex, 95
  progesterone, 131
  receptors, 131
  surface antigen, 95
  tumor typing, 15
Tumor necrosis, 15
Tyrosine kinase family, 106

Urinary clearance, 239
Urinary mucins, 51

v-H-ras and v-erbB, 111
Volume of distribution, 239

Western blotting, 14, 19, 134